ESSENTIALS OF CLINICAL DENTAL ASSISTING

ESSENTIALS OF
CLINICAL DENTAL ASSISTING

JOSEPH E. CHASTEEN, D.D.S., M.A.

Associate Dean for Clinical Affairs,
School of Dentistry, University of Colorado
Health Sciences Center, Denver, Colorado;
Formerly Director and Associate Professor,
Dental Auxiliary Utilization Program,
University of Michigan School of Dentistry,
Ann Arbor, Michigan

THIRD EDITION

with **880** illustrations

The C. V. Mosby Company

ST. LOUIS • TORONTO • PRINCETON   1984

MOSBY

A TRADITION OF PUBLISHING EXCELLENCE

Editor: Darlene Warfel
Assistant editor: Melba Steube
Manuscript editor: Robert A. Kelly
Design: Staff
Cover design: Gail Morey Hudson
Production: Carol O'Leary, Barbara Merritt, Teresa Breckwoldt

THIRD EDITION

The C.V. Mosby Company
11830 Westline Industrial Drive, St. Louis, Missouri 63146

Library of Congress Cataloging in Publication Data

Chasteen, Joseph E., 1943-
  Essentials of clinical dental assisting.

  Includes bibliographies and index.
  1. Dental assistants. 2. Dentistry. I. Title.
[DNLM: 1. Dental assistants. 2. Dentistry. 3. Technology, Dental.   WU 90 C489e]
RK60.5.C45   1984   617.6   84-3431
ISBN 0-8016-1127-X

AC/VH/VH 9 8 7 6 5 4 3 2   02/D/260

FOREWORD

In the third edition of *Essentials of Dental Assisting* it is obvious that Dr. Chasteen's experience in teaching and working with dental assistants lends both academic and practical approaches to the profession and shows a keen sense of the dental assistants' needs and interests.

This edition does not attempt to include everything required in a dental assisting curriculum. Instead, it provides a clinical orientation to dental assisting. It has been reorganized into 26 smaller chapters for easier reading by the students.

Dental assisting educators are well aware that recent advances in the credentialing of dental assistants and the team concept of oral health care delivery have significantly altered the practice of dentistry and—even more so—dental assisting education.

Dental assisting education today demands excellent books for use both as texts in schools and as reference books in the dental office. One cannot teach for tomorrow using textbooks and techniques of yesterday. Education should become a lifelong pursuit. To go on learning, as well as to go on sharing that learning with others, is one of the major responsibilities of a professional.

This book should prove valuable not only to the students who use it but also to all dental assisting educators engaged in raising the standards of our profession.

Doni Wingate Bird, C.D.A., R.D.A.
University of New Mexico

PREFACE

The intent of this text is to present the fundamentals of common clinical procedures that a dental assistant would most likely encounter in general dental practice. A notable exclusion is the area of dental radiographic technique, which is a subject for an entire text in itself. The writing style has been geared to the prospective dental assistant who has very little or no previous knowledge of dentistry. A great number of illustrations are included in an effort to add clarity to the instruction.

Essentials of Clinical Dental Assisting represents a point of beginning for the prospective clinical dental assistant. On completion of the reading of the text the student should be motivated to build on the fundamentals presented through both clinical experience and participation in continuing education programs. No text can or should be the last word on any subject, but rather a step in the development of the subject at a given point in time.

The third edition has undergone substantial revision and reorganization. More emphasis has been placed on four-handed dentistry, and new treatment techniques have been added. Reorganizing subjects into sections with smaller chapters should assist students in their study.

No one writes a book alone, although the writer's existence can be lonely at times. This textbook was written by several people, not by one person. Although my hand produced the words herein, my mind was guided by contributions from students, colleagues, and friends. My deepest gratitude is extended to everyone who contributed to the contents of the book.

Special thanks are due to the following individuals who willingly helped with this third edition. The laborious task of typing the manuscript was accomplished by Beth Demkowski. The photography was done by Kerry Campbell and his colleagues in the Photography Department at the University of Michigan School of Dentistry. New graphics were created by the talented Chris Jung. Nancy Wolter gave willingly of her time and expertise in the preparation of materials for illustrations and served as a model dental assistant. Marti Diederich was a tolerant and understanding model for new photographs.

Additional appreciation is extended to all publishers, authors, and manufacturers who graciously granted permission to reproduce materials used in this text.

Joseph E. Chasteen

CONTENTS

ESSENTIALS OF CLINICAL DENTAL ASSISTING

PREVENTIVE DENTISTRY

CHAPTER 1

PREVENTION OF DENTAL CARIES

It was recognized long ago that the best treatment for any disease is to prevent it from occurring. The alternative to controlling disease is to treat it after it occurs. This alternative is less desirable by far because of the destructive nature of dental disease. The two most common dental diseases, dental caries and periodontal disease, result in the loss of normal tissue. In both disease categories the damaged tissue can never be regained. At best, dentists can only halt the progress of the disease before more damage occurs. The damaged tissue is gone forever. It seems reasonable to approach the establishment of dental health by protecting the hard and soft tissues one is given in the first place. This is the basis for the concept of preventive dentistry.

The dental assistant is a key person in the incorporation of prevention programs in private practice. An increasing number of dental practices are establishing formal prevention programs for their patients. The dental assistant is frequently placed in charge of this important function. It is therefore essential that the fundamentals of prevention be clearly understood before the assistant assumes these responsibilities.

DENTAL PLAQUE
Nature of dental plaque

In a discussion of the prevention of dental disease, the first order of business is to identify one of the prime culprits in the cause of both dental decay and periodontal disease. This culprit is plaque—a soft, adherent collection of salivary products and bacterial colonies on the teeth. It accumulates on the surface of the teeth continuously throughout the life span of most people in varying degrees. The only hope a patient has in eliminating this disease-producing material is to continually remove it by toothbrushing and dental-flossing.

Plaque growth begins approximately 6 hours after a thorough cleaning of the teeth. The first phase of plaque development is the deposition of adherent products from the saliva. These products are primarily composed of mucin, which forms a thin, adherent layer on the teeth called the *pellicle*. Once the pellicle has been deposited on the clean tooth surface, bacteria that inhabit the oral cavity attach themselves to the pellicle. After attachment, the bacteria multiply to form large masses of bacterial colonies. This begins to occur approximately 18 hours after a thorough cleaning of the teeth and continues until the plaque is fully matured by the end of 3 weeks.

Mature plaque consists primarily of bacteria of various types. Each type of organism functions in a different way. Some bacteria produce harmful chemical substances, and others produce substances that are needed by neighboring bacteria to survive. Still other organisms produce adherent substances that are interspersed with the bacteria and hold the plaque intact on the tooth surface. Additional minor components of plaque include salivary mucin, dead epithelial cells, and food debris. Mature plaque is in reality a microscopic community of different bacteria and other substances that function to produce dental disease.

Research has revealed that plaque that is located above the gingiva (supragingival plaque) consists of a different combination of bacteria than does plaque that is located below the free gingival margin (subgingival plaque) (Fig. 1-1). In patients who experience dental decay, caries, the bacteria found in supragingival plaque are capable of producing acids that can erode the surface of the tooth. These bacteria also tend to thrive in an acidic environment. On the other hand, subgingival plaque consists of bacteria that do not grow well in the presence of acid. These organisms do not produce acids, but rather other chemical

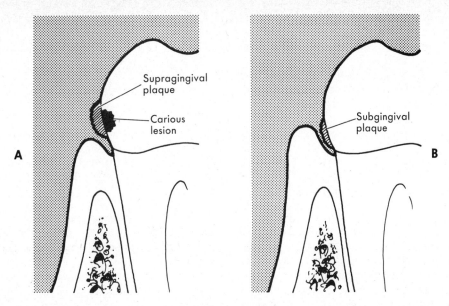

Fig. 1-1. Common sites for the accumulation of dental plaque. **A,** Supragingival plaque. **B,** Subgingival plaque.

compounds that penetrate the soft gingival tissue and cause it to become inflamed. Therefore current thinking regarding the disease-producing potential of dental plaque is that supragingival plaque, because of its acidic nature, is responsible for the production of dental caries. Subgingival plaque, because of its capacity to produce substances that are toxic to soft tissue, is responsible for periodontal disease (gum disease). Plaque is extremely adherent and cannot be washed away by simply rinsing the mouth. More vigorous methods such as toothbrushing and dental-flossing are required to remove it. This will be discussed in detail in Chapter 2.

Dental plaque and dental caries

Streptococcus mutans is one of the first organisms to attach to the pellicle and multiply. The streptococci are capable of producing both polysaccharides and acids from carbohydrates that are consumed by the patient. This is important because the polysaccharides help to attach the streptococci to the pellicle. The acid that they produce is capable of demineralizing the enamel layer of the tooth. This demineralization is the first stage of dental caries.

Other organisms in dental plaque produce various substances that help the bacterial mass attach to the pellicle. The fact that acid-producing bacteria are at-

tached to the tooth surface contributes to a greater effectiveness of acid demineralization of tooth enamel. The plaque, because of its thickness and density, prevents acid produced within it from being either diluted by saliva or neutralized by chemicals contained in the saliva. Therefore the acid remains rather concentrated adjacent to the tooth surface and is able to break down the enamel more quickly.

Once the caries process has been initiated, another organism, *Lactobacillus,* can become retained in the decayed area (carious lesion). Since the lesion is acidic, these organisms thrive, and like those of *Streptococcus mutans,* they convert sugar to acid, which in turn attacks tooth structure. It is also believed that *Lactobacillus* organisms can become lodged in the retentive pits and fissures in the tooth surface, where they multiply and the acid they produce attacks tooth structure (p. 15).

Dental plaque and periodontal disease

The irritating effect of subgingival plaque on the soft gingiva that surrounds the teeth is rather profound. If the plaque is allowed to remain in contact with this delicate tissue for prolonged periods of time, the gingiva becomes inflamed. The potential for serious damage to all the supporting structures around the teeth exists when the gingiva is inflamed for sustained periods of time. Thus the initiation of two of the most common periodontal diseases, gingivitis and periodontitis, is caused by the presence of plaque. The present strategy for the prevention of these periodontal diseases is the continuous removal of plaque from the surfaces of the teeth through various oral hygiene methods such as toothbrushing and flossing between the teeth.

A discussion of periodontal disease and its treatment is presented in Chapter 21.

Dental plaque and mouth odors

Dental plaque, besides being a factor in dental disease, is also a major contributor to breath odors. In fact, most mouth odors stem from the accumulation of dental plaque. The plaque mass has an unpleasant odor. If it is allowed to accumulate on the teeth and tongue, it will create an unpleasant mouth odor. This can be easily demonstrated by brushing the teeth without the use of dentifrice and then smelling the bristles of the brush. The unpleasant odor is readily detectable.

DIETARY CONTROL OF DENTAL CARIES

Although there is continuous research into the cause of dental caries, a basic understanding of the disease can be explained by the use of the following formulas:

1. Carbohydrates + Bacteria → Acids
   (Dental plaque)

2. Acids + Susceptible tooth structure → Decay

In essence, the first formula states that some bacteria living in the oral cavity can convert carbohydrates to organic acids. When these acids are produced in close contact with the tooth, as would be the case in a plaque mass or in pit and fissure areas, they are capable of demineralizing tooth enamel. In other words, they cause tooth decay. The progress of dental caries continues through the enamel and into the dentin layer, and the tooth is progressively destroyed.

From a caries-prevention standpoint, plaque-control programs and periodic dental prophylaxis are both directed toward eliminating the plaque mass so that acids cannot be produced in significant quantities in contact with the tooth surface.

Because bacteria can be harbored in the many pits and fissures found in normal tooth anatomy and because plaque control may not be 100% effective, further attention has to be paid to controlling tooth decay

by other means. These include controlling the diet of the patient and by protecting the teeth through the use of fluoride and sealant materials.

One of the most effective ways to control dental caries is to regulate the dietary habits of the patient. Diet influences caries prevention in two ways:

1. *Tooth development and maturation.* Proper dietary intake of vitamins A, C, and D, calcium, phosphorus, and fluoride during tooth formation and maturation influences the resistance of tooth structure to future caries.
2. *Local effects of food on caries susceptibility.* Sticky foods, specifically carbohydrates, can be converted by certain bacteria into acids that demineralize the tooth structure. This local effect often overrides the resistance that the teeth acquire during their formation.

The local effect of food on the tooth surface is instrumental in initiating tooth decay, whereas the progress of decay in the tooth structure is greatly influenced by resistance the tooth acquired during its formation.

The thrust of dietary control of dental caries is primarily directed toward controlling the local effect that food has on caries production, since it tends to override the resistance of the tooth to decay to some degree. A reasonable approach to any dietary regimen requires that the basic nutritional needs of the patient be met while caries control is being accomplished. Therefore it is extremely important that the patient's present diet be analyzed for both its basic food value and carbohydrate intake.

Dietary analysis

Nizel* suggests a practical method for dietary analysis. His method includes a diet diary, a diet evaluation summary, and a sweets intake summary. From these documents valuable dietary information can be obtained.

Diet diary. The patient is given a form such as found in Table 1-1 and asked to fill it in over a 5-day period that includes a weekend day or a holiday. This is to obtain an adequate sampling of the patient's dietary habits. Encourage the patient not to alter the normal diet habits during this period. Absolutely everything that is placed in the patient's mouth should be recorded in the diary. This includes medications, cough drops, breath mints, gum, sugar-cured chew-

---

*Nizel, A.E.: The science of nutrition and its application in clinical dentistry, ed. 2, Phildelphia, 1966, W.B. Saunders Co.

Table 1-1. Food intake diary for 5 days (include one weekend day or a holiday)

Name: _____

Instructions

1. Record every type of food consumed, solid or liquid, at mealtime, between meals, at the soda fountain, while watching television. Record also candies, Lifesavers, gum, cough drops or syrups.
2. For each meal, list the food preparation (fried, boiled, etc.), and amount in household measures (1 tsp, 1 tbsp, 1 cup [8 oz], 4 oz glass, number of pieces).
3. For fruits and vegetables, record whether raw, fresh, frozen, or canned.
4. Record amount of sugar or sugar products and cream or milk added to cereal, beverages, or other foods.
5. Record foods in the order in which they are eaten.
6. Particular information on extras is most important to us. *Do not leave out* the smallest detail.

	Fourth day*			Fifth day		
	Food	Quantity	Prepared	Food	Quantity	Prepared
Breakfast						
10:00 A.M.						
Lunch						
3:00 P.M.						
Dinner						
Extras						

From Nizel, A.E.: The science of nutrition and its application in clinical dentistry, ed. 2, Philadelphia, 1966, W.B. Saunders Co.
*Preceded by same setup for first, second, and third days.

Table 1-2. Diet evaluation summary; sample analysis of a child patient

Food groups	First day	Second day	Third day	Fourth day	Fifth day	Average servings per day	Recommended average number of servings			Difference
							Child	Adolescent	Adult	
Milk group	I	II	III	I	II	2	3-4	4 or more	2	Child: −2
Meat group	II	I	0	II	I	1+		2 or more		−½
Vegetable-fruit group (total number of servings, including those rich in vitamins C and A)	II	I	III	ⅧⅬ	0	2		4 or more		−2
Bread-cereal group (enriched or whole grain)	ⅧⅬ	ⅧⅬ II	IIII	ⅧⅬ I	III	5		4 or more		Ok

Modified from Nizel, A.E.: The science of nutrition and its application in clinical dentistry, ed. 2, Philadelphia, 1966, W.B. Saunders Co.

Table 1-3. Foods and mixed dishes classified according to food group and amounts commonly considered as one serving

Foods and mixed dishes	Amount commonly considered as one serving	Food group	Foods and mixed dishes	Amount commonly considered as one serving	Food group
Apple	1 medium size, 3-4 oz.	Veg.-fruit	Cocoa, made with milk	1 cup	Milk
			Collards	½ cup (4 oz)	Veg.-fruit
Apple juice	½ cup	Veg.-fruit	Corn	½ cup (4 oz)	Veg.-fruit
Apricots	3-4 oz, 2-3 medium	Veg.-fruit		1 ear, 5 inches	
Asparagus	½ cup (4 oz)	Veg.-fruit	Crackers, round, thin	6 crackers	Bread-cereal
Avocado	½ cup (4 oz)	Veg.-fruit	Saltines	3 crackers	Bread-cereal
Bacon	2 slices	Fat	Graham	3 crackers	Bread-cereal
Bananas	1 medium	Veg.-fruit	Oyster	24 crackers	Bread-cereal
Beans (dry)	½ cup cooked	Meat	Cress	½ cup (4 oz)	Veg.-fruit
Beans (fresh), green or wax	½ cup cooked (4 oz)	Veg.-fruit	Cucumbers	½ cup (4 oz)	Veg.-fruit
			Custard pudding	½ cup	Milk (½) Sugar, 3 tsp
Beef	2-3 oz, cooked hamburger	Meat			
			Dandelion greens	½ cup (4 oz)	Veg.-fruit
Beet greens	½ cup (4 oz)	Veg.-fruit	Duck	2-3 oz, cooked	Meat
Beets	½ cup (4 oz)	Veg.-fruit	Egg, in any form	2	Meat
Berries	½ cup (4 oz)	Veg.-fruit	Eggplant	½ cup (4 oz)	Veg.-fruit
Biscuits (baking powder)	1 medium, 2-inch diameter	Bread-cereal	English muffins	1 muffin	Bread-cereal
			Escarole	½ cup (4 oz)	Veg.-fruit
Blancmange	½ cup	Milk (½) Sugar, 3 tsp	Figs (fresh)	3 small	Veg.-fruit
			Fish—cod, haddock, bass, mackerel, flounder, halibut	3-4 oz, cooked	Meat
Bread, corn	1 piece, 2-inch square	Bread-cereal			
Bread, all varieties	1 slice (1 oz)	Bread-cereal	Fish chowder	1⅓ cup	Meat (½) Milk Veg.-fruit (½)
Broccoli	½ cup (4 oz)	Veg-fruit			
Brussels sprouts	½ cup (4 oz)	Veg.-fruit			
Butter	1 tsp	Fat	Grapefruit	½ medium	Veg.-fruit
Buttermilk	1 cup	Milk	Grapes	3-4 oz, 22 Tokay, 60 green, seedless	Veg.-fruit
Cabbage	½ cup (4 oz)	Veg.-fruit			
Cantaloupe	¼ medium melon	Veg.-fruit	Greens, all kinds, cooked	½ cup	Veg.-fruit
Carrots	½ cup (4 oz)	Veg.-fruit			
Cauliflower	½ cup (4 oz)	Veg.-fruit	Grits	½ cup (1 oz)	Bread-cereal
Cereals, cooked (oatmeal, corn meal, Cream of Wheat, etc.)	½ cup (1 oz)	Bread-cereal	Guava	3 oz	Veg.-fruit
			Heart	2-3 oz, cooked	Meat
			Ice cream	½ cup	Milk (¼)
			Kale	½ cup (4 oz)	Veg.-fruit
Cereals, ready-to-eat, flaked or puffed	¾-1 cup (1 oz)	Bread-cereal	Kidney	2-3 oz, cooked	Meat
			Lamb	2 rib chops, ½ inch thick	Meat
Celery	½ cup (4 oz)	Veg.-fruit			
Chard	½ cup (4 oz)	Veg.-fruit	Lentils, dried	½ cup, cooked	Meat
Cheese, cheddar, American, Swiss	1 oz	Milk	Lettuce	½ cup (4 oz)	Veg.-fruit
			Liver	2-3 oz, cooked	Meat
Cheese, cream	2 tbsp.	Fat	Lobster	2-3 oz, cooked	Meat
Cheese, soft type, cottage	½ cup	Milk (⅓)	Macaroni	½ cup	Bread-cereal
			Macaroni and cheese	1 cup (8 oz)	Bread-cereal Milk
Cheese bits	½ cup (10-20 crackers)	Bread-cereal			
			Mango	3-4 oz	Veg.-fruit
Cherries	3-4 oz, 15 large	Veg.-fruit	Margarine	1 tsp	Fat
Chicken	½ breast or 1 leg and thigh (4 oz)	Meat	Mayonnaise	1 tbsp	Fat
			Meat loaf	3-4 oz	Meat Bread-cereal (¼)
Chickory	½ cup (4 oz)	Veg.-fruit			
Clams	3-4 oz, cooked (½ cup)	Meat	Meat stew	1 cup (8 oz)	Veg.-fruit Meat

From Nizel, A.E.: The science of nutrition and its application in clinical dentistry, ed. 2, Philadelphia, 1966, W.B. Saunders Co.

Table 1-3. Foods and mixed dishes classified according to food group and amounts commonly considered as one serving—cont'd

Foods and mixed dishes	Amount commonly considered as one serving	Food group	Foods and mixed dishes	Amount commonly considered as one serving	Food group
Meat, lean—beef, lamb, pork, veal	3-4 oz	Meat	Salmon	2-3 oz, cooked	Meat
Melons, honeydew	1/4 melon; 1/2 cup diced	Veg.-fruit	Sandwiches	2 slices bread	Bread-cereal
			Filling:		
Milk (fresh, diluted, evaporated, reconstructed, or dried)	1/2 cup	Milk		2 oz. meat, fish, chicken, egg, or peanut butter	Meat (1/2)
				1 slice cheese	Milk
Muffins	1 medium	Bread-cereal		lettuce, tomato	Veg.-fruit
Mushrooms	1/2 cup	Veg.-fruit	Sardines	2-3 oz	Meat
Nectarines	1 medium	Veg.-fruit	Sauerkraut	1/2 cup	Veg.-fruit
Noodles	1/2 cup	Bread-cereal	Sausage (bologna, frankfurters, liverwurst, etc.)	2-3 oz, 3 slices	Meat
Nuts	2 tbsp, 1/2 oz	Meat (1/4)		1 large or 2 small frankfurters	
Okra	1/2 cup (4 oz)	Veg.-fruit			
Olives	10-12	Fat	Shredded Wheat	3/4-1 cup, 1 oz	Bread-cereal
Onions	1/2 cup (4 oz)	Veg.-fruit	Shrimp	2-3 oz, cooked	Meat
Oranges	1 medium, 3-4 oz	Veg.-fruit	Soup, vegetable	1 cup	Veg.-fruit
Oysters	6-8 medium	Meat	Soup—cream of tomato, asparagus, corn	1 cup	Milk (1/2)
Pancakes	1, 4-inch pancake	Bread-cereal			
Papaya	3-4 oz (1/2 cup)	Veg.-fruit	Soup, clear—chicken or beef bouillon	1 cup	Meat (1/2)
Parsnips	1/2 cup (4 oz)	Veg.-fruit			
Peaches	1 medium, 3-4 oz	Veg.-fruit	Soup—noodle, rice, or barley	1 cup	Bread-cereal (1/2)
Peanut butter	2 tbsp	Meat (1/2)			
Pears	1 medium, 3-4 oz	Veg.-fruit	Spaghetti	1/2 cup	Bread-cereal
Peas, fresh or canned	1/2 cup, cooked	Veg.-fruit	Spaghetti (Italian style with meat sauce)	1 cup spaghetti	Bread-cereal (2)
Peas, dried	1/2 cup, cooked	Meat		1/2 cup meat sauce	Meat (1/2)
Peppers	1/2 cup (4 oz)	Veg.-fruit	Spinach	1/2 cup (4 oz)	Veg.-fruit
Pineapple	3-4 oz, 1/2 cup diced	Veg.-fruit	Squash	1/2 cup (4 oz)	Veg.-fruit
Plums	1/2 cup (1 medium)	Veg.-fruit	Strawberries	3-4 oz (1 cup)	Veg.-fruit
Popcorn	3/4-1 cup	Bread-cereal	Swordfish	2-3 oz, cooked	Meat
Pork	1 chop, 1 inch thick	Meat	Tangerines	3-4 oz, 1 medium	Veg.-fruit
Pies, fruit—2 crusts (apple, berry, peach, cherry, etc.)	1/6 of a pie	Bread-cereal Veg.-fruit Sugar, 2 tbsp	Tapioca pudding	1/2 cup	Milk (1/2) Sugar, 3 tsp
Pies, cream—1 crust (custard, squash)	1/6 of a pie	Bread-cereal (1/2) Milk (1/2) Sugar, 2 tbsp	Tomatoes	1 medium, 3-4 oz	Veg.-fruit
			Tortillas	1 medium	Bread-cereal
			Tuna	2-3 oz, cooked	Meat
			Turkey	2-3 oz, cooked	Meat
Pie, lemon meringue—1 crust	1/6 of a pie	Bread-cereal (1/2) Sugar, 3 tbsp	Turnips	1/2 cup (4 oz)	Veg.-fruit
			Turnip greens	1/2 cup (4 oz)	Veg.-fruit
Popovers	1 popover	Bread-cereal	Veal	2-3 oz, cooked	Meat
Potato chips	8-10 pieces	Bread-cereal	Venison	2-3 oz, cooked	Meat
Potatoes	1 medium, 3-4 oz	Veg.-fruit	Waffles	1/2 medium	Bread-cereal
Pretzel sticks	1/2 cup (10-20 crackers)	Bread-cereal	Watermelon	1/16 of a melon, 1/2 cup diced	Veg.-fruit
Prunes	4 medium	Veg.-fruit	White sauce for creamed chicken, meat, fish, or vegetables	1/2 cup	Milk (1/2)
Rabbit	2-3 oz, cooked	Meat			
Radishes	1/2 cup (4 oz)	Veg.-fruit			
Rice	1/2 cup	Bread-cereal			
Rolls, plain	1 roll, medium, Parker House, or cloverleaf	Bread-cereal	Yams	1 medium	Veg.-fruit
			Yoghurt	1 cup	Milk
Rutabaga	1/2 cup (4 oz)	Veg.-fruit			
Ry-Krisp	4 crackers	Bread-cereal			

ing tobacco, as well as food items. Sugarless gum and candies should also be included.

The method of preparation of each food must be listed as well. It is important to know whether the food was boiled, fried, raw, canned, or baked. The quantity of food should be estimated with household measures (cups, tablespoons, ounces). Do not forget to have the patient include between-meal treats!

Diet evaluation summary. After the diary is completed for a 5-day period, it is evaluated with the form shown in Table 1-2. This form is intended to evaluate the diet from a nutritional value standpoint. This is a simplified way of checking to see if the patient is getting an adequate amount of food from each of the four basic food groups (milk, meat, vegetable-fruit, and bread-cereal). Table 1-3 can be used to determine the food group and normal serving values.

The entries are made in the dietary evaluation form by simply placing a mark in the appropriate box to indicate a serving in that food group. (Place ½ in the column if only a half-portion is consumed.) The servings per day are averaged over the 5 days. If the daily serving average meets the recommended levels, no changes are made with respect to nutritional value of the diet. Increases in amounts of foods in any food group that is below the recommended levels are certainly in order. These are recorded as minus values in the difference column. In the example in Table 1-2, the child patient is not receiving the recommended number of servings in milk, meat, and vegetable-fruit groups. However, the patient's diet is more than adequate in the bread-cereal group.

This diet evaluation summary is a good service to provide to the dental patient. Besides being useful

Table 1-4. Sweets intake summary

Form and when eaten	First day	Second day	Third day	Fourth day	Fifth day	Total number of exposures	Classification of sweets as to form	
Sugar in solution							***Sugar in solution***	***Retentive sweets***
During meal		✔		✔	✔	3	Cough medicines	Cakes
End of meal						0	(sweetened)	Sugar-coated chewing gum
Between meals		✔		✔		2	Soft drinks, pop, tonic	Cookies
Solid sweets							Sweetened condensed milk	Doughnuts
During meal			✔			1	Sweet sauces—	Dried fruits
End of meal		✔				1	chocolate, butterscotch, etc.	Fruits cooked in sugar
Between meals	✔		✔		✔	3		Ice cream
Retentive sweets							***Solid sweets***	Jams
During meal				✔		1	Candy	Jellies
End of meal	✔	✔	✔		✔	4	Cough drops	Marshmallows
Between meals				✔		1	Frosting	Muffins
GRAND TOTAL						16	Lifesavers	Pies

Classification of sweets as to form (continued):

Solid sweets
- Candy
- Cough drops
- Frosting
- Lifesavers

Retentive sweets
- Cakes
- Sugar-coated chewing gum
- Cookies
- Doughnuts
- Dried fruits
- Fruits cooked in sugar
- Ice cream
- Jams
- Jellies
- Marshmallows
- Muffins
- Pies
- Pastries
- Puddings
- Sugar-coated cereal
- Sweet rolls
- Vegetables glazed with sugar, e.g., candied sweet potatoes
- Vegetables cooked with sugar or molasses, e.g., Boston baked beans

16 × 20 minutes = 320 minutes or 5.3 hours

Modified from Nizel, A.E.: The science of nutrition and its application in clinical dentistry, ed. 2, Philadelphia, 1966, W.B. Saunders Co.

Table 1-5. Examples of hidden sugars in food

Food item	Size of portion	Approximate sugar content in teaspoons	Food item	Size of portion	Approximate sugar content in teaspoons
Beverages			*Candy*		
Coca-Cola	12 fl oz	3	Baby Ruth	2 oz bar	3
Dr. Pepper	12 fl oz	$2\frac{1}{2}$	Chunky	1 oz bar	$2\frac{1}{2}$
Fanta Root Beer	12 fl oz	$4\frac{1}{2}$	Fudge	1 oz square	4
Grape Tang	12 fl oz	$7\frac{1}{4}$	Hershey (plain)	$1\frac{1}{20}$ oz bar	$2\frac{1}{4}$
Hawaiian Punch	12 fl oz	5	Marathon	$1\frac{1}{4}$ oz bar	$2\frac{3}{4}$
Koolaid Punch	12 fl oz	6	Milky Way	$1\frac{1}{2}$ oz bar	4
Pepsi Cola	12 fl oz	$1\frac{3}{4}$	Munch	$1\frac{3}{16}$ oz bar	$1\frac{1}{4}$
7-Up	12 fl oz	3	Nestle's Crunch	$1\frac{1}{16}$ oz bar	3
Sprite	12 fl oz	$6\frac{1}{2}$	Peanut brittle	1 oz piece	$3\frac{1}{2}$
			Snickers	$1\frac{1}{2}$ oz bar	$2\frac{1}{2}$
Cakes, cookies, and doughnuts			Three Musketeers	$1\frac{3}{4}$ oz bar	$2\frac{1}{2}$
Angle food cake	4 oz piece	5-7	Tootsie Roll	$1\frac{3}{8}$ oz bar	$1\frac{3}{4}$
Applesauce cake	4 oz piece	4-5			
Banana cake	2 oz piece	2	*Canned fruits and juices*		
Cheesecake (plain)	4 oz piece	2	Canned apricots	4 halves and 1 tbsp syrup	$3\frac{1}{2}$
Chocolate cake (plain)	4 oz piece	5-6	Canned fruit juice	12 fl oz	1-2
Chocolate cake (iced)	4 oz piece	8-10	Canned fruit cocktail	1 cup	9-12
Pound cake	4 oz piece	5	Canned peaches	2 halves and 1 tbsp syrup	$3\frac{1}{2}$
Brownies	$\frac{3}{4}$ oz piece	2			
Gingersnaps	1	2			
Macaroons	1	4	*Dairy products*		
Oatmeal cookies	1	2	Chocolate milk	1 cup	3
Doughnut (plain)	1	3	Cocoa	1 cup	3-4
Doughnut (glazed)	1	4-5	Ice cream (vanilla)	$\frac{1}{3}$ pt ($3\frac{1}{2}$ oz)	2
			$\frac{1}{2}$% white milk	1 cup	$2\frac{1}{2}$
Jams and jellies			Skim milk	1 cup	—
Apple butter	1 tbsp	1	Whole milk	1 cup	—
Jelly	1 tbsp	4-6			
Strawberry jam	1 tbsp	4	*Bread*		
			Hamburger bun	1 bun	$\frac{1}{8}$
Desserts			White bread	1 slice	$\frac{1}{8}$
Apple pie	1 slice (average)	7			
Berry pie	1 slice	10	*Cereals* (with $\frac{1}{2}$ cup $\frac{1}{2}$% milk)		
Mincemeat pie	1 slice	4	40% Bran Flakes	1 oz	$3\frac{1}{2}$
Pumpkin pie	1 slice	5	Corn Flakes	$\frac{3}{4}$ oz	3
Banana pudding	$\frac{1}{2}$ cup	2	Frosted Flakes	1 oz	$5\frac{1}{4}$
Chocolate pudding	$\frac{1}{2}$ cup	4	Fruit Loops	$\frac{3}{4}$ oz	$4\frac{3}{4}$
Tapioca pudding	$\frac{1}{2}$ cup	3	Product 19	1 oz	$2\frac{3}{4}$
			Raisin Bran	$1\frac{1}{4}$ oz	$3\frac{1}{4}$
			Rice Krispies	$\frac{5}{8}$ oz	3
			Special K	$\frac{5}{8}$ oz	$2\frac{3}{4}$

information to the patient, it is also an expression of concern for the patient's well-being by the dental health team.

Sweets intake summary. The essence of dietary analysis in caries control is to determine the intake of sugars in the oral cavity. The more frequently decay-producing (cariogenic) bacteria are exposed to sugars, the more acid they can produce. This implies that frequency of sugar intake is more significant than the total amount of sugar consumed, which is actually the case. One candy bar eaten all at one time will produce less acid than the same candy bar consumed in small quantities throughout the day. The reason is that the cariogenic bacteria can convert only so much carbohydrate (sugars) to acids at one time. The first few bites of the candy bar saturate the capacity of the bacteria. The remainder of the candy bar has little effect on acid production if it is eaten immediately. It has been demonstrated that the acid produced during meal time tends to be buffered by the increased flow of saliva during a large meal. This concept explains why patients who snack a lot and have between-meal treats tend to have a greater decay experience.

The sweets intake summary (Table 1-4) is used to determine the frequency of sugar intake. The diet analyzer must take care in examining the diet for sweets because they are often hidden in the diet in the form of condiments, sauces, batters, breads, and canning syrups. This is why the method of preparation is important in recording the diet diary. Table 1-5 can be used as a guide to typical sugar content of various common foods.

Foods containing refined sucrose have consistently demonstrated a higher potential for contributing to tooth decay. However, other sugars, such as glucose, fructose, maltose, and lactose, also have caries-producing potential, although perhaps to a lesser degree than does refined sucrose. Even some sugar substitutes such as mannitol and sorbitol are suspected of having some caries-producing potential when consumed in sufficient quantity with sufficient frequency.

Nizel suggests that the diet analyzer (dental assistant) circle in red all foods in the diet diary that contain sugar so that the patient can see how sugars are spread throughout the diet. These sugar exposures are entered in the sweets intake summary (Table 1-4).

The number of exposures is totaled in the right-hand column. The total number of exposures can be multiplied by 20 minutes to determine the actual number of minutes of acid production the patient experienced during the 5-day period. It has been shown that cariogenic bacteria produce acid for approximately 20 minutes after exposure to sugar. This is valuable information to give to patients to impress them with the damaging effect sugars have on teeth. The example shown in Table 1-4 demonstrates that the patient experienced approximately 5.3 hours of acid attack on his teeth during this 5-day period. The fact that retentive and solid sweets remain on the surfaces of teeth longer certainly makes matters worse, since acid production continues for 20 minutes after all traces of sugar have been removed from these tooth surfaces. If a patient has traces of a sugar-laden food such as cake remaining on his or her teeth for 30 minutes after eating, acid production continues for 30 minutes plus 20 minutes after the food particles are removed. Thus a total of 50 minutes of acid production is possible. This raises the importance of avoiding solid and retentive sweets whenever possible. It also indicates the need for brushing and flossing the teeth as soon as possible following the ingestion of these foods to reduce the acid production time.

Some dentists suggest another method of impressing patients with sugar intake, which employs a small fishbowl and a box of half-teaspoon–sized sugar cubes. Patients are asked to assist in determining the sugar exposures in the diet diary. Each time a sugar exposure is discovered, the quantity is determined from Table 1-5, and patients are instructed to drop the same quantity of sugar into the fishbowl. At the end of their dietary analysis patients have a good visual display of their sugar intake by looking at the level of sugar cubes in the fishbowl (Fig. 1-2).

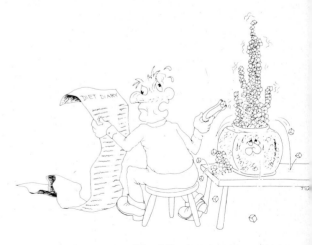

Fig. 1-2

Diet control

After the dietary data are collected and analyzed, the diet must be altered to meet the patient's nutritional needs when necessary. If levels of sugar intake are unacceptable, they should be reduced.

One simple method of reducing the frequency of acid production is to limit eating to three meals a day. If sweets are eaten, they should be consumed at mealtime. Some research has indicated that certain chemicals contained in the saliva actually help repair or remineralize softened enamel. This phenomenon occurs principally between meals. Snacking between meals not only adds to the frequency of acid production by bacteria but also interferes with the process of remineralization by the saliva. Thus between-meal snacking with foods containing sugar has a twofold negative effect. If a patient insists on snacking between meals, it should at the very least be limited to sugar-free foods.

For more severe cases, more vigorous control is required. Patients are placed on a rigid dietary regimen such as the Oregon diet plan (Table 1-6). This plan maintains rigid control of carbohydrate intake, which results in the reduction of the numbers of cariogenic bacteria in the mouth as well as a reduction in acid production.

The effectiveness of a diet plan is measured by a reduction in the *Lactobacillus* count taken from various saliva samples as the diet progresses. The ultimate measure of effectiveness of diet control is, of course, the reduction or elimination of caries.

DIAGNOSTIC SALIVA TESTS

Since dental caries is a complex disease that is influenced by many factors, no single diagnostic test has been developed to absolutely predict the current caries activity of a patient. However, some tests have been developed to examine individual factors in this complex disease process. These tests have proven to be of assistance in predicting the susceptibility of some patients to dental caries.

The *Lactobacillus* count

The *Lactobacillus* count is a test designed to determine the number of *Lactobacillus* organisms per milliliter of saliva. A sample of the patient's saliva is collected by having the patient chew a soft piece of paraffin 3 to 4 hours after eating. This stimulates salivary flow. The patient then expectorates into a sterile collection bottle until approximately 5 to 10 ml of saliva has been collected.

Table 1-6. Oregon plan for caries control

Part I

Diet plan follows the basic four food groups pattern.

Calories, fat, carbohydrate and protein are calculated for each individual, considering age, height, bone structure, etc.

Diet is restricted in carbohydrates in that allowance is lowered at least one fourth to one third below recommended allowances.

The protein allowance is calculated *at least* 10% above the recommended allowances.

All free sugar and concentrated sweets are excluded—in other words, no sugar or foods prepared with sugar are allowed. This also means no honey, molasses, raw sugar, or the like.

Length of time on the diet as planned is variable, depending on individual differences and on each individual's cooperation.

Part II

Patients are kept on the diet as planned until *at least three consecutive sets of zero counts (or very low level—100 to 300) are received* (*Lactobacillus* counts). *Then* and *only then* is the patient allowed to add sugar in desired amounts at *one meal* only—*none between meals.* When several sets of counts show no increase, the patient is then allowed to go off the diet regimen. At that time the patient should be cautioned to keep concentrated sweets to a minimum and preferably at mealtimes.

It is well to recheck the patient in 3 to 6 months, by checking the oral cavity and taking additional saliva samples to determine the count. If the count is again high, the patient should be so advised and asked to return to the diet regimen.

Advantages

1. This plan is economically feasible for the average family at the present time.
2. The plan sets forth a good procedure and background for future use in developing a better understanding of a well-balanced diet. Following the "Basic 4" makes for better dietary habits for both general health and, specifically, dental health.
3. The Oregon plan is a well-balanced diet and adaptable to a long-range program.
4. Good food habits are more firmly established by a long-range program. "Breakovers" may occur, but to a lesser degree than in a short-range program.

Disadvantage

The *Lactobacillus* count lowers slowly.

The sample is prepared in a microbiology lab and incubated on a specially prepared medium in a Petri dish for 4 days. At the end of the incubation period the Petri dish is examined for the presence of colonies of *Lactobacillus*. These colonies are counted, and the number of organisms per milliliter of saliva can be determined.

There is a strong correlation between the *Lactobacillus* count and sugar retention in the mouth, since these organisms depend on sugar for their survival. Therefore the higher the *Lactobacillus* count, the greater the retention of sugar in the patient's mouth. Because *Lactobacillus* organisms convert sugar to acids that can demineralize tooth structure, *Lactobacillus* counts have been of interest to dentists for some time.

The modified Snyder test

Another saliva test used to demonstrate the acid production potential of oral bacteria is the modified Snyder test. This simple test involves the addition of a sample of the patient's oral bacteria to a test tube of blue-green colored Snyder Test Agar.* As the tube is incubated over a 72-hour period, it is examined for color changes at various intervals. As the incubation progresses, acid-producing bacteria lower the pH of the agar, which causes the color to change. The more acid-producing bacteria present in the sample, the more rapidly the color change occurs during incubation.

The dental assistant can conduct the modified Snyder test as follows:

1. Collect approximately 10 ml of the patient's saliva in a sterile bottle or test tube 3 to 4 hours after a meal.
2. Stir the sample vigorously with a sterile cotton tip applicator.

*Difco, Detroit, Michigan.

3. Push the cotton tip into the blue-green Snyder Test Agar. Break off the portion of the stick that has been handled. Replace cap of tube.
4. Incubate the tube at 37° C, and record the color of the agar at 24, 48, and 72 hours from the start of incubation.

A positive test is indicated when the color of the agar changes from blue-green to yellow. The more rapidly this color change occurs, the greater the potential of the patient's oral bacteria to produce acid.

Table 1-7 can be used as a guide to interpretation of the color changes in the modified Snyder test.

The dramatic color change associated with this test is helpful as a visual aid that can be used as a motivational tool in the patient education phase of a prevention program. A patient with a Snyder test result such as example 4 in Table 1-7, in which the agar turns yellow after only 24 hours, would probably be much more susceptible to caries than a patient with a test result such as example 2, in which it took 72 hours for the agar to turn yellow.

The saliva flow-rate test

It has been fairly well established that saliva constitutes an efficient defense system against dental caries. This defense mechanism works in the following ways:

1. Saliva has a cleansing effect on nonsheltered areas of the teeth.
2. Teeth take up calcium from the saliva they are bathed in, and the enamel becomes more resistant to acid demineralization with age.
3. Saliva decreases the rate of development of carious lesions by supplying calcium and phosphorus, which are required to reharden acid-softened enamel.
4. Bicarbonates, phosphates, and some proteins in saliva act as buffers to neutralize acid produced in the caries process.

Table 1-7. Color changes in the modified Snyder test

Example	Starting color	Color at 24 hours	Color at 48 hours	Color at 72 hours	Suggested degree of caries susceptibility
1	Blue-green	Green	Green	Green	Little or none
2	Blue-green	Green	Light green	Yellow	Slight
3	Blue-green	Green	Yellow	—	Moderate
4	Blue-green	Yellow	—	—	Excessive

Modified from Wilkins, E.M.: Clinical practice of the dental hygienist, Philadelphia, 1976, Lea & Febiger.

5. Saliva has some antibacterial effect that suppresses cariogenic bacteria.

Studies have shown that patients with little or no saliva flow often have extremely high caries rates, presumably because of the loss of this valuable defense mechanism.

A simple test to determine the saliva flow-rate in an individual is as follows:

1. In a 30-ml graduated cylinder, collect all the saliva that a patient can expectorate in 5 minutes.
2. Record the amount collected and divide by 5 minutes to determine the flow rate in milliliters per minute.
3. Compare the result with the normal range of 0.5 ml to 1.0 ml per minute.
4. Determine the relative viscosity of the saliva using the following descriptions:
   A. Serous (watery)
   B. Mucous (thick and stringy)
   C. Frothy (sudslike)

The results of the test should reveal the viscosity of the patient's saliva as well as the flow rate compared with normal. Normally the saliva should be rather serous. A markedly diminished flow rate may result in a reduction in the natural cleansing action of saliva as well as a reduction in the acid-neutralizing effect. Thick mucous or frothy saliva also results in a reduction in the natural cleansing action. These conditions not only diminish the defensive system provided by normal saliva but also may cause patients to drink beverages containing sugar to relieve the associated feeling of a dry mouth.

FLUORIDE

Probably no single public health measure has been as effective in reducing dental caries as the use of fluoride. Fluoride compounds such as sodium fluoride, stannous fluoride, and acidulated phosphate fluoride react with tooth enamel to make it more resistant to demineralization by bacterial acid. In other words, fluorides make teeth less vulnerable to decay.

Fluorides are incorporated into the crystal structure of tooth enamel. The existence of fluoride in the crystal structure makes the enamel less soluble in bacterial acids. Furthermore, recent studies have revealed that the presence of fluoride in the enamel layer of a tooth may actually inhibit acid-producing bacteria in dental plaque. A tooth whose enamel contains no fluoride will be far more vulnerable to caries than a fluoridated tooth. There are three ways in which a tooth can have fluoride incorporated in the enamel crystal structure:

(1) ingestion, (2) topical application, or (3) both ingestion and topical application.

Ingestion

The history of fluoride is a long and interesting one. The first indication that some substance (later found to be fluoride) could inhibit or eliminate dental caries was discovered in 1916 in Colorado. Residents of certain areas in Colorado had a curious stain in their enamel, but at the same time, the teeth were resistant to dental caries. This aroused the curiosity of researchers to determine what caused this phenomenon. After a great deal of research, it was discovered that all these patients with stained teeth and resistance to dental caries drank ''well water'' most of their lifetime. Continued research demonstrated that if persons consumed fluoride during the years of tooth development and for a few years after eruption, their teeth would be more resistant to dental caries.

During the course of experiments to determine the favorable effect of fluoride on tooth enamel, it was also discovered that excessive ingestion of fluoride could result in staining (fluorosis) and pitting of the teeth (mottling) (Fig. 1-3). The Colorado residents were found to have consumed excessive concentrations of fluorides in their water supply. Through experimentation it was discovered that a concentration of 1 part fluoride in 1 million parts of water (1 ppm) was the most favorable concentration. This 1 ppm concentration makes the caries resistance effective without causing staining and pitting of the teeth.

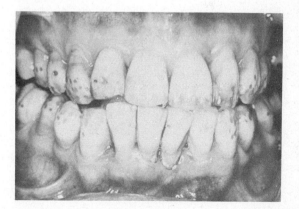

Fig. 1-3. Consumption of excessive concentrations of fluoride can result in both fluorosis (dark-stained areas) and mottling of enamel (pitted areas).

Most communities now provide their residents with the 1 ppm fluoride concentration in the city water supply so that they can benefit from this caries-prevention phenomenon. In rural areas where well water is consumed or in cities without fluoridated water supplies, children should be given dietary supplements of fluoride during the tooth-developing years (birth to 21 years of age). The water supply should be tested for its present level of fluoride, and the dietary supplement prescribed to adjust the concentration up to the equivalent of 1 ppm. This testing service is provided by most state laboratories. If the well water contains a natural fluoride concentration of 1 ppm, no supplemental fluoride should be ingested so as to avoid staining (fluorosis) and possible mottling.

Repeated studies on the effectiveness of ingested fluorides have indicated that there is approximately a 60% reduction in caries in patients who have consumed 1 ppm fluoride during the tooth-developing years. The reason for such a high reduction in caries is that the fluoride is incorporated throughout the entire layer of enamel. This renders the entire enamel layer more resistant to demineralization by bacterial acids.

Topical application

After the discovery of the effectiveness of ingested fluoride on inhibiting dental caries, other ways of using fluoride in caries prevention were explored. It was discovered that patients who did not benefit from ingested fluoride could receive some caries-inhibiting effect by painting a clean tooth with a high concentration of fluoride. A reduction of approximately 40% in caries experience can be achieved with this topical application method.

Topically applied fluoride penetrates only the outermost portion of the enamel layer, and hence it is less effective than ingested fluoride. Newly erupted teeth allow better incorporation of fluoride in the crystal structure than do more mature teeth. Topical fluoride must be applied to a clean tooth and on a semiannual or annual basis to achieve maximum effect.

Some of the agents that are used today are 2% sodium fluoride, 8% to 10% stannous fluoride, and 1.23% acidulated phosphofluoride gels. The gels are probably the most widely used today because of their convenience and pleasant taste.

The gel technique of accomplishing a "fluoride treatment" is rather simple. The teeth are polished with a rubber cup and polishing paste and flossed to remove any plaque and stain. The teeth are dried, and

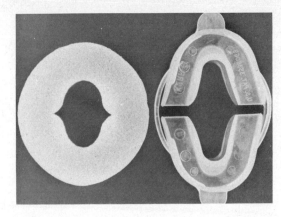

Fig. 1-4. Tray with foam-rubber liner for topical application of fluoride gel.

the gel is placed in a polyvinyl tray that will cover the teeth. The gel-filled tray is placed over the dry teeth and left in place for approximately 4 minutes. Maxillary and mandibular arches can be done at the same time. It is advisable to pump the trays up and down upon insertion, to force the gel into the less accessible areas in and around the teeth. One manufacturer provides trays with foam-padding liners and instructs the patients to bite up and down on the trays after insertion to accomplish this task (Fig. 1-4).

After the 4-minute waiting period is complete, the trays are removed, and the mouth is evacuated but not rinsed. The patient can expectorate the excess gel but is cautioned not to eat or drink for 30 mintues after the fluoride application.

Topical fluorides applied at home

In addition to periodic fluoride treatments done in the dental office, there is rather strong evidence that supplemental applications of fluoride are beneficial to patients with a high caries rate. Daily use of fluoridated toothpastes approved by the American Dental Association (ADA) has proven to be effective in the prevention of caries. To date these approved products include Crest, Colgate, MacLeans, Aqua-Fresh, and Aim.

Patients with severe caries susceptibility also benefit from the use of daily rinses with mouthwashes containing either 0.05% sodium fluoride or 0.1% stannous fluoride. The ADA to date has approved two products for over-the-counter purchase by patients. These products are Fluoriguard (0.05% sodium fluoride) and Stan-Care (0.1% stannous fluoride).

The use of various forms of fluoride seems to additionally benefit caries-susceptible patients. However, use of these fluoride-containing agents should be under the guidance of the dentist.

Combined ingestion and topical application

There has been some debate as to whether patients who have ingested fluoride throughout their lifetime would benefit from topical fluoride applications. Recent research indicates that some additional benefit can be derived from this practice. The benefit is minimal but probably worthwhile.

ENAMEL PIT AND FISSURE SEALANTS

The enamel layer of the tooth does not provide a perfect covering for all teeth. Particularly in posterior teeth, the occlusal surfaces contain several voids in the enamel called *enamel pits and fissures* (Fig. 1-5). These pits and fissures vary in extent from one tooth to another. Some teeth do not contain any.

Teeth that do contain rather deep pits and fissures have been shown to be more vulnerable to dental caries in these voids. Oral bacteria and their nutrients can easily enter the fissures and initiate decay. It is nearly impossible to adequately clean these voids by toothbrushing or conventional prophylaxis procedures. Hence the bacteria are harbored in the pits and fissures and can create the acid environment that initiates dental caries. Dental caries studies have demonstrated that approximately 44% of all carious lesions in young patients occur in occlusal surfaces with deep pits and fissures.

Although fluorides have significantly reduced the overall decay experienced by individuals, they have done so primarily by reducing caries on smooth surfaces. Close analysis of studies of caries reduction with the various fluoride methods clearly demonstrates that tooth surfaces with pits and fissures do benefit from the fluoride protection, but not as much as smooth tooth surfaces. It is this fact that has stimulated interest in research of a method of preventing tooth decay in enamel pits and fissures, in addition to the fluoride methods.

In 1965 the first report of a clinical trial using an occlusal sealing technique was presented. The objective of occlusal sealing was to establish a physical barrier over the openings of the enamel pits and fissures (Fig. 1-6). The sealing of these voids would then prevent oral bacteria and their nutrients from collecting in the voids. Furthermore, these agents would seal in any bacteria already in the fissure. Thus

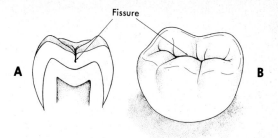

Fig. 1-5. Enamel pits and fissures. **A,** Longitudinal section. **B,** Buccal view.

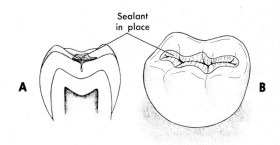

Fig. 1-6. Pit and fissure sealant in place. **A,** Longitudinal section. **B,** Buccal view.

the bacteria would be cut off from their nutritional supply and die. This basic concept has proved to be highly successful. Research on pit and fissure sealants so far seem to indicate that as much as an 80% to 90% reduction in occlusal caries is possible when sealants are used.

Materials

The success of any procedure is greatly dependent on the technique and materials that are used. The most successful materials seem to be adhesive resins containing bisphenol-A, glycidyl methacrylate, and methyl methacrylate. These acrylic-like resins must meet the following criteria to be successful:

1. Must completely bond to the enamel to form an adequate seal
2. Must resist biting forces to prevent fracture and subsequent leakage
3. Must resist wear
4. Should be esthetically pleasing to the patient

Two commercially available products (Fig. 1-7)

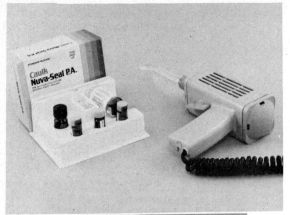

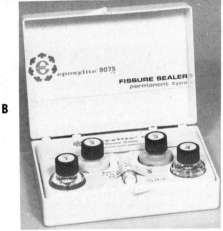

Fig. 1-7. Pit and fissure sealing agents. **A,** Sealant base material used with light source. **B,** Self-curing kit. (**A** courtesy Caulk Dental Mgf., Milford, Del.; **B** courtesy Lee Pharmaceuticals, S. El Monte, Calif.)

utilize two different methods of hardening the sealant after it is applied to the tooth. One product depends on chemicals within the product to harden the material. The other utilizes an ultraviolet light to activate the chemical within the product to form a hard, glass-like seal.

One common problem that has persisted until recently is that of bonding the sealant to the enamel to form an adequate seal. A solution seems to be to condition the tooth by cleaning it with a pumice polishing paste, followed by an etching procedure. Etching is accomplished by applying to the enamel a 50% solution of phosphoric or citric acid, which will form pores in the enamel surface. The sealant pene-

trates these pores and bonds to the enamel when it hardens.

Technique of application

The armamentarium for application of pit and fissure sealants is shown in Fig. 1-8.

The following description of the step-by-step procedure is given to emphasize the fundamentals of the technique. The directions given by the manufacturer of the sealant should be followed.

1. The teeth to be treated should be polished with a rubber cup and a paste consisting of water and flour of pumice. (Avoid prophylaxis paste containing oils or glycerin.)
2. The teeth are isolated and dried thoroughly.
3. The etching agent is applied with cotton pliers and cotton pellets, by gently moving the cotton over the enamel surface to be covered by the sealant. Vigorous rubbing will defeat the purpose of the etching by collapsing the microscopic pores being formed by the etching agent.
4. The teeth are rinsed and dried thoroughly. The teeth to be treated must remain completely dry after the etching process until the sealant is applied and hardened.
5. The sealant is prepared and applied to a thickness that will just clear the occlusion.
6. The sealant is allowed to harden if it is a self-curing type, or it is hardened using the appropriate light source.

The patient should be checked at 6-month intervals to evaluate the sealant. If there is evidence of loss or damage to the seal, the sealant is replaced in the manner just described.

Indications and contraindications

Not all posterior teeth are candidates for the sealing procedure. The selection of teeth to be treated should be based on the following considerations:

1. *Patient's oral hygiene.* Pit and fissure sealants should be considered as only one part of a total prevention scheme. It would be futile to protect the pit and fissure areas of teeth while the other tooth surfaces and oral tissues are neglected.
2. *Patient's caries activity.* Sealants would be helpful in patients with high caries rates and deep occlusal fissures. However, it again would be futile without other preventive measures such as fluorides, diet control, and proper oral hygiene.
3. *Caries susceptibility of individual occlusal surfaces.* Only deep enamel pits and fissures need to be treated. Occlusal surfaces with shallow grooves do not harbor caries-producing bacteria and are far more resistant to decay.

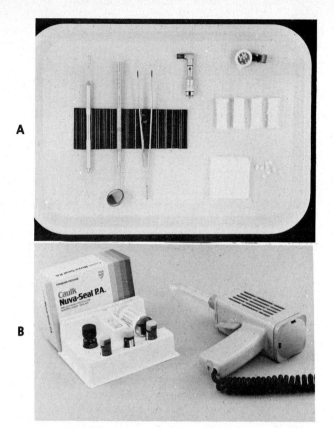

Preset tray

Cowhorn explorer, No. 3
Mouth mirror, No. 4
Cotton pliers
Prophylaxis angle and rubber cup
Paste of flour of pumice
2x2 inch gauze sponges
Cotton pellets

Add-on items

Sealant kit
Ultraviolet light

Fig. 1-8. Armamentarium for application of pit and fissure sealants. **A,** Preset tray. **B,** Sealant kit and light source.

4. *Caries history of the individual tooth.* There is little reason to seal a tooth that has been in the mouth 4 years or more without developing occlusal decay. Chances are minimal that it will develop occlusal decay if it has not already done so by this time.

Newly erupted posterior teeth should be sealed routinely if they have deep pits and fissures because of their known vulnerability to occlusal decay.

Role of the dental assistant

The specific role of the dental assistant in this procedure will depend greatly on the laws governing dental practice in each state. For the present, most states will allow the assistant to assist the dentist in this procedure. There is obvious need for an extra pair of hands during the prophylaxis and isolation phases. However, this procedure is an ideal candidate for consideration as an expanded duty for dental auxiliaries.

SUMMARY

The ability to control common oral disease requires the utilization of several prevention tactics. All tactics discussed here complement each other. Plaque control, diet control, fluorides, and pit and fissure sealants are the essential elements of prevention. Proper use of these elements is the real challenge of preventive dentistry.

BIBLIOGRAPHY

Bagchi, M.K., et al.: Salivary flow rate in relation to dental caries, J. Indian Dent. Assoc. **43:**131-134, 1971.

Dreizen, S.: Mechanisms of dental caries. In Lazzari, E.P., editor: Dental biochemistry, ed. 2, Philadelphia, 1976, Lea & Febiger.

Dreizen, S.: Salivary protection against cariogensis. In Rowe, N.H., editor: Proceedings of symposium on incipient caries of enamel, Ann Arbor, Mich., November 1977, University of Michigan School of Dentistry and The Dental Research Institute.

Englander, H.R., et al.: Dental caries activity and the pH: titratable alkalinity and rate of flow of human parotid saliva, J. Dent. Res. **37:**906-911, 1958.

Englander, H.R., et al.: Incremental rates of dental caries after repeated topic sodium fluoride applications in children with life-long consumption of fluoridated water, J. Am. Dent. Assoc. **82:**354-358, 1971.

Gwinett, A.J.: The bonding of sealants to enamel, J. Am. Soc. Prev. Dent. **3:**21-29, January 1973.

Heigetz, S.B.: Self-applied fluorides for use at home, Clin. Prevent. Dent. **4**(2):6-10, 1982.

Horowitz, H.S., and Doyle, J.: The effect on dental caries of topically applied acidulated phosphate–fluoride: results after three years, J. Am. Dent. Assoc. **82:**359-366, 1971.

Horowitz, H.S., and Heifetz, S.B.: Evaluation of topical applications of stannous fluoride to teeth of children born and reared in a fluoridated community: final report, J. Dent. Child. **36:**355, 1969.

Horowitz, H.S., and Heifetz, S.B.: The current status of topically applied fluorides in preventive dentistry. In Newburn, E., editor: Fluorides and dental caries, Springfield, Ill., 1975, Charles C Thomas, Publisher.

Loesche, W.J.: The bacteriology of dental decay and periodontal disease, Clin. Prev. Dent. **2**(3):18-24, 1980.

Newburn, E.: Sugar and dental caries. Clin. Prevent. Dent. **4**(3):11-13, 1982.

Nizel, A.E.: The science of nutrition and its application in clinical dentistry, ed. 2, Philadelphia, 1966, W.B. Saunders Co.

Parker, R.B.: Our common enemy, J. Am. Soc. Prev. Dent. **1:**14-17, January-February 1971.

Ripa, L.W.: Occlusal sealing: rationale of the technique and historical review, J. Am. Soc. Prev. Dent. **3:**32-38, January 1973.

Shannon, I.L., et al.: Inorganic phosphate concentration in body fluids as related to dental caries status, J. Dent. Res. **41:**1373-1379, 1962.

Trimble, H.C., et al.: Rates of secretion of saliva and incidence of dental caries, J. Dent. Res. **17:**299, 1938.

Wei, S.H.Y., and Wefel, H.S.: Topical fluoride in dental practice, J. Prev. Dent. **4**(4):25-32, 1977.

CHAPTER 2

ORAL HYGIENE PROCEDURES AND AIDS

DENTAL PROPHYLAXIS

The term *prophylaxis* means the prevention of disease. A dental prophylaxis is a procedure that is done to prevent dental disease. The objective of the procedure is to identify and eliminate undesirable substances from the surfaces of the teeth. These substances include plaque, stain, calculus, and food debris. Patients refer to this procedure as a "cleaning of the teeth." It is indeed a cleaning of the teeth that has as its primary purpose the prevention of periodontal disease and dental caries.

The need for this valuable service varies with the individual. To a great extent, the frequency of needing a prophylaxis is determined by the effectiveness of a patient's own personal oral hygiene efforts. Generally speaking a majority of patients require this service twice a year. On the other hand, some patients require it only on a yearly basis, and still others should have a prophylaxis done every 2 to 4 months.

Armamentarium

A suggested setup for performing the prophylaxis is shown in Fig. 2-1.

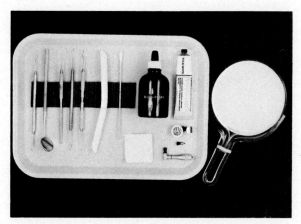

Preset tray

Cowhorn explorer, No. 3
Mouth mirror, No. 4
Periodontal probe, 0
Curette scaler, No. 13 and No. 14
Modified sickle scaler, double-ended
Oral evacuator tip
Cotton swab
Disclosing solution
Silicate lubricant
Gauze sponges, 2 × 2 inch
Dental floss
Prophylaxis paste
Polishing brush
Prophylaxis angle and rubber cup

Add-on items

Hand mirror
Fluoride (optional)
Dappen dish (may be a part
  of preset tray)

Fig. 2-1. Prophylaxis armamentarium: preset tray. (Optional fluoride setup not shown.)

Technique

Generally the methods used to perform the prophylaxis contain the following phases.

1. *Disclosing phase.* The patient's lips are coated with silicate lubricant to prevent staining. Disclosing solution is painted on the patient's teeth with the cotton swab. After the solution is rinsed off with the air-water syringe and oral evacuator, the areas of plaque accumulation appear as stained areas on the teeth (Fig. 2-2). This is an opportune time to demonstrate the results to the patient with the hand mirror and a mouth mirror.

   Some prevention assistants and hygienists like to demonstrate brushing techniques after using the disclosing solution. Using the hand mirror, the patient can see the disclosed plaque being removed with the toothbrush. This patient education effort clearly demonstrates that the toothbrush will do the job if it is used properly.

   The disclosing phase is also helpful as an aid to the operator in scaling and polishing.

2. *Scaling phase.* Scaling is the process of scraping adherent substances off the surface of the teeth. There are many designs of scalers. These instruments are introduced into the gingival crevices and interproximal areas to remove irritating debris (Fig. 2-3). Visibility and access are important during this phase. Efficient use of the oral evacuator and retraction of the lips and cheeks is of great assistance to the operator.

   As debris is removed from the teeth, the dental assistant should quickly remove it from the scaler with either the oral evacuator or the 2×2 gauze sponges. Accumulations of blood and saliva must be constantly removed during the scaling phase.

   The explorer is a valuable instrument for checking the presence of calculus in subgingival areas.

   As with toothbrushing techniques, a pattern should be established for scaling and polishing. This is helpful to the assistant in anticipating the operator's needs.

3. *Polishing phase.* After all areas of the mouth have been scaled, the teeth are polished using a slow-moving prophylaxis angle with a rubber cup. The rubber cup is filled periodically with a fine abrasive polishing paste.

   Polishing is primarily a "super toothbrushing" of the teeth. Polishing removes residual plaque and stain and leaves a smooth surface on the enamel.

   Constant oral evacuation by the assistant is usually needed during this phase to prevent spattering of polishing paste and saliva. Patients tend to salivate more during polishing procedures. This calls for an increase in evacuation of the lowest posterior regions of the mouth. A good oral rinse with the syringe and evacuator is helpful at this point, before flossing.

4. *Flossing phase.* Dental flossing is the best way to be sure that plaque is removed from between the teeth. Neither rubber cup nor scalers can completely clean the tight

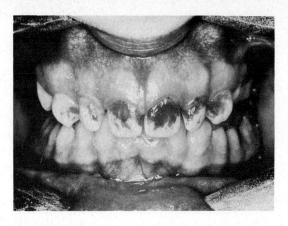

Fig. 2-2. Disclosed dental plaque on maxillary anterior teeth.

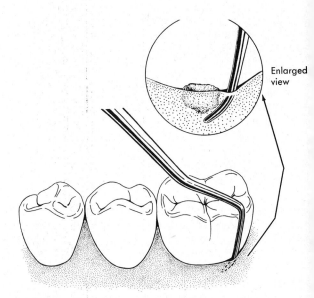

Fig. 2-3. Curette scaler placed in gingival crevice to remove existing calculus.

contact area between the teeth. A thorough cleaning should include the flossing phase.

Once again, with the patient using a hand mirror to observe his own mouth, a flossing demonstration can be given by either the prevention assistant or the hygienist. Following the demonstration it is advisable to have the patient floss various areas of the mouth while the assistant holds the mirror. This offers the assistant an opportunity to evaluate the patient's technique and to correct any mistakes.

Dental assistant's role

As was mentioned in the description of the procedure, the assistant is of great value in retraction and oral evacuation. The necessary instrument exchanges are accomplished through standard exchange techniques (Chapter 14).

Both the disclosing phases and the flossing phase can and should be done by the assistant. If a topical fluoride treatment is desired after the flossing phase, the assistant can accomplish this task as well if the state dental law allows assistants to provide this service.

TOOTHBRUSHING TECHNIQUES

Dental assistants are frequently called on to provide oral hygiene instructions for patients. Therefore the "prevention assistant" should be well informed regarding common techniques that can be used by patients to clean their teeth on a daily basis.

During the instructional phase of the plaque-control program, a specific technique of brushing the teeth should be taught for the individual patient's needs. There are only two guidelines to toothbrushing: (1) the method should remove plaque from the teeth and (2) the method should not harm the patient's tissues. Beyond that, several methods can be used. Select the method that works best for the patient you are teaching.

Probably the best starting point is to have patients demonstrate the method they are presently using. Evaluate the effectiveness of the method by the use of a disclosing agent followed by a thorough examination. Key areas that are often missed are the cervical areas and interproximal regions. This is especially true on the lingual surfaces of all teeth and the most posterior teeth. Never make a final judgment of the effectiveness of any toothbrushing technique by looking only at the anterior teeth. These areas are easiest to reach and therefore are usually better cared for than the less accessible areas of the mouth.

An intelligent approach to proper oral hygiene instruction is to recognize that often patients already possess the ability to adequately care for their teeth. It is not unusual to discover that many patients already meet the two guidelines previously mentioned. They thoroughly remove plaque from their teeth without harming their tissues. These patients need no further instruction. They should be encouraged to keep on with their own method for continued success.

A second group of patients may accomplish plaque removal fairly well but may be skipping a few areas. Teaching efforts should be directed toward telling them how well they are doing generally and where they can perfect their technique. Emphasis should be on the positive side by encouraging patients to continue their successful technique with a few helpful improvements.

Another group of patients who make a valiant effort at oral hygiene are the overzealous brushers. These patients do an excellent job of plaque removal but, in doing so, damage their own tissues. Help from the dentist in making this judgment is essential, since some of the early signs of tissue damage are often too subtle to be recognized by the dental assistant. Some obvious signs of tissue damage are soft tissue laceration, gingival recession, and tooth abrasion. Since this technique does not meet the two criteria of toothbrushing, a more favorable method should be taught to prevent further tissue damage while continuing successful plaque removal. Study models are helpful because they record the present condition of the tissues for future reference and also because a judgment can be made in the future as to whether or not tissue damage has been halted with the new brushing technique.

Still another group of patients are those who do not meet either brushing guideline adequately. This group should be taught a safe, effective brushing technique. Unfortunately, there is an abundance of people in this category. Most patients in plaque-control programs start in this category.

The key to all effective oral hygiene instruction is to recognize the plaque status of each patient, then proceed according to his or her needs. Proper recording of the plaque status of each patient should be done as a part of the individual's permanent dental record for future reference. This is essential for the evaluation of patients on future recall visits.

Several techniques can be employed to brush the teeth. The key to success is to choose a specific technique to meet the patient's needs. Generally speaking, most dentists agree that a brush with soft nylon bristles should be used to accomplish adequate plaque removal without tissue damage (p. 27). After toothbrush selection the brushing technique should be taught. Popular techniques that are taught currently are primarily directed toward ensuring adequate cleaning of the cervical and interproximal areas of the teeth. These are the areas most commonly missed by the patient. The following methods achieve this goal if they are properly done. Remember that variations of the basic techniques must be employed to meet the special needs of individual patients resulting from differences in dexterity, arch form, tooth position, missing teeth, and the presence of restorative devices.

Bass method

The Bass toothbrushing technique has gained great popularity in recent years because it is effective in cleaning the cervical and much of the interproximal areas of the teeth. Any portion of the interproximal area not cleaned by this technique is cleaned with dental floss and interdental stimulators.

The technique requires the use of a toothbrush with soft nylon bristles. The bristles should be 0.007 inch in diameter with rounded ends. The collection of bristles should be in a straight line (Fig. 2-4, *A*). These characteristics allow proper bristle action on the tooth surface without harming the delicate gingiva.

The bristles are placed at a 45-degree angle to the long axis of the tooth. The bristle tips are directed toward the gingiva (Fig. 2-4, *B*). The brush is then "shimmied" or worked vigorously in tiny circles. This action forces the bristle tips into the gingival sulcus to remove the adherent plaque. Fig. 2-4, *C* to *E*, shows proper brush placement. If the patient has difficulty moving the brush in tiny circles, a modified Bass technique can be used. This method simply calls for moving the bristles back and forth across the tooth surface using extremely short strokes.

Rotary scrub method

The rotary scrub technique is really a composite of several other toothbrushing techniques. The basic idea is to use a soft nylon brush as previously described. Place the bristle at a right angle to the facial and lingual surfaces and scrub the tooth surface using small, gentle circular strokes. Only gentle pressure is

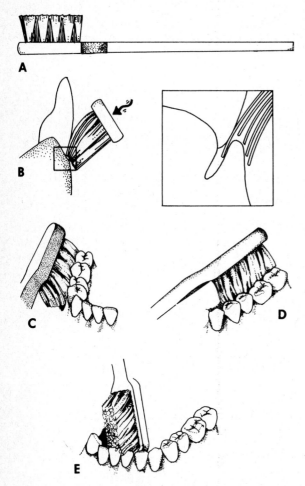

Fig. 2-4. Bass toothbrushing technique. **A,** Favorably designed toothbrush. **B,** Proper placement of bristles against buccal (and lingual) aspects of teeth so that bristles slip into gingival crevice. **C,** Proper buccal position of brush. **D,** Proper lingual position of brush. **E,** Proper lingual position for upper and lower anterior areas.

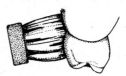

Fig. 2-5. Brush placement for rotary scrub toothbrushing technique.

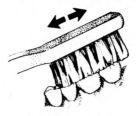

Fig. 2-6. Brush placement and action for cleaning occlusal surfaces.

applied. Care must be taken to avoid strong horizontal scrubbing motions, which can cause tooth abrasion and gingival trauma. This is an easy technique to learn. Therefore it is an excellent choice to teach children and adults who lack the necessary dexterity to use the Bass method. See Fig. 2-5 for brush placement.

General toothbrushing considerations

The brushing methods just described are not foolproof. Their effectiveness depends primarily on the skill of the individual patient. Although there are dif-

ferences in techniques, they all have the following steps in common:

1. *Brushing the occlusal surfaces.* Any technique requires that the biting surfaces be cleaned as well as the facial and lingual surfaces. This can be done by placing the bristle tips on the occlusal surfaces (Fig. 2-6) and scrubbing with forceful horizontal strokes. The action drives the bristle tips into the pit and fissure areas.

2. *Overlapping brush strokes.* Regardless of what technique is used or what area is being brushed, it is wise to brush an area approximately the length of the

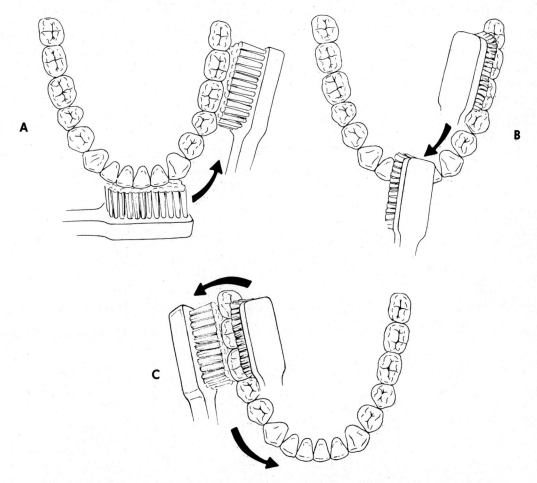

Fig. 2-7. Suggested toothbrushing pattern for upper and lower dental arches. **A,** Start on facial aspect and proceed posteriorly. **B,** Brush occlusal surfaces on left side; then brush lingual surfaces as brush is advanced around arch. **C,** Brush occlusal surfaces on right side, then facial surfaces as brush is advanced anteriorly to starting point.

brush head at a time. When this area is cleaned, move the brush ahead to the next area by two thirds the length of the brush head. This produces an overlapping of the cleaning effect. Overlapping helps to prevent areas from being skipped.

3. *Number of brush strokes.* Most techniques call for six to eight strokes on each area before moving on to the next. It is a good idea to have patients mentally count the strokes during the early learning phase for any technique.

4. *Brushing pattern.* One of the most important fundamentals of toothbrushing and flossing is to develop a pattern of cleaning the mouth that will be repeated each and every time. This is essential so that no areas are skipped because the patient forgets that an area has not been brushed. The order in which areas are cleaned is not critical, but the repetition of whatever pattern is selected is essential for a successful result.

Fig. 2-7 suggests a pattern of brushing that begins on the facial surfaces of the lower anterior teeth and proceeds posteriorly. When the last molar is reached, the occlusal surfaces are brushed. The position of the brush is then changed as shown, and the lingual surfaces are brushed around the entire arch. After the last molar on the opposite side is reached, the occlusal surfaces are brushed. The brush position is changed again, and the facial surfaces are brushed as the brush is moved anteriorly back to the starting point. The same sequence is followed in the upper arch. Repeating this pattern each time the teeth are brushed will help to avoid skipping areas where the brush is repositioned or entire segments of the mouth, which often happens when haphazard patterns are used. After the teeth are brushed, the upper surface of the tongue should be brushed to remove debris that accumulates on its rough surface.

5. *Rinsing.* The patient should always rinse with mouthwash or warm water after brushing and flossing to remove loose debris.

6. *Time of day for oral hygiene.* The practicalities of everyday life often interfere with ideal timing of when to brush. It is unrealistic to expect patients to carry out oral hygiene procedures during the busiest times of the day. A more effective approach is to suggest a thorough morning cleaning before beginning daily activities. Oral rinsing can easily be accomplished throughout the day to remove loose food debris after a meal. A brushing session should be suggested after the evening meal and before retiring at night. A close look at the patient's daily schedule should serve as a guide as to when the individual should brush and floss.

Problem solving

Patients encounter difficulties with virtually every technique. The following are some common problems that are encountered, and their solutions:

Problem: Skipping the last maxillary molar on the facial aspect

This problem is usually caused by the coronoid process of the mandible moving forward when the jaws are open. Simply place the brush in the approximate area. Then close the jaws nearly together. The coronoid process will move out of the way so that the brush can be properly positioned for adequate cleaning.

Problem: Skipping the distal surfaces of last molars

The tufts at the tip of the boothbrush should be "dangled" onto the distal surface by raising the handle of the brush relative to the biting surfaces (Fig. 2-8). Use a buccolingual sweeping motion to clean the distal surface.

Problem: Inadequate space on the facial surfaces for brush placement and proper movement

Usually the lingual surfaces present little problem insofar as gaining access to cleaning is concerned. Occasionally patients will complain that they do not have enough space to maneuver their brush on the facial aspects of the teeth. Closing the jaws together partially or completely after placing the brush in the buccal area will give greater access to the facial surfaces. This maneuver gives greater slack to the cheek to allow more movement. In cases where the lip interferes (usually the lower lip), the patient can be instructed to hold down the lip with one hand while manipulating the brush with the other.

Problem: Gaining access to the lingual surfaces in patients with narrow arches

Brushing the lingual surfaces is usually accomplished with the top two thirds of the brush head. In patients with

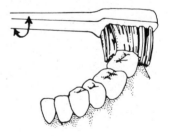

Fig. 2-8. Cleaning distal surfaces of last molars. Brush is swept back and forth in buccolingual direction.

narrow arches, a standard brush will not allow access on the lingual aspect of anterior teeth. Two suggestions to solve this problem are (1) cutting off three or four tufts from the handle-end of the brush head to shorten it or (2) using a standard-size brush in a vertical position and a circular scrubbing motion.

Problem: Missing the gingival portion of the teeth in various areas

The patient should feel the bristles of the brush contact the gingiva while brushing the entire arch, except while brushing the occlusal surfaces. This will help to ensure that the gingival or cervical areas of the teeth are cleaned, which is critical for the prevention of periodontal disease (Fig. 1-1). Caution should be exercised so that *gentle* brush movement is used, to avoid damage to the soft tissue. In addition, the brush should not be placed too far down on the gingiva, so that damage to the unattached gingiva can be avoided (Fig. 2-4, *B*).

DENTAL FLOSSING TECHNIQUES

The two vulnerable areas on the tooth surface where plaque accumulation can cause irritation of the gingiva are the cervical region and the proximal surfaces. The cervical areas on the facial and lingual aspects of the tooth are cleaned effectively with one of the toothbrushing methods just described. However, brushing does not clean the proximal surfaces adequately. The most effective way to clean the proximal surfaces is through the use of a durable string called *dental floss* (Fig. 2-9, *E*).

Dental floss is placed between the teeth in the interproximal areas, then rubbed against the two proximal surfaces on each side of the space. The floss acts as a scraping device to "shave" the plaque off the tooth surfaces. Since most periodontal disease begins in the interproximal area as a result of plaque accumulation, flossing is an extremely important preventive measure.

The key to learning proper flossing technique is to maintain control of the floss. This control begins by dispensing an adequate length of floss. Approximately 24 inches of floss is required. The strand of floss is then wrapped around the first joint of the middle finger of each hand (Fig. 2-10, *A*), with approximately 4 inches of floss extending between the two hands. This allows a positive grip on the floss. The 4-inch portion of floss can then be guided between the teeth in each quadrant of the mouth by using the index fingers of each hand, the thumbs, or a combination of a finger and a thumb (Fig. 2-10, *B*). These then become the

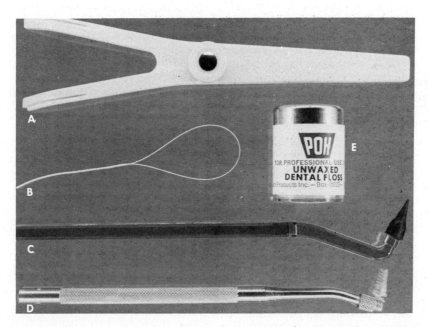

Fig. 2-9. Oral hygiene aids. **A,** Floss holder. **B,** Floss threader. **C,** Gingival stimulator. **D,** Proxobrush. **E,** Unwaxed dental floss.

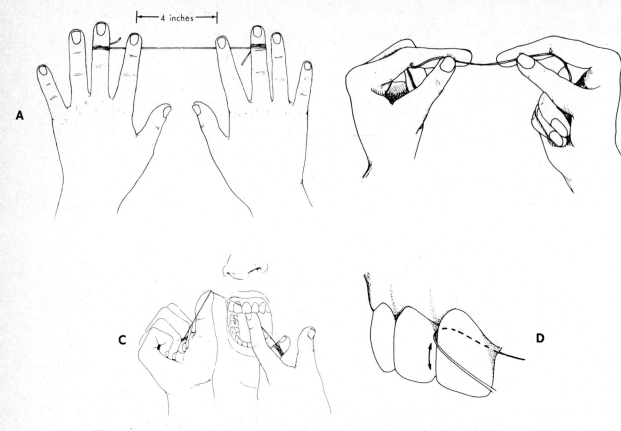

Fig. 2-10. Method of dental flossing. **A,** Wrap floss around middle finger of each hand, leaving approximately 4 inches of floss between index fingers. **B,** Use index fingers, thumbs, or a finger and a thumb to guide floss between teeth. **C,** Keep guide fingers (thumbs) as close to teeth as possible to avoid "snapping" floss through contact area. **D,** Once floss is below contact area, wrap it around proximal surface of each adjacent tooth and move it in an occlusal (incisal)-cervical direction to scrape surface clean.

guiding fingers to force the floss through the contact area. The choice of which combination of guiding fingers to use is left to the patient, based on convenience.

Passing the floss through the contact area should be done with great care so that the floss does not snap through the contact area and injure the interdental papilla. This is painful and discouraging to the patient. Place the guiding fingers on each side of the teeth to be flossed. The fingers should be as close to the teeth as possible. The floss is pulled back and forth in a buccolingual direction as the floss is forced toward the gingiva (Fig. 2-10, *C*).

Once the floss is through the contact area, it is pulled against the proximal surfaces to be cleaned. It is most important that the floss be "wrapped around" the tooth surface to ensure effective cleaning (Fig. 2-10, *D*). When the floss is properly positioned, it should be moved up and down to shave away the plaque. The wrapping and cleaning movements are repeated for each of the two proximal surfaces bordering the interproximal space.

The floss can be removed by gently pulling it in an occlusofacial direction with a back-and-forth motion. If a tight contact makes this difficult, simply unwind the floss from one hand and pull the free end in a facial direction to remove it from the interproximal area.

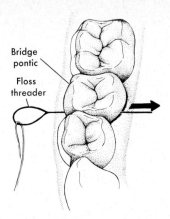

Bridge
pontic

Floss
threader

Fig. 2-11. Floss threader in use. A flexible plastic loop is used to guide floss under fixed bridges and splinted contacts.

Flossing is recommended at least once a day. Patients can do this while watching television or during other relaxation periods.

If patients have difficulty in using the hand method just described, a floss-holding device can be used as a substitute for the fingers. (See discussion of oral hygiene aids.)

Patients having fixed bridges in the mouth will find bridge-cleaning aids helpful in threading floss under these appliances (Fig. 2-11).

ORAL HYGIENE AIDS

Since the basis for oral health is the patient's ability to maintain adequate oral hygiene, some guidance should be offered on the selection and use of various oral hygiene aids. Patients can make a more intelligent approach to maintaining a high level of oral hygiene if they understand the purpose and use of these aids.

The selection of an oral hygiene regimen depends greatly on the individual patient's needs. A great deal has been written about various hygiene aids. The effectiveness of most devices can be debated, since there is wide variability in patients' utilization of these devices. Generally speaking, most dentists agree that any device is acceptable as an oral hygiene aid if it aids in plaque control and does so without harming the patient.

Toothbrushes. A common question posed by dental patients is "What is the best toothbrush to use?" There is no simple answer to this fundamental question. Although dentists themselves have varying opinions on the subject, they agree that it is the action of the bristles on the tooth surface that cleans the tooth and not the toothpaste. Dentifrices only assist in the cleaning process, although those containing fluoride preparations have proven effective in helping to prevent dental caries.

Research on toothbrushes has revealed two interesting facts. Many people purchase hard-bristle brushes. Evidence of damage to the teeth, surrounding soft tissues, or both exists in almost all patients who insist on using hard-bristle brushes. Second, soft-bristle brushes clean more inaccessible areas on and around the teeth. Far less tissue damage from toothbrushing is seen in patients using soft-bristle brushes.

Since a wide variety of toothbrushes and toothbrushing techniques have been recommended over the years, patients are often confused as to what is best for them. Each toothbrushing technique has advantages and disadvantages. The Bass method of toothbrushing has many advantages, and its only disadvantage is that it is somewhat difficult to learn and is more time-consuming. However, the dividends of optimum oral health from this method far outweigh the disadvantages. Since the dental profession is becoming increasingly united in this opinion, an intelligent selection of the type of toothbrush to use in this technique can be made.

In 1948 Dr. C.C. Bass developed a method of controlling bacterial plaque using a toothbrush with fine nylon bristles for maximum cleaning with minimal damage to the tooth and surrounding soft tissue. The characteristics of the toothbrush that he described are still found desirable today:

1. A straight, plain handle about 6 inches in length
2. Three rows of six tufts each
3. Bristles (a) of nylon, (b) of 0.007 inch in diameter, (c) of $^{13}/_{32}$ inch in length, (d) with rounded bristle ends, and (e) with 80 to 86 filaments per tuft

Several brushes meet most of the basic criteria Bass described. The only great variation in brush design seems to be the preference of some dentists for more tufts than Dr. Bass recommended. It appears that the most important features are that the bristles be nylon and have uniform diameters and rounded ends. The 0.007-inch diameter of nylon allows the best flexibility when gentle forces are applied to the brush. This produces a thorough cleaning action by the brush without laceration of the gingiva. The rounded bristle reduces the abrasiveness of the brush and protects the soft cementum and surrounding soft tissue. This type of brush is suitable for any controlled scrub technique as well as for the Bass method.

Electric toothbrushes need far more study before final conclusions can be drawn about their effectiveness. Generally speaking, none of the presently available brushes meets the Bass criteria of design and movement required for cervical cleaning. However, some generalizations can be made regarding electric toothbrushes. They are an extremely valuable aid in maintaining oral hygiene in patients who cannot adequately operate a manual toothbrush. These patients include the physically handicapped, young children, elderly patients, and mentally handicapped patients. If patients can maintain their oral hygiene to a higher degree with an electric brush than a manual brush without doing harm to their oral tissues, they should use the electric brush. Several studies have indicated that this is not usually the case, except in the groups of patients mentioned previously.

Dentifrice. There are several agents marketed presently to use in conjunction with the toothbrush to clean the teeth. Before selecting one of these agents, one should keep its purpose clearly in mind. Toothpastes, toothpowders, and toothpolishes are only aids to the process of toothbrushing. Flavoring agents in the dentifrice make toothbrushing a more pleasant experience. The action of the bristles of the toothbrush on the surface of the teeth is the principal factor in cleaning the teeth. The mild abrasive in dentifrice certainly assists in the cleaning process, but is useless when proper toothbrushing methods are not used.

Generally speaking, most dentists prefer to have their patients select a dentifrice that has a relatively low abrasive effect on the tooth surface and one that contains an effective topical fluoride.

Dental floss. The most efficient person with a toothbrush can only clean approximately 25% of the *proximal* surface area with the brush. Hence the remaining 75% of the *proximal* surface area has to be cleaned by some other means. Dental floss is the best agent for most patients.

Presently there are three basic products available for flossing: (1) waxed dental tape, (2) waxed dental floss, and (3) unwaxed dental floss.

The trend seems to be in favor of encouraging patients to use unwaxed dental floss of a high quality. Floss is thinner than dental tape and is usually easier to pass through the contact area between the teeth. The wax coating on dental floss has helped make passing the floss through the contact area a little easier. In addition, waxing helps to prevent fraying of the floss. However, several new brands of unwaxed floss have an improved method of winding the floss strands, so that the floss is less apt to fray when passed through the contact area between teeth.

Some disagreement exists among dentists as to whether unwaxed floss is the product of choice over waxed floss for effective plaque removal. The choice of the product to use should be left to the discretion of the dentist. Studies have confirmed that the effectiveness of removal of interproximal plaque depends on the patients' dedication to routine flossing rather than on the specific product that is used. However, if a patient has rough areas that cause unwaxed floss to fray or break, waxed floss should be recommended to avoid the frustration that could discourage the patient from flossing at all. These rough areas, usually caused by defective restorations, should be eliminated by the dentist so that the patient can use the unwaxed floss and benefit from its superior cleaning quality.

Disclosing agents. The key to the success of any preventive regimen is to educate the patient as to the presence of dental plaque on his teeth. Since plaque is usually a white material, it is difficult to see on the white tooth surface. Disclosing solution and tablets are principally vegetable dyes, which are absorbed by the plaque when they are applied to the teeth. These dyes are usually red or blue in color and give the patient an excellent color display of the accumulated plaque on his teeth. A plaque-free tooth will not stain. The patient can use these disclosing dyes as a guide for brushing and flossing. The patient simply brushes until the color is gone from the teeth.

Disclosing dyes are available in three forms: (1) disclosing solutions visible under normal light, (2) disclosing solutions visible under ultraviolet light, and (3) disclosing tablets visible under normal light. Disclosing solutions are generally more effective because they penetrate plaque better than the dissolved disclosing tablet. Disclosing solutions are usually limited to use in the dental office because they are more difficult for the patient to apply and they can be rather messy. Disclosing tablets, on the other hand, are very convenient for home use. The patient simply chews and dissolves the tablet in his mouth. He or she then swishes the dissolved tablet around the teeth and expectorates the excess.

The principal complaint of patients about disclosing solution and tablets that are visible under normal light is that they also stain the tongue, lips, and gingiva. A patient who has to be out in public after using these disclosing agents can find the stain somewhat embarrassing. A good recommendation is to advise a patient to use these agents before bedtime. The stain is usually gone by morning.

An alternative to this problem is a disclosing solution that is applied to the teeth and absorbed by the plaque but is not visible under normal light. The dye is only visible when it is exposed to ultraviolet light. Thus any inadvertent staining of the soft tissue is not visible under normal lighting conditions. However, because these disclosing solutions are visible only under ultraviolet light, the less accessible posterior areas of the mouth are sometimes overlooked.

Common green food coloring also works quite well as a disclosing agent. A few drops of the dye in approximately ½ inch of water in an ordinary drinking glass will reveal the presence of plaque quite dramatically after the patient has swished the solution around the mouth for a moment. The green stain on soft tissue fades rather rapidly, which is a distinct advantage of this method.

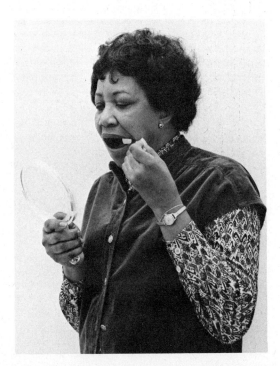

Fig. 2-12. Patient can examine her own teeth by standing in front of good light source and using hand mirror and mouth mirror simultaneously.

Mouth mirrors. For patients to be able to accurately assess their effectiveness in oral hygiene procedures, they must be able to inspect their teeth thoroughly. This is accomplished by using disclosing agents and a mouth mirror (Fig. 2-12). Inexpensive plastic mouth mirrors can be obtained through various companies. Some of these mirrors are available with flashlights built into the handle to make it easier for the patient to see into the posterior region of the mouth.

Bridge cleaners. Patients with fixed bridges and splints in the mouth should be encouraged to clean around and under these restorations. Plaque accumulates on these restorations as it does on natural teeth.

There are specially designed brushes for this purpose (Fig. 2-9, *D*). These brushes can be introduced under some bridges and adequately clean them. Other bridge designs require the use of dental floss to clean the gingival surface of the bridge. Floss has to be threaded under the bridge with a floss threader (Fig. 2-9, *B*) because of the soldered contacts present in a bridge (Fig. 2-11). After the floss is threaded under the bridge, the gingival surface of the restoration can be cleaned with the floss.

Floss holders. A somewhat frequent complaint voiced by patients is the difficulty of getting both hands in the mouth to introduce floss between the teeth. Other patients find placing their fingers in their mouths objectionable for various reasons, which discourages them from flossing routinely. Several manufacturers have attempted to circumvent these problems by designing a floss-holding device (Fig. 2-9, *A*) to guide the floss between the teeth, instead of the fingers.

Care should be exercised when these devices are used so that the floss does not lacerate the interdental papilla.

Gingival stimulators. Several devices are available for patient use to encourage an increase in circulation of blood to the gingiva. These are referred to as gingival stimulators (Fig. 2-9, *C*). They are in the form of rubber tips, soft wooden sticks, and toothpicks in plastic holders. Circulation of blood to the soft tissue is encouraged by massage of the gingiva with these devices. They are not in widespread use, and the selection of these devices should be made by the dentist in specific cases.

Irrigation devices. Another development in oral hygiene devices is the oral irrigator (Fig. 2-13, *A*). This device is designed to force pulsations of water between the teeth, under dental appliances, and

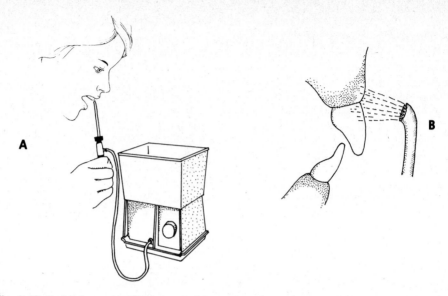

Fig. 2-13. Oral irrigator. **A,** Water-reservoir type that pumps an intermittent water spray on teeth. **B,** Nozzle guides water spray to remove loose debris.

around orthodontic bands and archwires (Fig. 2-13, *B*). The object of this is twofold. The primary objective is to remove food debris and bacterial plaque from these areas. Secondarily, the pulsating spray massages the gingival tissue to encourage circulation.

The use of oral irrigators is till somewhat controversial. Questions remain regarding their overall effectiveness and safety. The choice of whether or not to recommend them to individual patients is left to the discretion of the dentist.

Mouthwashes. The public has been besieged with advertisements on the effectiveness of mouthwash in eliminating mouth odors. The cause of most mouth odors is the presence of dental plaque and oral disease. Mouthwash will not completely eliminate either of these causal factors.

Mouthwash should be viewed as an agent to rinse away loose debris *after* brushing and flossing. This can be accomplished with warm tap water. Commercial mouthwashes, by and large, act as oral perfumes that mask odors only temporarily. They do leave a fresh taste in the patient's mouth, which gives the patient a comfortable feeling. Relatively new fluoride mouthwashes are available for use by caries-prone patients. The choice of using these products should be made with the advice of the dentist.

SUMMARY

To prevent any disease, the patient must understand the basic mechanism of the disease and what has to be done to prevent it. Guidance must be offered on prevention methods that will work for the patient as an individual. Overloading the patient with a barrage of gadgets, devices, and duties is self-defeating and ineffective. Offer what the patient genuinely needs to prevent disease—no more and no less.

BIBLIOGRAPHY

Diefenbach, U.: Why preventive dentistry? J. Am. Soc. Prev. Dent. **1**:26-29, July-August 1971.

Gilson, C.M., Charbeneau, G.T., and Hill, H.C.: A comparison of physical properties of several soft toothbrushes, J. Mich. Dent. Assoc. **51**:347-361, 1969.

Goldman, H.M., and Cohen, D.W.: Introduction to periodontics, ed. 5, St. Louis, 1977, The C.V. Mosby Co.

Jerman, A.C., and Christen, A.G.: Floss holders: what do periodontists think of them? Clin. Prevent. Dent. **3**(1):5-7, 1981.

Lobene, R.R., et al.: Use of dental floss: effect on plaque and gingivitis, Clin. Prevent. Dent. **4**(1):5-8, 1982.

Parker, R.B.: Our common enemy, J. Am. Soc. Prev. Dent. **1**:14-17, January-February, 1971.

Schmid, M.D., et al.: Cleaning effect of four different types of dental floss, J. Dent. Res. **60**(Special issue A):122, 1981.

Wunderlich, R., et al.: The effect of waxes and unwaxed dental floss on gingival response, J. Dent. Res. **60**(Special issue A): 862, 1981.

GENERAL DENTISTRY

CHAPTER 3

ORAL DIAGNOSIS AND TREATMENT PLANNING

The concept of all health treatment is to first identify and then eliminate disease. The identification of a disease is called a *diagnosis*. This chapter will deal with the diagnosis of oral disease and systemic conditions that relate to it.

The accuracy of a diagnosis is greatly dependent on the dentist's knowledge of anatomy and physiology as well as understanding of oral and systemic disease. To diagnose a disease of a part of the body, the dentist must know how the body part looks and functions normally. Identification of what is the "normal condition" for a patient is the basis for comparison in defining any abnormality. Another important aspect of diagnosis is the collection and analysis of data concerning the patient's general health as well as dental health. This information is obtained by an assortment of data-collecting techniques and devices referred to as *diagnostic tools*. The dental assistant plays an active role in the collection and recording of the diagnostic information that is used in arriving at a diagnosis and formulating a plan of treatment.

DIAGNOSTIC TOOLS
Medical-dental history

The medical-dental history gives patients an opportunity to contribute information regarding their general health, dental health, and attitude toward treatment. Since the history is usually obtained on the first office visit, this also gives the dentist an opportunity to establish rapport with the patient by an expression of interest in the total health of the patient. The history should be updated periodically as the patient's health status changes.

Histories are usually obtained by using a combination of a health questionnaire and personal interview. A health questionnaire is an orderly list of questions directed toward specific areas of interest to the dentist. These questions relate to the status of general health and dental health and draw out information regarding the patient's personal habits, attitudes, concerns, and family status. Fig. 3-1 is an example of a thorough health questionnaire. The personal interview portion of history taking is usually based on the positive, or "yes," responses on the health questionnaire and allows the patient to explain the "yes" responses in detail. It is this detail that is of greatest interest to the dentist.

A general outline of a medical-dental history is shown in Fig. 3-2. The questions on the health questionnaire apply to the various categories shown. A case history form can be used to record the valuable details of the patient history.

A summary of the value of a thorough medical-dental history is listed as follows:

1. Information is provided on general health that may influence the choice of treatment methods and drugs used and relates general health to oral conditions.
2. The history provides information on the patient's general health that can be of great value in treating a medical emergency in the dental office. This will be discussed further in Chapter 9.
3. Diagnostic information regarding the patient's oral health is provided.
4. The history is a valuable legal document to protect the dentist in medicolegal cases in which professional competence is questioned.
5. The process of history taking should improve the dentist-patient relationship, since it demonstrates the dentist's concern for the total patient and not just the patient's teeth.

Text continued on p. 37.

THE UNIVERSITY OF MICHIGAN
SCHOOL OF DENTISTRY

FORM #3A

Reg. No. ....

INSTRUCTIONS TO PATIENTS

If your answer is YES to the question asked, put a circle around (Yes).
If your answer is NO to the question asked, put a circle around (No).

Answer all questions. You may comment on answers which require explanation by writing in the space between questions.

Answers to the following questions are for our records only and will be considered confidential.

1. Do you think that your teeth are affecting your general health in any way? Yes No
2. Are you dissatisfied with the appearance of your teeth? Yes No
3. Are you worried about receiving dental treatment? Yes No
4. Do you have difficulty in chewing your food? Yes No
5. Are you being treated for any condition by a physician now? Yes No
6. Have you ever experienced a bad reaction to a dental anesthetic? Yes No
7. Do you bleed for a long time when you cut yourself? Yes No
8. Have you ever had any injury to your face or jaws? Yes No
9. Have you ever had surgery or x-ray treatment for a tumor, growth or other condition in your mouth or on your lips? Yes No
10. Are you taking any medicines now? Yes No
11. Have you been examined by your physician within the last year? Yes No
12. Has there been any change in your general health in the last year? Yes No
13. Have you lost weight without dieting in recent months? Yes No
14. Have you ever been seriously ill? Yes No
15. Have you ever been hospitalized? Yes No
16. Have you ever had a major operation? Yes No
17. Have you had any of the following:
    - Rheumatic Fever .... Yes No
    - Inflammatory Rheumatism .... Yes No
    - Jaundice (yellow skin and eyes) .... Yes No
    - Diabetes (sugar disease) .... Yes No
    - High Blood Pressure .... Yes No
    - Tuberculosis .... Yes No
    - Venereal Disease .... Yes No
    - Heart Attack .... Yes No
    - Stroke .... Yes No
    - Heart Murmur .... Yes No
18. Have you ever had a blood transfusion? Yes No
19. Do you ever have asthma or hay fever? (Underline which one) .... Yes No
20. Do you ever have hives or skin rash? Yes No

HEALTH QUESTIONNAIRE

FORM #3A

Form 9497

Continued.

Fig. 3-1. (Courtesy, School of Dentistry, University of Michigan, Ann Arbor, Mich.)

21. Have you ever experienced a bad reaction to any of the following drugs:

Aspirin .... Yes   No

Penicillin .... Yes   No

Iodine .... Yes   No

Sulfonamides (sulfa) .... Yes   No

Barbiturates (sleeping pills) .... Yes   No

Other medicines .... Yes   No

22. Do you have frequent, severe headaches?   Yes   No

23. Do you have any complaints regarding your eyes?   Yes   No

24. Do you have sinus trouble?   Yes   No

25. Do you have nosebleeds?   Yes   No

26. Are you a mouth breather?   Yes   No

27. Do you have any sensitive teeth?   Yes   No

28. Have you had a toothache recently?   Yes   No

29. Do you have bleeding gums?   Yes   No

30. Do you have frequent canker sores or cold sores?   Yes   No

31. Have you ever had a severe sore mouth?   Yes   No

32. Is it difficult for you to open your mouth as wide as you would like?   Yes   No

33. Does your jaw click when you chew?   Yes   No

34. Do you have any chest pain on exertion?   Yes   No

35. Are you ever short of breath on mild exertion?   Yes   No

36. Do your ankles swell?   Yes   No

37. Do you have a persistent cough?   Yes   No

38. Do you ever cough blood?   Yes   No

39. Are there any foods you cannot eat?   Yes   No

40. Do you have any difficulty swallowing?   Yes   No

41. Do you have frequent indigestion   Yes   No

42. Do you vomit frequently?   Yes   No

43. Do you urinate more than six times a day?   Yes   No

44. Are you thirsty much of the time?   Yes   No

45. Have you ever had painful and swollen joints?   Yes   No

46. Do you ever have fits or convulsions?   Yes   No

47. Do you have a tendency to faint?   Yes   No

48. Do you bruise easily?   Yes   No

49. Do you have any blood disorder such as anemia (thin blood)?   Yes   No

50. Are you excessively nervous?   Yes   No

51. Do you get tired easily?   Yes   No

52. *Women.* Are you pregnant at the present time?   Yes   No

Date .... Patient's Signature ....

       year   month   day

Examiner ....

Checked by Dr. ....

Fig. 3-1, cont'd

THE UNIVERSITY OF MICHIGAN
SCHOOL OF DENTISTRY

FORM #3B

HISTORY

History of the Chief Complaint

Reg. No. ....

Present Illness

Dental History

Dental examination (frequency):—

Approximate date of last dental examination:—

Dental prophylaxis (frequency):—

Approximate date of last dental prophylaxis:—

Date of last extraction:—

reason for extractions (caries, periodontal disease):—

complications:—

Orthodontic treatment: dates (inclusive):—

correction for:—

Periodontal treatment: dates:—

condition treated:—

surgery:—

occlusal adjustment:—

Prosthesis (fixed and removable):—

date made:—

modifications:—

Endodontic treatment:—

tooth no.:—

date completed:—

apical surgery:—

Medical History and Review of Systems

Amplify positive answers from Health Questionnaire
(include question number; use reverse side of sheet also)

Physician's name and address:—

HISTORY

FORM #3B

Form 9498

Continued.

Fig. 3-2. (Courtesy, School of Dentistry, University of Michigan, Ann Arbor, Mich.)

Family History

Health of parents, sibs, children

Familial diseases:—

    Oral:—

    Systemic:—

Family dental experience:—

Personal History

Oral hygiene:

    brushes when?...............................   brushing method:—

    number and type of brushes owned:—

    previous toothbrush instruction:—

    dentifrice:—   mouthwash

    tape or floss:—   stimulators

    toothpicks:—

    appliance care:—

Habits: bruxism:—   clenching:—   nail biting:—

    smoking (quantity, type):—   alcohol (quantity/day):—

    other:—   sugar in diet (all sources):—

Dietary habits (summary):

DATE...

Fig. 3-2, cont'd

6. All dental personnel may benefit from information obtained in the history regarding contagious disease. Protective masks, gloves, and possibly delaying treatment until the disease is cured are ways in which the dental team can protect themselves against infection from the patient.

The dental assistant may be called on to provide the patient with the health questionnaire and inspect it for proper completion. Be sure all questions are answered and that it is dated and signed by the patient. Assistants are often asked to record the pertinent details during the personal interview with the dentist.

Clinical examination

Clinical examination of a patient calls on the dentist to use some of the physical senses to aid in the diagnosis of oral disease. The senses of sight, sound, and touch are all used during a clinical examination.

A visual inspection of the patient's hard and soft tissues can reveal changes in color, shape, and size of oral structures. Abnormal function can be detected by watching the patient's face, eyes, and mouth during conversation. Unusual movements of the facial muscles, tongue, and eyes are often signs of neuromuscular disease. Observation of a patient's reaction to various diagnostic tests is helpful in arriving at an accurate diagnosis.

Unusual sounds are beneficial in diagnostic procedures. Clicking of the patient's temporomandibular joint may be a clue to the presence of joint disease.

Abnormal speech patterns may lead the examiner to investigate possible oral causes of the abnormality, such as abnormal positioning of the teeth and "tongue-tie." Tapping on teeth with the handle of a mirror produces a rather sharp sound in normal teeth and a rather dull sound in certain dental disease. This procedure of tapping tissues as a part of the examination is called *percussion*.

Palpation is the use of the examiner's sense of touch to reveal abnormalities. The tissues of the body all have a certain texture under normal circumstances. Often one of the first signs of disease is a change in texture of a tissue. It may be more or less firm, larger or smaller, and possibly tender to the touch.

The medical-dental history and the clinical examination as well as the other diagnostic tools yet to be discussed reveal signs and symptoms of disease. Generally these two terms are used together to describe the characteristics of a disease. Specifically, a sign is a characteristic that is observable by either the patient or the examiner. Examples of clinical signs are swelling, ulcerations, fever, and change in the color, texture, and position of structures. A symptom is a characteristic of a disease that the patient feels and relates to the examiner. Some examples of symptoms include pain, dizziness, nausea, bad taste, and difficulty in chewing or swallowing.

Clinical examination of a patient should include the inspection of the following three general areas:

1. *Extraoral structures.* These structures include general shape of the face and head, skin texture

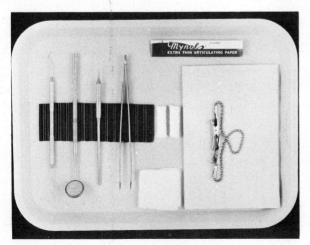

Preset tray

Cowhorn explorer, No. 3
Mouth mirror, No. 4
Periodontal probe, 0
Cotton pliers
Cotton rolls
Articulating paper
Patient napkin
Neck chain
Gauze sponges, 2 × 2 inch

Add-on items

Dental records
Radiographs
Pencils, colored
Pulp testing devices (as needed)
Alginate impression setup
  (as needed)

Fig. 3-3. Armamentarium for clinical examination.

and color, eye size and color of the sclera (white of the eye), the temporomandibular joint, and the shape of the jaws.

2. *Intraoral soft tissues*. The entire oral mucosa and submucosal structures such as glands, lymph nodes, and muscles should be examined.
3. *Intraoral hard tissues*. The intraoral portion of the bone of the jaws and the teeth should be examined for abnormalities.

The dental assistant is called on to record the clinical findings as they are dictated by the dentist, in addition to standard chairside duties described in Section 3. The armamentarium for a clinical examination is shown in Fig. 3-3.

Dental radiographs

Radiographs, or x-ray films, of the teeth and bone are perhaps the most valuable diagnostic tool the den-

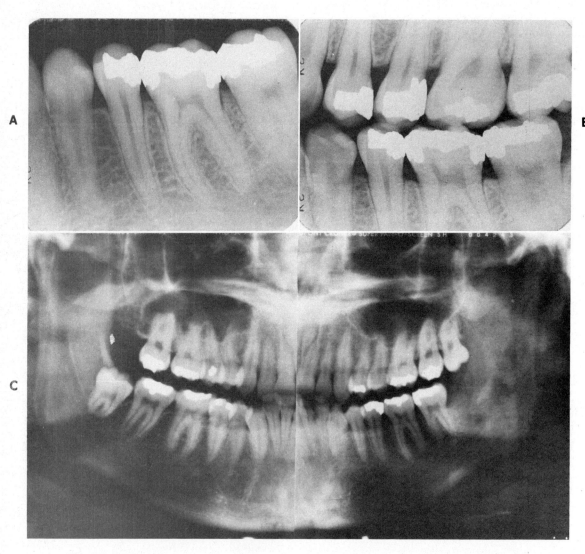

Fig. 3-4. Radiographs commonly used for oral region. **A,** Periapical view. **B,** Posterior bite-wing view. **C,** Panoramic radiograph, approximately one third normal size (Panorex).

tist has to evaluate structures that cannot be seen by clinical observation. The information revealed by the radiograph, correlated with the patient history and clinical findings, constitutes a major source of diagnostic information.

The value of a radiograph depends on the quality of the picture itself and the ability of the dentist to interpret it. Modern dental practice calls on dental auxiliaries to take the radiographic pictures. Needless to say, it is a great responsibility to be delegated to assistants and hygienists. Without a good-quality radiographic survey of the patient, the dentist's ability to interpret diagnostic findings is greatly limited. An auxiliary who can provide this valuable service to the dentist is truly an important asset to a dental practice.

Two classes of radiographs are used in oral diagnostic procedures: intraoral and extraoral views. Intraoral radiographs are taken with the film placed in the patient's mouth, and extraoral radiographs are taken with the film held outside the mouth. Fig. 3-4 demonstrates some examples of these two classes of radiographs.

Intraoral radiographs are in greater use than extraoral types. The extraoral radiograph is generally considered to be a supplemental film that is taken in special cases. A typical, routine, complete radiographic survey of a patient includes a series of 14 periapical and four bite-wing radiographs. Periapical views reveal discrepancies in both the crown and root portion of the teeth as well as the surrounding supporting tissues of the teeth. Bite-wing views provide information primarily in the area of the crowns of teeth. Table 3-1 demonstrates some common radiographic findings found on the various views.

There are several excellent texts on dental radiography available for dental auxiliaries who want to review this subject in detail.

Proper processing of x-ray films in the darkroom will provide the dentist with a permanent radiographic record of the patient's condition. This is important as a future reference to determine the progress of disease or healing. Radiographs are valuable in medicolegal cases that may occur against the dentist.

Pulp tests

A common supplemental diagnostic tool is a battery of tests that will determine the health status of the pulp of a tooth. These tests are discussed in detail in Chapter 22.

Plaque disclosure

The application of disclosing agents on the patient's teeth reveals the status of the patient's oral

Table 3-1. Common findings on radiographs

Type of radiograph	Findings
Posterior bite-wing	Interproximal caries
	Restorative contour
	Integrity of cervical margins of restoration
	Pulp size and relationship to caries and restorations
	Height of alveolar crest
	Location of calculus
Periapical	Pathological changes in periapical area
	Integrity of supporting bone
	Root size and shape
	Integrity of periodontal space and lamina dura
Panorex	Entire dentition in view on one film
	Pathology in bone and the temporomandibular joint
	Development of dentition (children)
	Position of impacted teeth
	Jaw fractures
	Location of foreign bodies

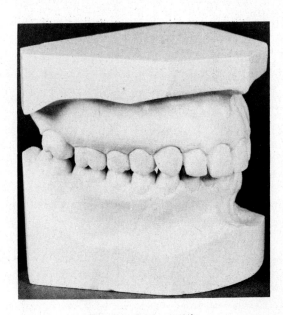

Fig. 3-5. Study models.

hygiene (Chapter 2). The dentist can correlate the presence of dental plaque with oral conditions that may be damaging to the patient.

Study models (Fig. 3-5)

Study models (casts) are plaster reproductions of the patient's teeth and surrounding tissues. They are obtained by an impression-taking procedure, described in Chapter 24, using alginate impression material.

Study models give the dentist a permanent record of the three-dimensional condition of the patient's teeth and jaws at the time the impression is made. Study models provide information on the position, size, and shape of teeth. The size, shape, and contour of the surrounding soft tissues and jaws are also recorded on the study model.

The study models give dentists a unique opportunity to study a patient's *occlusion,* or biting relationship, in detail. They can view the teeth and jaws from angles that are not possible by only looking into the mouth.

In addition to their diagnostic value, study models are beneficial in planning treatment for the patient. After treatment has been completed, a new set of models can be made to demonstrate the improvements obtained through treatment. Orthodontists use this "before-and-after" idea to demonstrate the improvements in appearance and function of the teeth after treatment.

Photographs

Dentistry is utilizing the time-honored photograph more and more in everyday practice. Colored prints and slides are excellent ways to record the progress of treatment of many oral conditions. Again, the before-and-after idea can be accomplished with pictures.

Photographs are excellent ways for the dentist to consult with specialists to arrive at a diagnosis and plan treatment. The old adage that "a picture is worth a thousand words" applies in dentistry as well.

Manufacturers of photographic equipment have developed many easy-to-use cameras for intraoral photography. The assistant should not be surprised to find photographing patients a part of daily tasks.

Photographs should become a part of the patient's permanent record.

Bacterial analysis

The determination of specific types of organisms present in the oral cavity in special situations is help-

ful to the dentist in arriving at an accurate diagnosis and treatment plan. Bacterial studies are done by collecting samples of material from suspicious areas in the oral cavity and placing them in sterile containers. The samples can be incubated and studied to determine what type of organism may be present and in what quantity. Three common uses of bacterial studies in dentistry are in caries prevention, endodontic procedures, and treating infections.

Patients who have evidence of an oral infection that persists even when an antibiotic has been administered are candidates for a bacterial analysis of the infection. The bacterial analysis will reveal the specific organism that is the offender, and a specific drug can be selected to eliminate it.

Vigorous caries-control measures have been developed (Chapter 1) that are based on the elimination of certain *Streptococcus* and *Lactobacillus* organisms from the oral cavity. Saliva samples are taken and analyzed to determine the presence and quantities of these organisms in the saliva. If the quantity is high, a vigorous diet-control plan may be indicated.

Endodontic (root canal) procedures use bacterial analysis to determine the status of contamination that may exist in a pulp chamber of a tooth that is being treated. Such information is valuable in the diagnosis and treatment of these endodontically involved teeth. This matter is discussed in Chapter 22, which deals with the subject of endodontics.

Biopsy

Biopsy is the surgical removal of a piece of tissue from the body for examination under the microscope to help in establishing an accurate diagnosis. The tissue sample usually consists of both diseased and some normal adjacent tissue for comparison. The common biopsy techniques will be discussed in Chapter 25.

Exfoliative cytology

Cytology is the study of cells. Exfoliation means the process of shedding, in this instance, of tissue cells. Some suspected soft-tissue diseases such as oral cancer can be detected by (1) scraping the surface of the lesion with a tongue blade and (2) examining the scrapings under a microscope for abnormal tissue cells, which will confirm the diagnosis.

Medical tests

On occasion, certain medical tests are indicated to establish a diagnosis and to protect the patient from unnecessary harm during treatment. Some of these are listed as follows:

1. Blood pressure determination
2. Blood tests when clinical signs and symptoms indicate them
3. Vitamin C test

DENTAL RECORDS

Record keeping is an essential part of dental practice. The dental record is the entire collection of information that has been obtained from the patient. In essence, the dental record is a library on the patient to which the dentist and staff refer repeatedly. Records should be complete and in neat order for easy reference. It is a wise practice to preserve dental records as long as possible for medicolegal reasons such as lawsuits and assisting law enforcement agencies in identification procedures.

Dental records vary widely in format from one practice to another, yet they all contain basically the same elements. The specific design of the record is determined according to the personal preference of the dentist. The basic elements of a typical dental record include the following:

1. Patient information section
2. Medical-dental history
3. Dental chart
4. Treatment plan
5. Radiographs
6. Envelope

Patient information section

Every business that has an appointment and billing system requires certain information about its customers to conduct orderly business practices. Dental offices are no exception. Patients must be contacted by telephone and by mail. Insurance forms have to be filled out correctly, and other business procedures have to be carried out that require personal information about the patient.

Some offices use a separate form such as the one in Fig. 3-6 to record information, and others utilize a

MR. MRS. MISS	REGISTRATION DATE	DATE OF BIRTH	S M W D
HOME ADDRESS		HOME TEL.	
		SOC. SEC. NO.	
EMPLOYER	ADDRESS		
OCCUPATION	BUS. TEL.		
PREVIOUS ADDRESS	CITY	STATE	
PERSON RESPONSIBLE FOR ACCOUNT			
ADDRESS			
REFERRED BY	PHYSICIAN		
DENTAL INSURANCE PROGRAM		LOCAL NO.	
PURPOSE OF CALL			
PREFERRED DAY FOR APPTS.	TIME	AM PM	
REMARKS			
		FORM 1063 COLWELL CO., CHAMPAIGN, ILL.	

Fig. 3-6. Patient registration form. (Courtesy Colwell Inc., Champaign, Ill.)

combination health questionnaire–patient information form.

Patient information should be updated periodically because addresses, telephone numbers, employers, and marital status change.

Medical-dental history

The details of the medical-dental history were discussed previously. This information should be updated periodically as the patient's health status changes. The history should be placed in a prominent place (on top of the dental chart) when the patient record is laid out before treatment. This serves as a reminder to the dentist to review it as needed before beginning treatment.

Dental chart (Fig. 3-7)

The dental chart serves as a convenient form for recording clinical data acquired during both the oral and radiographic examinations. Although there are many different chart designs available, almost all of them contain a schematic drawing of the dentition on one side and a services-rendered section on the other side.

The schematic drawing of the dentition helps the assistant to quickly record information as it is dictated during the examination appointment. Various charting symbols are used to expedite the recording process. Afterward the dentist has a pictorial display of the needed treatment that can be referred to at a glance. The dental chart used along with the treatment planning sheet affords the dentist the opportunity to create a detailed analysis of the patient's condition and plan of treatment.

There are several auxiliary uses of the dental chart besides recording the treatment to be done. The following list represents some of the more common kinds of information that can be included on the chart.

1. *Patient information section.* The dentist may find it helpful to review some of this personal information to facilitate conversation with the patient as well as conduct favorable business practices.
2. *Medical precaution section.* Whenever the medical-dental history reveals a systemic condition that the dentist must be aware of before and during treatment, such information can be written in a special area on the chart. This serves as an added reminder to exercise precaution.
3. *Radiographic history.* A listing of the radiographs the patient has had taken can be displayed in this area on the chart. This helps the

dental staff to locate the most recent radiographs quickly. Such a listing also allows the dentist to quickly review which radiographs are available for reference.

4. *Remarks.* Probably every chart should have an area on it designated for personal notations the dentist wants to make regarding treatment or characteristics of the patient. This type of information is helpful in future appointments. If a dentist has already discussed the need for a bridge with a patient at a previous appointment, this notation would prevent unnecessary repetitions. It is nice to know in advance if a patient is apprehensive or uncooperative. This can be noted in a remarks section on the chart for future reference.
5. *Fee estimates.* If the dentist has discussed treatment with the patient and established the fee for the service, it is helpful to record this on the chart for easy reference at the completion of treatment. The treatment planning sheet can be used to itemize the treatment in detail if it is extensive.
6. *Completed treatment.* Opinions vary on the use of the dental chart to record treatment that has been completed. Almost all dentists record the completed treatment and fees assessed on the "services rendered" side of the chart (Fig. 3-7, *B*), using some verbal description or code. Some dentists wish to use the drawing side of the chart to indicate the completion of restorative procedures in addition to the verbal description.

Certainly not all dentists include the entire list of items on dental charts; however, it can be done as shown in Fig. 3-8. It is very convenient for the entire staff to have this information available at a glance. Figs. 3-8 and 3-9 demonstrate the recording of diagnostic and treatment information on the schematic drawings of the teeth.

Treatment planning sheet (Fig. 3-10)

After all the diagnostic information has been obtained and analyzed, the dentist will arrive at a diagnosis. More correctly, the dentist will probably arrive at more than one diagnosis. Patients often have more than one condition afflicting them at one time. It is not uncommon to see caries, periodontal disease, and some soft tissue lesions all at the same time in the same patient.

The dentist then assembles all the information

Text continued on p. 48.

A

Name ____________________ Home Phone ______ Business Phone ______ Date ______
LAST FIRST MIDDLE

Home Address ______ City ______ Date of Birth ______ Age ______ Referred By ______

Occupation ______ Employer ______ Employer Address ______ City ______

Marital Status ______ Spouse Name ______ Spouse's Occupation ______

Employer ______ Employer's Address ______ City ______ Credit Rating ______

Person Financially Responsible ______ Relationship to You ______ Recall ______

Billing Address ______ City ______ Zip ______ Dental Insurance ______

Physician ______ Phone ______ Former Dentist ______ Address ______

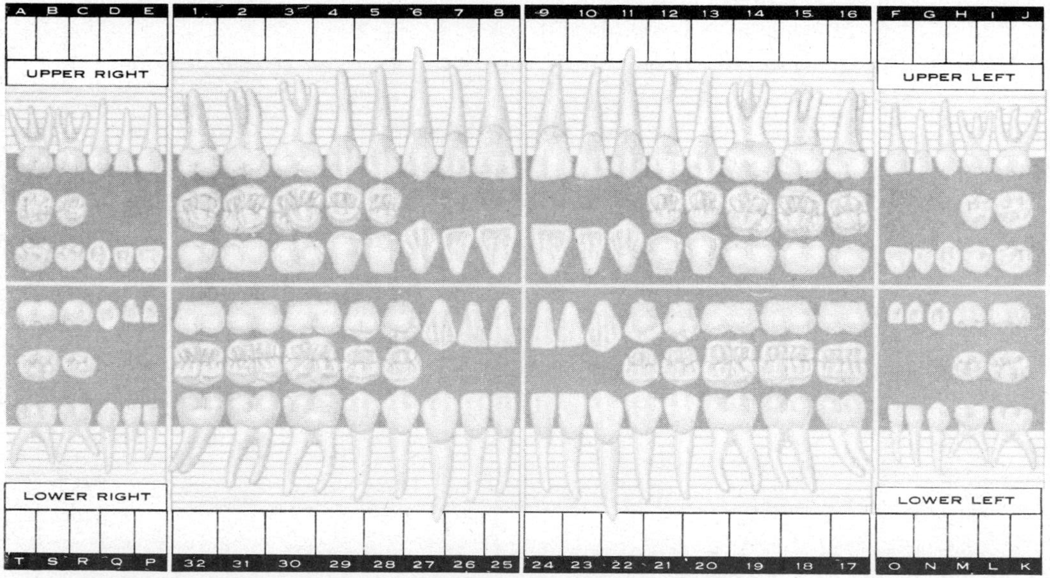

A B C D E
1 2 3 4 5 6 7 8
9 10 11 12 13 14 15 16
F G H I J
UPPER RIGHT
UPPER LEFT
LOWER RIGHT
LOWER LEFT
T S R Q P
32 31 30 29 28 27 26 25
24 23 22 21 20 19 18 17
O N M L K

MEDICAL PRECAUTIONS:

ANESTHESIA: YES [ ] NO [ ]

REMARKS ______

RADIOGRAPHIC HISTORY:

Date	Survey	Date	Survey

REMARKS: ______

FEE ESTIMATES

DATE	TREATMENT	FEE

FORM C - 103 -B

Continued.

Fig. 3-7

PATIENTS NAME _____

BILLING NAME _____

ADDRESS _____

_____

_____

_____

FINANCIAL ARRANGEMENT

_____

_____

_____

_____

_____

1 - 2 - 3 - 4 - 5

DATE	SERVICES	CHARGES	PAID	BALANCE

B

FORM C - 103 - C

Fig. 3-7, cont'd

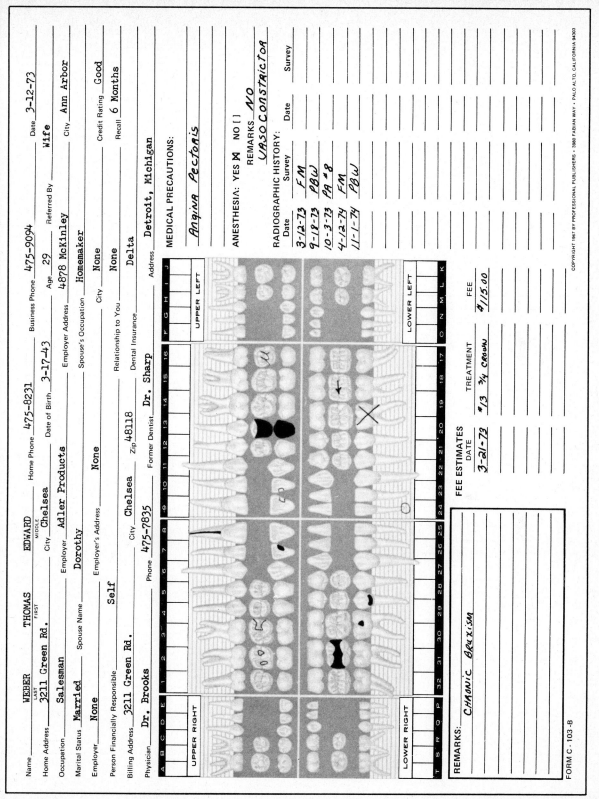

Name _____ WEBER _____ THOMAS _____ EDWARD _____ Home Phone 475-8231 _____ Business Phone 475-9094 _____ Date 3-12-73
                    LAST   FIRST   MIDDLE
Home Address 3211 Green Rd. _____ City Chelsea _____ Date of Birth 3-17-43 _____ Age 29 _____ Referred By Wife
Occupation Salesman _____ Employer Adler Products _____ Employer Address 4878 McKinley _____ City Ann Arbor
Marital Status Married _____ Spouse Name Dorothy _____ Spouse's Occupation Homemaker
Employer None _____ Employer's Address None _____ City _____ Credit Rating Good
Person Financially Responsible Self _____ Relationship to You _____ Recall 6 Months
Billing Address 3211 Green Rd. _____ City Chelsea _____ Zip 48118 _____ Dental Insurance Delta
Physician Dr. Brooks _____ Phone 475-7835 _____ Former Dentist Dr. Sharp _____ Address Detroit, Michigan

MEDICAL PRECAUTIONS:

Angina Pectoris

ANESTHESIA: YES ☒ NO [ ]
REMARKS No
VASO CONSTRICTOR

RADIOGRAPHIC HISTORY:

Date	Survey	Date	Survey
3-12-73	FM		
9-19-73	PBW		
10-3-73	PA #8		
4-12-74	FM		
11-1-74	PBW		

FEE ESTIMATES

DATE	TREATMENT	FEE
3-21-73	#13 ¾ Crown	$115.00

REMARKS: CHRONIC BRUXISM

FORM C - 103 -B

Fig. 3-8

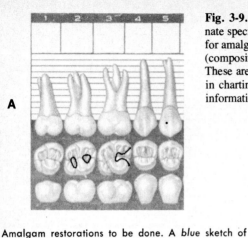

Fig. 3-9. Colored pencils are helpful in charting to designate specific types of restorations. A suggested code is blue for amalgam restoration, red for esthetic restorative material (composite, silicate, acrylic), and gold for gold restoration. These are only examples of some symbols that can be used in charting. Each dentist has a system of charting clinical information.

Amalgam restorations to be done. A *blue* sketch of the outline form of the restoration to be placed indicates specifically what is to be done.

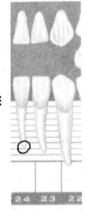

Esthetic restorations to be done. A *red* sketch of the outline form of the restoration indicates what is to be done.

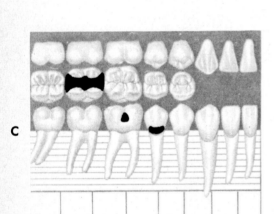

Completed restorations. After the tooth has been restored, the outline of the restoration is filled in with the appropriate color that represents the type of restorative material used.

Gold restorations can be represented by coloring the surfaces covered by the restoration with gold pencil. Example is a three-quarter crown on tooth no. 13.

Circle around the root apex indicates endodontic treatment to be done.

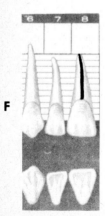

The *u* on the occlusal view of a tooth indicates that it is *unerupted.*

Solid blue line through the center of the root indicates a filled root canal.

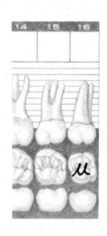

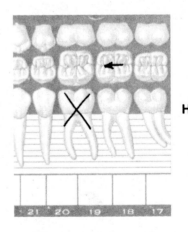

Arrow on the occlusal view indicates that a tooth is malposed or drifted out of normal position in the direction of the arrow. X on the facial view indicates a missing tooth.

ESTIMATE SHEET

PATIENT'S NAME

TOOTH OR SURFACE	DESCRIPTION OF SERVICE	NO. APPTS.	TIME REQUIRED	FEE
	PROPHYLAXIS	1	30	25.00
	X-RAYS	1	15	15.00
	DIAGNOSTIC MODELS			
17	Extract	1	30	90.00
17	Suture removal	1	5	N/C
$3^{5,6}$	Amalgam	1		
$7,8^2$	Composite	1	30	40.00

DATED 11-4-83

ACCEPTED K.S.

_____ DENTIST

CASE PLANNING TIME 10 min.

James Boyd PATIENT

—

HUSBAND _____ FATHER

ACTUAL PRESENTATION TIME 5 min.

FORM 9400 COLWELL CO., CHAMPAIGN, ILLINOIS

Fig. 3-10. Treatment plan. (Courtesy Colwell Inc., Champaign, Ill.)

available regarding the diagnosis and formulates a plan of treatment in detail. Treatment plans can vary from planning a single restoration to planning multiple-treatment regimens. If the treatment plan is extensive, it is helpful to use a treatment planning sheet to describe the entire sequence of the treatment.

The treatment planning sheet can be thought of as an extension of the dental chart in which extensive treatment plans can be recorded. Smaller treatment plans can be simply indicated on the drawing side of the chart. Also, for clinical convenience, some phases of the more extensive treatment plans can be recorded on the chart in addition to the treatment planning sheet.

Radiographs

Radiographs can be stored either in the same envelope with the rest of the dental record or in a separate radiographic file. The individual office system and personal preferences will determine the appropriate filing of radiographs.

TREATMENT PLANNING

Probably one of the most challenging areas for the dentist is planning the appropriate treatment for a patient. Treatment plans vary from simple to complex. The more complex the diagnosis, the more the dentist must call on a variety of resources to formulate an acceptable treatment regimen.

The treatment plan is essentially a "game plan" for the dentist, which is established after careful study of the diagnostic information. Then the dentist can begin treatment in a well-organized pattern. A treatment plan establishes the following basic patient information:

1. A description of the proposed treatment
2. The sequence in which treatment will be done
3. The approximate number of appointments that will be needed for treatment
4. The treatment to be done at each appointment
5. The time required for each appointment
6. Interval of time needed between appointments for healing or completion of laboratory procedures
7. A fee estimate for the service to be performed

The basic information in the treatment plan is of benefit for both dental personnel and the patient because appointment scheduling is based on the treatment plan. The information helps the dental staff to arrange appropriate times for appointments in a pre-

planned manner. It is also of great assistance to the patients to be able to plan appointments around their personal activities such as vacations, job interviews, or speeches when the aftereffects of treatment might impinge on these events. The best time for the extraction of an impacted third molar is definitely not the day before the senior prom!

Factors influencing treatment planning

The format of a treatment plan is influenced by several factors. These factors may alter the entire treatment plan, or a portion of it, or simply change the sequence of treatment. Following are some of the common factors to be considered:

1. *Patient attitude.* The patient must have an interest in receiving care. This may be influenced by the patient's personal background, oral hygiene, priorities in life, and fears.
2. *Economics.* The question of cost is a major factor in patients' acceptance of a proposed treatment plan. Fees are far more acceptable to patients when well-organized treatment plans are presented to them in an understandable way. Patients can then begin to appreciate the time and effort that will be devoted to their well-being. This is called case presentation (Fig. 3-11).
3. *Presence of systemic disease.* The influence of systemic disease may cause a delay of treatment or even make some aspects of treatment impos-

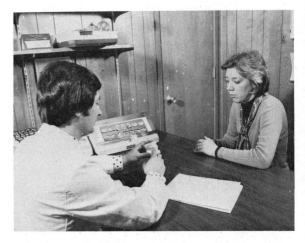

Fig. 3-11. Case presentation. Diagnosis, treatment, and fee estimates are discussed with patient.

sible because of the systemic risks involved. Terminal illnesses certainly influence the dentist's thoughts on choosing a reasonable plan.

4. *Chief complaint.* The reason for the patient's seeking treatment in the first place must be considered strongly in the sequence of treatment. A patient with a throbbing abscess on a lower molar is not particularly interested in having a teeth cleaning or other treatment performed until the pain in the offending tooth is treated.

5. *Age of the patient.* Age often has a strong influence on treatment planning. The child who has a loose primary tooth with decay would be better served by extraction of the tooth than by restoration, since it is about to be shed anyway. An elderly patient who is near death poses the question of whether extensive treatment will be useful to the individual.

These factors may be present individually or in various combinations. It is not unusual for the dentist to create alternate treatment plans based on the factors just discussed. Modification of a selected treatment plan may have to be made as treatment progresses, because of unforeseen circumstances.

Format of the treatment plan

Kerr and associates suggest a general outline for treatment planning that is rather widely used in general practice*:

I. Systemic treatment
 A. Referral to a physician for systemic evaluation and treatment as indicated by history and clinical findings
 B. Appraisal of the influence of systemic treatment on the dental treatment plan
 C. Premedication with antibiotics or sedatives as indicated by the history
 D. Corrective therapy for oral infection

*From Kerr, D.A., Ash, M.M., and Millard, H.D.: Oral diagnosis, ed. 6, St. Louis, 1983, The C.V. Mosby Co.

II. Preoperatory treatment
 A. Oral surgery
 B. Endodontic therapy
 C. Caries control
 D. Periodontal therapy
 E. Orthodontic treatment
 F. Occlusal adjustment
III. Corrective treatment
 A. Operative dentistry
 B. Prosthetic dentistry
IV. Periodic recall examinations and maintenance treatment

Essentially, what the format suggests is that the general well-being of patients be considered above all else. The next priority is to establish a proper foundation for restoring the mouth by eliminating pain, diseased tissue, progressive disease, and malocclusion. After the foundation is sound, restoration of the mouth with various dental restorations and prosthetic appliances can begin. After the corrective phase of treament patients must maintain their healthy state by proper home care procedures and routine recall examinations.

SUMMARY

This chapter is intended to give the assistant a basic understanding of the process of collecting and recording clinical information through various diagnostic methods. The appreciation for the value of accurate dental records should be clear in the mind of dental assistants, since they play a significant role in record keeping. The analysis, diagnosis, and orderly approach to treatment through a well-organized treatment plan contribute not only to the health of the patient but also to the maintenance of a well-organized office that is a pleasure for everyone who works there.

BIBLIOGRAPHY

Kerr, D.A., Ash, M.M., and Millard, H.D.: Oral diagnosis, ed. 6, St. Louis, 1983, The C.V. Mosby Co.

CHAPTER 4

TOOTH NUMBERING AND
SURFACE ANNOTATION

TOOTH NUMBERING SYSTEMS

Since the use of proper names for each tooth can be cumbersome, numbering systems have been developed that simplify the identification of individual teeth. These systems are extremely helpful in charting information on records, in verbal communication, and in correspondence such as referral letters. The following numbering systems are in common use.

American Dental Association (ADA) sequential numbering system

The ADA has adopted a standard sequential numbering system for all 32 teeth in the permanent dentition. Each tooth is assigned a number so that whenever that number is used it will indicate a specific permanent tooth.

Fig. 4-1 demonstrates this system. Tooth No. 1 represents the patient's maxillary right third molar. The numbering progresses toward the anterior teeth and continues through the patient's maxillary left quadrant where the maxillary left third molar is assigned the number 16. The mandibular teeth are numbered starting in the mandibular left quadrant, with the third molar being assigned the number 17. Numbering continues around the arch to the mandibular right third molar, which becomes tooth No. 32.

This system has widespread use in the dental profession because it is extremely simple. It avoids confusion when reference is made to specific teeth or areas around specific teeth. It is much simpler to refer to tooth numbers than to refer to teeth by their somewhat cumbersome anatomical names.

ADA sequential lettering (A-T) system for primary teeth

The same basic system is used to identify the primary teeth, except that they are identified with the upper-case letters A through T (Fig. 4-2). Tooth A represents the primary maxillary right second molar. The lettering progresses just as in the numbering system described for permanent teeth. The use of letters to designate *primary* teeth avoids confusion with the identification of permanent teeth, which are assigned individual numbers.

Zsigmondy/Palmer system

The Zsigmondy/Palmer system identifies specific teeth by assigning a number (for a permanent tooth) or a letter (for a primary tooth) to teeth in each of the four quadrants of the mouth.

The permanent dentition is identified by assigning a number of teeth from 1 through 8 within each quadrant. In this system, the number 8 represents third molars, whereas the number 1 represents central incisors (Fig. 4-3, *A*). A grid system is used to identify specific teeth in the mouth. Fig. 4-3, *B*, represents the grid that is used for the permanent dentition. The grid represents the patient's mouth as the operator or assistant views it. To specifically designate the maxillary right third molar, the symbol $\underline{8}\rfloor$ is used. The bracket around the tooth indicates the quadrant in which the tooth is located. For example, the number 8 is placed above the horizontal line, which indicates that it is a maxillary tooth. Since the number 8 is located to the left of the vertical line as it is viewed, the tooth is located in the patient's right quadrant. Hence this tooth is the maxillary right third molar.

The quadrant symbols are as follows:

$\rfloor$ = Maxillary right

$\lfloor$ = Maxillary left

$\ulcorner$ = Mandibular left

$\urcorner$ = Mandibular right

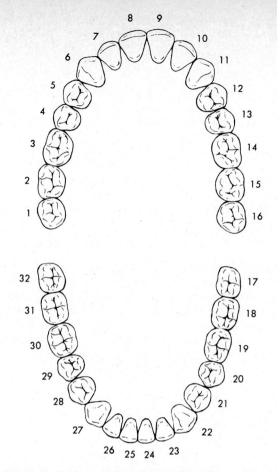

Fig. 4-1. American Dental Association (ADA) sequential numbering system of permanent dentition.

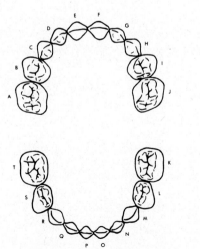

Fig. 4-2. ADA sequential lettering system for primary teeth.

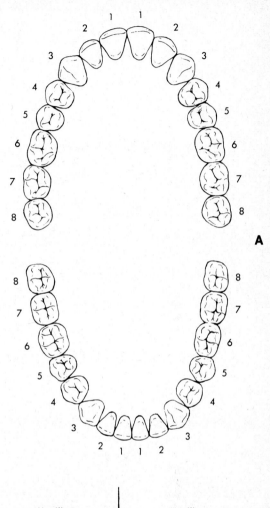

Fig. 4-3. Zsigmondy/Palmer numbering system for permanent dentition. **A,** Anatomical arrangement. **B,** Schematic arrangement.

Maxillary right		Maxillary left
87654321		12345678
87654321		12345678
Mandibular right		Mandibular left

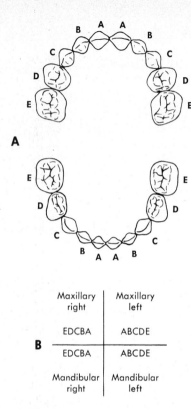

A

B

Maxillary right	Maxillary left
EDCBA	ABCDE
EDCBA	ABCDE
Mandibular right	Mandibular left

Fig. 4-4. Zsigmondy/Palmer numbering system for primary dentition. **A,** Anatomical arrangement. **B,** Schematic arrangement.

6EDCBA	ABCDE6
6EDCB1	1BCDE6

Fig. 4-5. Schematic display of mixed dentition using Zsigmondy/Palmer tooth identification system.

The primary teeth can be identified using this same basic system. The teeth in the quadrant are labeled with letters A through E. The primary second molars are assigned the letter E, and the central incisors are assigned the letter A (Fig. 4-4, *A* and *B*). For example, the symbol ⌐c⌐ would represent the primary maxillary right cuspid in the primary dentition.

This system is frequently used by orthodontists because the entire dentition can be displayed on one grid regardless of whether the patient has a primary, mixed, or permanent dentition. The example shown in Fig. 4-5 is a mixed dentition. The patient has most of the primary teeth still present, as indicated by letters in all quadrants. However, the numbers in each quadrant indicate that some permanent teeth have erupted. Specifically, the 6s indicate that all four first permanent molars are present. The 1s in the lower arch indicate that both permanent central incisors have also erupted and have replaced the primary central incisors.

Federation Dentaire Internationale (FDI) system

The FDI system was designed to facilitate computer storage of records, which is often used in research as well as in some dental offices. The numbering system uses a two-digit number to identify each tooth. The first digit indicates the quadrant in which the tooth is located. The second digit identifies the specific tooth in that quadrant. The quadrants are numbered as follows:

Quadrant No. 1 = Maxillary right
Quadrant No. 2 = Maxillary left
Quadrant No. 3 = Mandibular left
Quadrant No. 4 = Mandibular right

As in the Zsigmondy/Palmer system, the teeth are assigned numbers 1 through 8 in each quadrant. Tooth No. 1 is the central incisor, and No. 8 is the third molar (Fig. 4-6). The following are random examples of the FDI tooth numbering system for the *permanent* dentition:

FDI number	Tooth name
15*	Maxillary right second premolar
22	Maxillary left lateral incisor
36	Mandibular left first molar
44	Mandibular right first premolar

The primary dentition is numbered in a similar fashion. The quadrants in the primary dentition are numbered as follows:

Quadrant No. 5 = Maxillary right
Quadrant No. 6 = Maxillary left
Quadrant No. 7 = Mandibular left
Quadrant No. 8 = Mandibular right

*Pronounce digits only, for example, "one-five," not "fifteen."

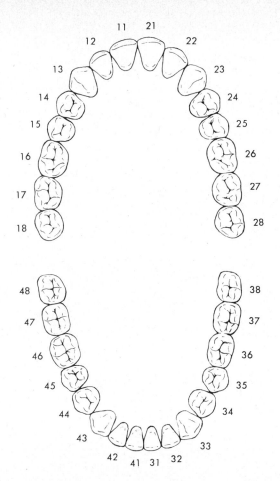

Fig. 4-6. Federation Dentaire Internationale (FDI) tooth numbering system for permanent dentition.

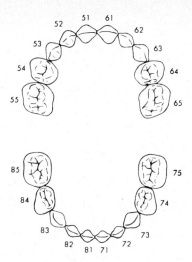

Fig. 4-7. FDI numbering system for primary dentition.

The teeth are numbered 1 through 5 in each quadrant, with tooth No. 1 being the central incisor and No. 5 being the second molar (Fig. 4-7).

The following are random examples of the FDI tooth numbering system for the primary dentition:

FDI number	Tooth name
54	Maxillary right first primary molar
63	Maxillary left primary cuspid
75	Mandibular left second primary molar
84	Mandibular right first primary molar

The choice of which specific tooth numbering system is used in a dental practice is left entirely to the preference of the dentist.

TOOTH SURFACE ANNOTATION
Tooth surface names

Each surface of the crown of a tooth is identified by a specific name (Fig. 4-8, *A* to *C*). These surface names are summarized in Table 4-1. Tooth surface names are used in clinical dentistry to describe locations of caries, defects, or restorations in a patient's teeth. It is imperative that the dental assistant learn these surface names and where to apply them.

Tooth surface designations

Tooth surface numbering and lettering systems have been used for years to simplify the recording of clinical information. In these systems each tooth surface is assigned a number or a letter to designate the surface so that surface names do not have to be written out on clinical records. These systems, when combined with tooth numbering systems, create a shorthand method for recording clinical information.

The two most common methods of designating tooth surfaces are as follows:

Tooth surface	Surface number	Surface abbreviation
Mesial	1	m
Distal	2	d
Facial (buccal, labial)	3	f (b = buccal, lab = labial)
Lingual (palatal)	4	l (p = palatal)
Occlusal (incisal)	5	o (i = incisal)

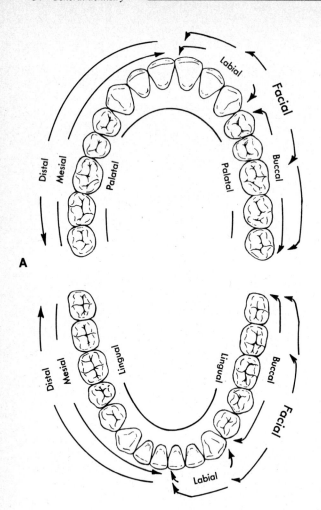

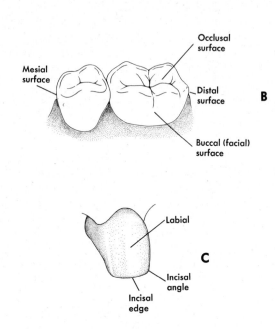

Fig. 4-8. Tooth surface names. **A,** Upper and lower arches. **B,** Anterior teeth. **C,** Posterior teeth.

Posterior teeth that have a prominent oblique or transverse ridge which divides the occlusal surface into two distinct sections have an additional designation:

Tooth surface	Surface number	Surface abbreviations
Mesial occlusal	5	o
Distal occlusal	6	o (no specific designation; therefore the number 6 is preferred)

These prominent ridges are typically found on the following teeth (Fig. 4-9):

Permanent dentition	Primary dentition
Maxillary first molars	Maxillary second molars
Maxillary second molars	Mandibular first molars
Mandibular first bicuspids	
Mandibular second bicuspids (15% of the population)	

Recording surfaces to be restored using the numbering systems

Tooth surface designations are used in combination with tooth numbers by writing the tooth number as a stem with the surface numbers as exponents to that stem. For example, tooth No. 18 (ADA system) is used to identify the mandibular left second permanent

Table 4-1. Summary of tooth surface names

Posterior teeth (pre-molars, molars)	Anterior teeth (cus-pids, incisors)	Description
Occlusal	Incisal edge	Horizontal biting surface
Mesial	Mesial	Vertical surface toward midline
Distal	Distal	Vertical surface away from midline
Buccal	Labial	Vertical surface toward cheek or lips
Lingual*	Lingual	Vertical surface of lower teeth toward tongue
Palatal*	Palatal	Vertical surface of upper teeth toward the palate
Facial†	Facial	Universal term for vertical surface of any tooth that is toward facial tissues (labial or buc-cal = facial)

*The terms *lingual* surface and *palatal* surface are often used inter-changeably.
†The term *facial* surface is often used in place of *buccal* surface (posterior teeth) or *labial* surface (anterior teeth) for convenience.

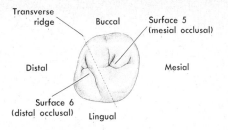

Fig. 4-9. Occlusal view of maxillary right first molar with surfaces 5 and 6 identified.

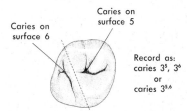

Fig. 4-10. Occlusal view of tooth No. 3 with caries present on surfaces 5 and 6.

molar. If caries is present on the mesial surface, the number 1 or the letter m is used to designate the mesial surface and is placed as an exponent to the number 18.

18^m or 18^1 = Caries present on the mesial surface of the mandibular left second permanent molar

The advantage of using this shorthand method of iden-tifying teeth and their surfaces is readily apparent when compared with the longhand method of record-ing the same information.

If more than one surface has caries present that will require more than one restoration, the tooth number is rewritten with the appropriate exponent. Another method is to write the tooth number once and place a comma between the exponents. For example:

$$18^1, 18^3 \text{ or } 18^{1,3}$$

If the abbreviations for tooth surfaces are preferred, they are used in a similar fashion. For example:

$$18^1 = 18^m$$
$$18^3 = 18^f$$
$$18^{1,3} = 18^{m,f}$$

On the other hand, if more than one surface of a tooth has caries that can be restored with only one restoration, the tooth number is written only once and without commas between the exponents. For ex-ample:

$$30^{152}$$

Teeth with transverse ridges such as the maxillary right first permanent molar (No. 3) that have caries present on both portions of the occlusal surface (Fig. 4-10) would be recorded as follows:

$$3^5, 3^6 = 3^{5,6}$$

The abbreviation method does not allow for a clear distinction between those portions of the occlusal sur-face separated by the transverse ridge, and these would have to be recorded as follows:

$$3^0, 3^0 = 3^{0,0}$$

When this system is employed by the operator, the operative phase of a treatment plan might appear as shown in Fig. 3-10.

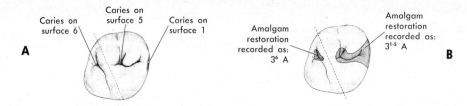

Fig. 4-11. Occlusal view of tooth No. 3. **A,** Caries present on surfaces 1, 5, and 6. **B,** Amalgam restorations used to restore tooth.

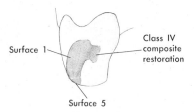

Fig. 4-12. Mesial lingual view of Class IV composite restoration on tooth No. 8.

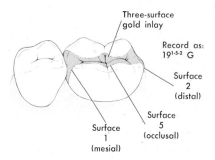

Fig. 4-13. Three-surface gold inlay on tooth No. 19.

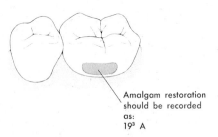

Fig. 4-14. Class V amalgam restoration located on buccal surface of tooth No. 19.

Recording restored teeth using the numbering systems

Once teeth have been restored, this information can be recorded graphically on dental charts (Fig. 3-8) or the same information can be placed in the "completed treatment" section under "services rendered" (Fig. 3-7, *B*) and on insurance forms using the numbering systems.

When numbering systems are used, the tooth number is repeated for each separate restoration done on that tooth. For example, if an occlusal amalgam restoration is placed on the distal occlusal portion of tooth No. 3 and a two-surface amalgam restoration is placed on the mesial and mesial occlusal portions of the same tooth, the information would be recorded as follows (Fig. 4-11, *A* and *B*):

$$3^6A, \ 3^{1\text{-}5}A$$

The letter A is used in this case to indicate the restorative material used. The hyphen in $3^{1\text{-}5}$ indicates that the surfaces 1 and 5 are connected by the restorative material. A composite restoration that restores both the mesial surface and a portion of the incisal edge of tooth number 8 would be recorded as follows (Fig. 4-12):

$$8^{1\text{-}5}C$$

The letter C is used here to indicate composite restorative material. A tooth restored with a gold inlay that covers three surfaces, such as the mesial, occlusal, and distal surfaces of tooth No. 19, would be recorded as follows (Fig. 4-13):

$$19^{1\text{-}5\text{-}2}G$$

The letter G may be used to indicate gold as the restorative material. A single surface that is restored with amalgam, such as the facial surface of tooth No. 19, would be recorded as follows (Fig. 4-14):

$$19^3A$$

SUMMARY

Charting clinical information, filling out insurance claim forms, and handling correspondence are all duties that may be delegated to the dental assistant. Therefore a working knowledge of various tooth numbering and tooth surface annotation systems is essential.

BIBLIOGRAPHY

Charbeneau, G.T., et al.: Principles and practice of operative dentistry, ed. 2, Philadelphia, 1981, Lea & Febiger.

CHAPTER 5

GENERAL OPERATIVE INSTRUMENTS AND SUPPLIES

The variety of instruments and supplies that are used in operative procedures is very large and continually growing as new products and techniques are developed. The selection of an armamentarium for a specific procedure is based on the personal preference of the dentist, which creates a problem for the beginning dental assistant in learning instrumentation. This chapter is intended to acquaint the beginning dental assistant with some of the more common instruments and supplies that are used in operative dentistry. Such a background will make it easier for the assistant to adapt to the individual dentist's armamentarium.

Instruments that are used for specific operative procedures will be discussed in later chapters.

DENTAL HANDPIECE

The dental handpiece is probably the most frequently used instrument in operative and restorative dentistry. Patients refer to this instrument as the "dentist's drill." The handpiece works on a similar principle as a drill in that cutting and polishing instruments are held in the handpiece and spun at various speeds to cut or polish tooth structure. Since the instrument is held in the hand to guide the cutting action, it acquired the name *handpiece*.

The two types of handpieces used in dentistry are the conventional-speed and the high-speed handpieces. The conventional-speed handpiece can turn a cutting instrument at speeds up to 25,000 rpm, and the high-speed handpiece can operate at 100,000 to 450,000 rpm. Both types are air driven and needed in modern dental practice.

Conventional-speed handpiece

The conventional-speed handpiece is a multipurpose instrument. Before the introduction of the high-speed handpiece in the 1940s, the conventional-speed handpiece was the only instrument available to cut cavity preparations, polish teeth, and finish dental restorations. Since the arrival of the high-speed handpiece, the use of the conventional-speed handpiece in cavity preparations has been reduced to caries removal and fine finishing of the detail of the preparation. The high-speed handpiece is used to do most of the bulk cutting of the preparation. Despite the fact that the conventional-speed handpiece is used to a lesser degree in cavity preparation, its overall importance in dentistry has not diminished. Its relatively slow speed range, coupled with favorable turning power (torque), makes it an ideal instrument for various finishing, polishing, and contouring procedures as well as caries removal. These procedures require maximum control by the dentist. The conventional-speed handpiece provides this control when it is used properly.

The basic conventional-speed handpiece is referred to as the "straight handpiece" because of its straight-line design with no bends in the working end of the instrument. The straight handpiece is used with various long-shafted cutting instruments (Fig. 5-1, *A*). This is a handy style for polishing, grinding, and adjusting dental restorations both in the oral cavity and in work at the laboratory bench. The cutting and polishing instruments that are used in the straight handpiece are designated HP (handpiece) style instruments. An HP designation means that the cutting or polishing instrument has a long, straight shaft that inserts into the staight handpiece (Fig. 5-2, *C*).

Attachments for conventional-speed handpiece. Attachments are available for the conventional-speed handpiece that expand its use considerably. Two of the most common attachments are the contra-angle and the prophylaxis angle (Fig. 5-1).

The contra-angle holds a variety of short-shafted

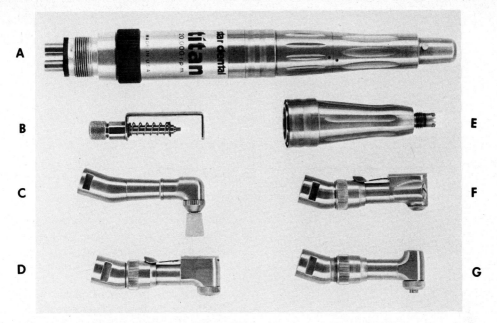

Fig. 5-1. Conventional speed handpiece (HP) and accessories. **A,** Handpiece motor with straight HP attachment. **B,** Bur changing tool. **C,** Prophylaxis angle. **D,** Latch-type (RA) contra-angle. **E,** Motor to angle adaptor. **F,** High-torque contra-angle. **G,** Friction grip (FG) contra-angle.

burs, grinding stones, and polishing disks for use intraorally. The slight bend in this attachment is the source of its name. This bend, plus the use of short-shafted cutting instruments, allows the dentist access to all areas of the mouth.

Contra-angles are available in both latch and friction-grip types. The difference between these is in the method used to hold the cutting instrument in the head of the contra-angle. The latch type holds the end of the cutting instrument by mechanically grasping a small groove on the end of the instrument shaft (Fig. 5-2, *B*). Cutting and polishing instruments that are used in the latch-type contra-angle are designated RA (right angle) instruments. An RA designation means that the shaft of the instrument has a retention groove on the end opposite the working end of the instrument. Friction-grip contra-angles hold the instrument by grasping the entire shaft by a friction chuck in the head of the contra-angle (Fig. 5-2, *A*). Instruments that are used in the friction-grip contra-angle are referred to as FG (friction-grip) instruments. An FG instrument has a short, smooth shaft with no retention groove on the end as the RA instruments have. It is

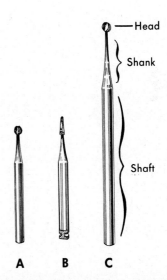

Fig. 5-2. Different styles of shafts on rotating cutting instruments. **A,** Friction grip (FG). **B,** Latch (RA). **C,** Handpiece (HP).

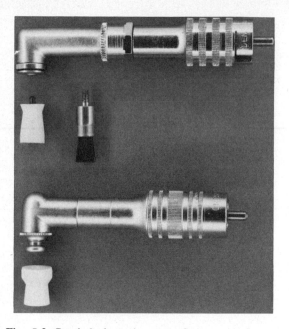

Fig. 5-3. Prophylaxis angles. *Top,* Screw type. *Bottom,* Snap-on type.

important to designate which style of cutting instrument is needed—HP, RA, or FG—when new instruments are ordered for the conventional-speed handpiece and its attachments.

Many FG burs are also available with shorter than normal shanks (short shank). These are useful in gaining access to confined areas of the oral cavity.

The prophylaxis angle is a standard attachment for the conventional-speed handpiece. It is used to hold polishing cups, disks, and brushes that are needed to remove plaque and stain during the dental prophylaxis procedure. Like the contra-angle, there are two types of prophylaxis angles available. One is a screw type, which holds the polishing instrument in place by a threaded shaft. A second type is referred to as a snap-on type, which has a smooth knob (Fig. 5-3). The assistant must designate which type of prophylaxis angle is in use when ordering replacements for the polishing instruments.

A rubber polishing cup is the most common device used on the prophylaxis angle. It is dipped in a polishing agent that lodges in the cup. The cup is then pressed against the surface to be polished and the handpiece is rotated at slow to moderate speeds to

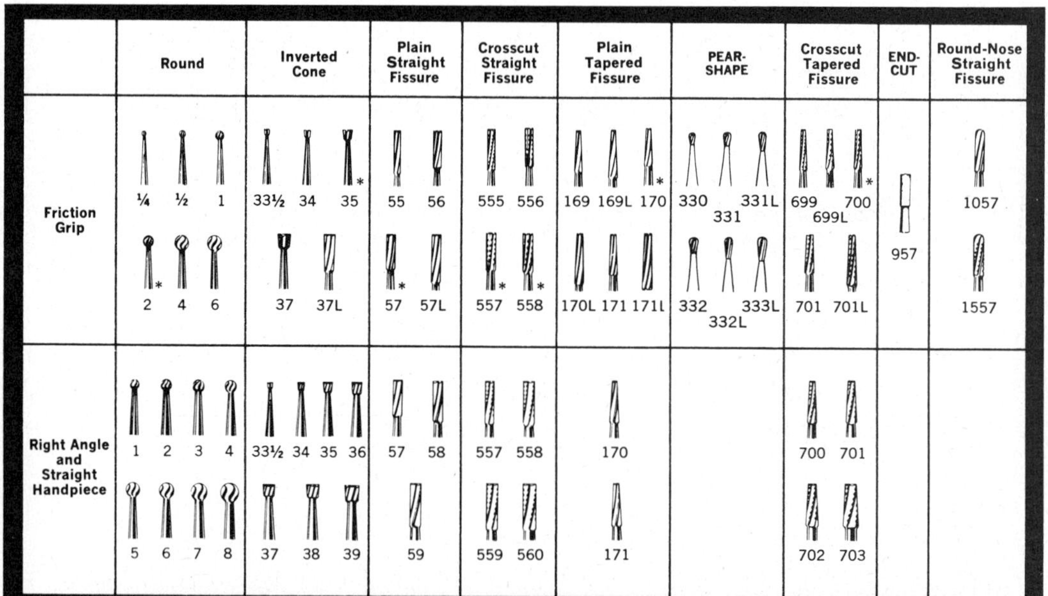

	Round			Inverted Cone			Plain Straight Fissure		Crosscut Straight Fissure		Plain Tapered Fissure			PEAR-SHAPE		Crosscut Tapered Fissure		END-CUT	Round-Nose Straight Fissure
Friction Grip	¼	½	1	33½	34	35*	55	56	555	556	169	169L	170*	330	331L / 331	699	700* / 699L		1057
	2	4	6*	37	37L		57*	57L	557*	558*	170L	171	171L	332	333L / 332L	701	701L	957	1557
Right Angle and Straight Handpiece	1	2	3	4	33½ 34	35 36	57	58	557	558	170					700	701		
	5	6	7	8	37	38 39	59		559	560	171					702	703		

*Available in short shank

Principal use: cavity preparation.

Fig. 5-4. Common bur styles used for cavity preparation. (Courtesy Kerr Manufacturing Co., Romulus, Mich.)

achieve the polishing action. The polishing agent used is determined by the polishing procedure to be accomplished. There are polishing pastes available for the prophylaxis procedure and still others for polishing various dental restorations.

Prophylaxis angles must be cleaned and lubricated frequently because the abrasive polishing agents cause excessive wear on all moving parts of the angle.

Handpieces, whether they are conventional- or high-speed types, are usually activated by a foot control. The foot control works like the accelerator of an automobile: the more it is depressed, the faster the handpiece will operate. The foot control frees the dentist's hands to operate the handpiece with greater ease and stability.

Maintenance of the conventional-speed handpiece and its attachments is important to ensure proper function and long instrument life. Manufacturer's instructions generally call for running the handpiece and attachments in a cleaning solution and then lubricating them with a special handpiece oil. Excess oil is drained off on paper towels, and then the instrument is wiped clean with an alcohol sponge. This procedure will prevent oil from leaking out of the instrument during its operation and alleviate the slippery feel on the surface of the instrument.

Rotary instruments for conventional-speed handpiece. A wide variety of instruments can be used in the conventional-speed handpiece. These include burs, diamond stones, polishing disks, grindstones, abrasive wheels, and burnishers. Some of these rotary instruments are available in all types of shafts—HP, FG, and RA—whereas others are only in one type or another. Figs. 5-4 to 5-8 show a variety of popular

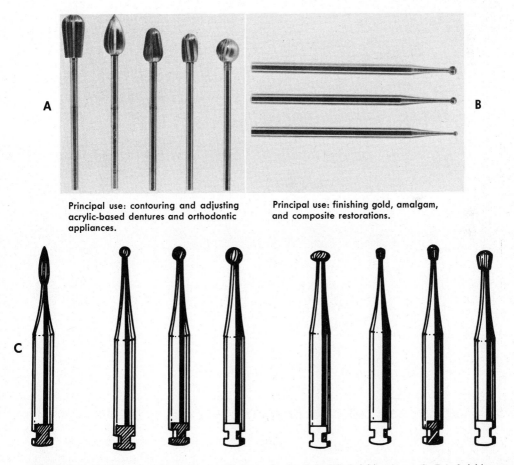

Principal use: contouring and adjusting acrylic-based dentures and orthodontic appliances.

Principal use: finishing gold, amalgam, and composite restorations.

Fig. 5-5. Commonly used burs. **A,** Acrylic burs. **B,** Straight HP finishing burs. **C,** RA finishing burs.

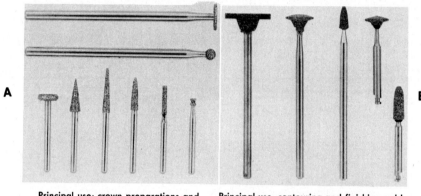

Principal use: crown preparations and occlusal equilibration.

Principal use: contouring and finishing gold, amalgam, and composite restorations; occlusal equilibration. (Also available in finer-grit white stones.)

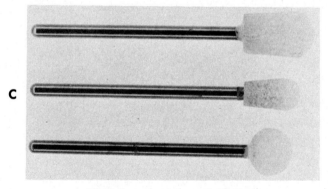

Principal use: contouring and adjusting acrylic-based dentures and orthodontic appliances.

Fig. 5-6. Commonly used stones. **A,** Diamond stones. *Top:* HP style. *Bottom:* FG style. **B,** Green stones. **C,** Acrylic stones.

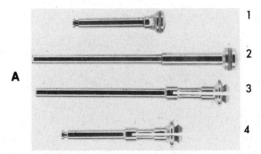

Principal use: attachment of various polishing
and cutting wheels and disks to handpiece.

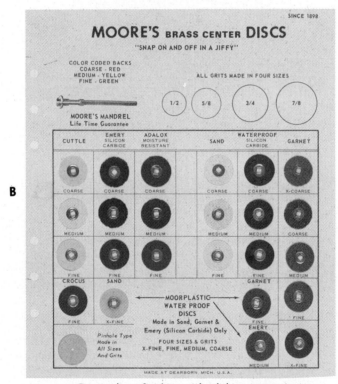

Principal use: finishing and polishing restorations.

Fig. 5-7. Commonly used finishing disks and mandrels. **A,** Mandrels. *1,* RA screw style; *2,* HP screw style; *3,* HP Moore's style; *4,* RA Moore's style. **B,** Assortment of sandpaper disks used with Moore's mandrels.

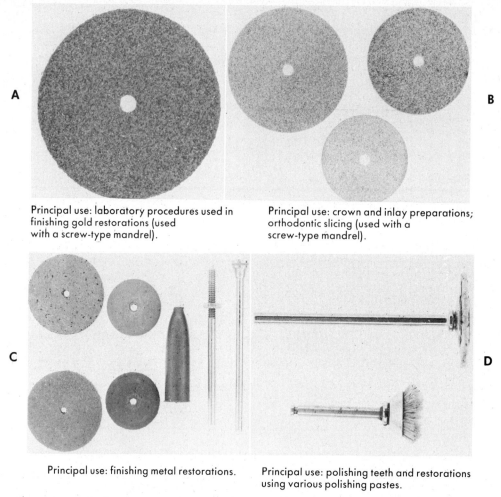

Principal use: laboratory procedures used in finishing gold restorations (used with a screw-type mandrel).

Principal use: crown and inlay preparations; orthodontic slicing (used with a screw-type mandrel).

Principal use: finishing metal restorations.

Principal use: polishing teeth and restorations using various polishing pastes.

Fig. 5-8. Commonly used finishing and polishing devices. **A,** Carborundum disk. **B,** Lightning disks. **C,** Abrasive impregnated rubber disks and point with mandrels (Craytex). **D,** Bristle brushes.

rotary instruments available and the common uses of the instruments.

Various mandrels are available to attach different replacement polishing and grinding devices to the handpiece. Some of the common devices used on these mandrels are polishing disks, rubber abrasive wheels, grinding stones, and separating disks (Figs. 5-7 and 5-8).

High-speed handpiece (Fig. 5-9)

The high-speed handpiece is one of the greatest advancements in dental equipment in recent dental history. This instrument allows the dentist to remove unwanted tooth structure rapidly and with great accuracy. Its use has expedited operative procedures considerably, with less fatigue for both the dentist and the patient. The use of this instrument has eliminated the excessive hand pressure that was required during cavity preparation when only conventional-speed handpieces were used.

The fundamental difference between high-speed and conventional-speed handpieces is, of course, how fast a cutting instrument can be spun in the handpiece. However, another significant difference should be

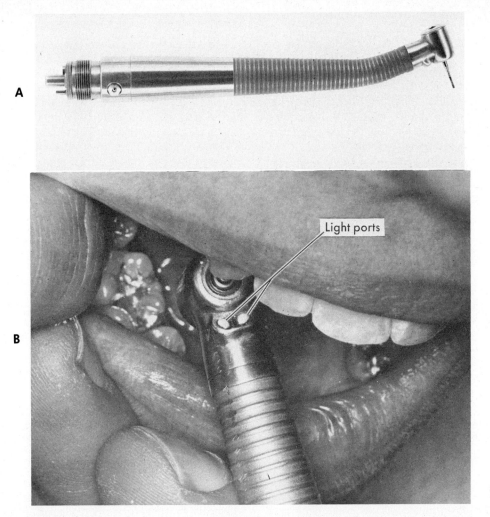

Fig. 5-9. High-speed handpieces. **A,** Regular style (nonfiberoptic). **B,** Fiberoptic style in use.

noted. High-speed handpieces operate at high speed, but they have very little torque. The opposite is true of conventional-speed handpieces. Torque is essentially the turning power of the instrument when pressure is applied during the cutting procedure. High-speed handpieces will stop operating if the dentist applies excessive pressure to the cutting instrument during a cavity preparation. Hence a light touch is required of the dentist so that the instrument can function properly.

The very high speed range of the high-speed handpiece permits rapid cutting of tooth structure. Most of

the bulk of tooth structure is removed with the high-speed handpiece during cavity preparations. Refinement of the detail of the preparation and caries removal is accomplished with both the conventional-speed handpiece and hand cutting instruments.

The extremely high speed of this handpiece created some new problems that were not as significant when only conventional-speed handpieces were used. Regular steel burs commonly used in conventional-speed handpieces had to be replaced with harder, carbon steel burs that would not dull as readily under high-speed use. A second problem was frictional heat. Carbide burs or diamond stones turning against extremely hard tooth structures at high speed generate a great deal of frictional heat. Research has indicated that this heat is significant enough to damage the delicate dental pulp. Water-spray devices were developed for all high-speed handpieces to combat frictional heat by constantly spraying the tooth and the cutting instrument with cool water during its use. The water spray also helps to remove debris from the cavity preparation in addition to cooling the tooth.

Use of the water-spray coolant with the high-speed handpiece created, in turn, two problems for the operating team. The accumulation of water necessitated the development of a high-velocity evacuator to remove the water from the mouth during cavity preparation. The second problem was interference with the dentist's vision while operating by indirect vision, that is, by looking in the mouth mirror. The water coolant drops water on the mouth mirror and obscures the operator's vision. Both of these problems have been solved to a great extent by the aid of a skillful chairside assistant. Careful placement of the oral evacuator tip during cavity preparation will remove the excess water coolant. Indirect vision is greatly improved if the dentist positions the mirror as far from the tooth to be prepared as possible and the assistant continuously sprays the surface of the mirror with air to blow water off the mirror surface. It is interesting to note that the need for the use of a water coolant with the high-speed handpiece has, in turn, created the need for an extremely skillful chairside assistant.

The high-speed handpiece utilizes the friction grip–type chuck; therefore all burs, diamond stones, and polishing devices intended for use in the high-speed handpiece must have the FG (friction grip) designation when they are ordered (Figs. 5-4 and 5-6, *A*). These handpieces are now also available with fiber optic lights that are mounted in the head of the instrument to assist in lighting the cavity preparation (Fig. 5-9, *B*).

Most manufacturers of high-speed handpieces recommend daily use of a spray lubricant to maintain the handpiece. These lubricants are available in aerosol cans with a long spray nozzle that can be inserted in the air tube of the handpiece. One or two applications of lubricant a day is usually sufficient. The surface of the handpiece should be wiped clean with a disinfectant between patients. Some modern handpieces can be autoclaved.

MISCELLANEOUS COMMON OPERATIVE INSTRUMENTS AND SUPPLIES

There are a number of different instruments and supplies that are used in operative and restorative dentistry. The instruments presented here are only the fundamental instruments found in most instrument setups for operative procedures. The first two are the most widely used. Virtually all instrument setups will include a dental mirror and an explorer.

Dental mirrors (Fig. 5-10). Dental mirrors are multipurpose instruments. Their principal use is to allow the dentist to see into the inaccessible areas of the mouth by indirect vision. When the operator can look directly at an area without looking in a mirror, this is called direct vision. Mirrors are also helpful in direct vision in that they can be used to reflect light into the details of the area being examined or treated.

The operating team should always remember that the dental mirror is an excellent retractor. Many problems that both the dentist and assistant encounter in terms of visibility and access to an area can be solved by use of the retraction function of the dental mirror.

Dental mirrors are available in sizes 2 to 6, with plane or magnifying surfaces. The cone-socket stem is the most popular type used today. This stem screws into a standard-size handle, which allows the dentist to replace a scratched or damaged mirror without having to purchase the still useful handle.

Dental explorers. The dental explorer is a hand instrument that is used primarily as a probe to examine the less accessible areas of the teeth. There are several styles of explorers available (Fig. 5-11). All the styles of explorers have a very fine tip on the working end of the instrument. This fine tip allows the dentist to feel various discrepancies on the surface of the teeth and around dental restorations. Thus the explorer actually becomes an extension of the dentist's hand.

The explorer is another multipurpose instrument. Dentists have discovered many uses for the instrument besides its examination function. Some of the more common auxiliary uses of the explorer are listed:

1. Excess cement that is used to seal gold restorations in place can be removed from between the teeth with the explorer.
2. The explorer is useful in carving small areas of amalgam restorations, such as overhangs on the cervical margin, and removing amalgam against a matrix band before the band is removed.

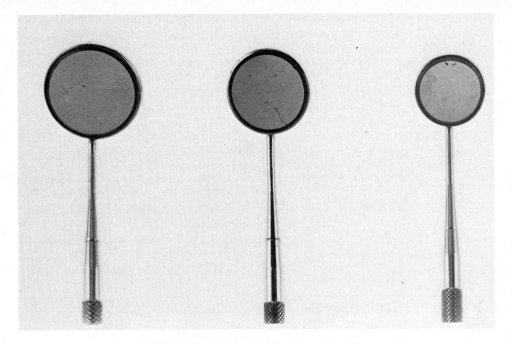

Fig. 5-10. Various sizes of mouth mirrors.

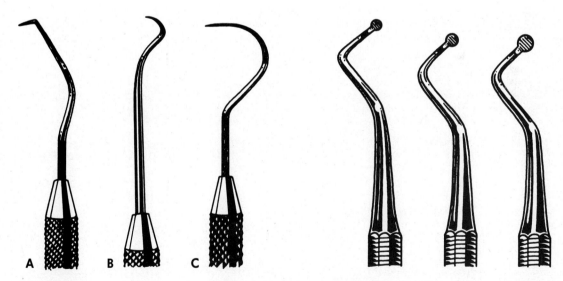

Fig. 5-11. Dental explorers. **A,** No. 17. **B,** Cowhorn No. 3. **C,** Shepherd's hook.

Fig. 5-12. Various sizes of spoon excavators.

3. Debridement of areas of food impaction is often easily accomplished with the explorer.
4. Some dentists find the explorer a convenient instrument to place gingival retraction cord prior to impressing taking.

Spoon excavator (Fig. 5-12). This hand instrument was originally designed to remove debris and caries from an extensively damaged tooth. However, like the explorer, the spoon excavator has been used for other tasks. Following are some of the more common auxiliary uses of this instrument:

1. The spoon excavator is a convenient instrument to use in placement and shaping of cavity liners and cement bases.
2. Like the explorer, the excavator is helpful in placement of gingival retraction cord.
3. Removal of excess cement after cementation of a gold restoration can be accomplished with the spoon excavator.
4. Both temporary and permanent restorations can be removed with the spoon excavator from a prepared tooth in gold and porcelain restorative procedures.
5. The excavator is a most helpful instrument to assist in placing amalgam matrix bands that are occasionally difficult to seat properly in the cervical area of a preparation.

The chairside assistant should always have a gauze sponge ready to wipe the working end of the excavator free of debris when the dentist is using it to debride an area or to place cavity medications.

Spoon excavators are available in small, medium, and large sizes and are usually double ended.

• • •

There are probably as many uses for both the spoon excavator and the explorer as there are dentists. The lists given represent only a few of the most common uses of these two popular instruments.

Cotton pliers (forceps) (Fig. 5-13). These are standard instruments found on operative and restorative instrument setups. They are used to place and retrieve small-sized materials in the oral cavity. Items such as cotton pellets, gingival retraction cord, cotton rolls, articulating paper, matrix bands, and wedges are commonly handled by cotton pliers. The dentist generally uses this instrument when it is more convenient than using the fingers to handle these items. Cotton pliers are available in both locking and nonlocking styles.

Straight-beaked forceps (thumb forceps) (Fig. 5-13, *C*) are used to retrieve other instruments, materials, and devices from sterile storage areas to avoid contamination with the fingers.

Ball burnisher (hand type). The ball burnisher is intended for use in smoothing the surface of dental restorations by rubbing the ball-shaped working end against the surface of the restoration (Fig. 5-14). The ball burnisher is also frequently used in placing cavity liners.

Filling instruments (Fig. 5-15). This group of small-bladed instruments is designed to place soft,

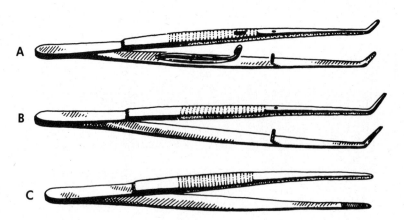

Fig. 5-13. Dental pliers (forceps). **A,** Locking style cotton pliers. **B,** Nonlocking style cotton pliers. **C,** Thumb-style cotton pliers.

moldable materials into cavity preparations. These materials include dental cements, composite materials, and acrylic. Filling instruments are also useful in filling gold and porcelain restorations with cement before seating. Some dentists find the smaller styles convenient for placing gingival retraction cord.

It is recommended that a plastic rather than a stainless steel type be used to place composites in anterior teeth. The coarse texture of composites can abrade the metal instrument and stain the restoration.

Cement spatulas (Fig. 5-15). A wide variety of cement spatulas is available for mixing dental cements and composite materials. A general guideline for selecting them is to be familiar with the mixing requirements for the material to be prepared. If the material is rather thin and must be mixed over a wide area, a narrow, more flexible spatula should be used for mixing. On the other hand, if the material is very thick and heavy textured, a spatula with a thicker blade is more helpful in mixing the material.

A special consideration in spatula selection centers around the preparation of composite materials. The abrasive nature of these materials requires the use of a Teflon spatula so that the material will not become discolored during the mixing process. Use of metal spatulas tends to impart a gray discoloration to the material.

Dappen dish (Fig. 5-16, *A*). The dappen dish is a handy item that is used to dispense various materials during a dental procedure. For convenience, the dish has a deep well in one end and a shallow well in the other. Materials that are often placed in dappen dishes for use during a given procedure are acrylics, alcohol, disclosing solution, various medicaments, amalgam, and tap water, just to mention a few.

Napkin holder (Fig. 5-16, *B*). This is a standard

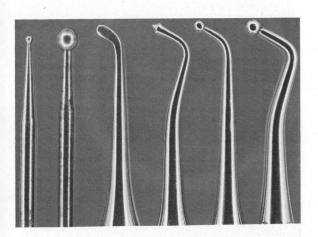

Fig. 5-14. Burnishers. *Left to right:* two ball burnishers (HP style), No. 4 SSW (hand), anatomic (hand), two ball burnishers (hand).

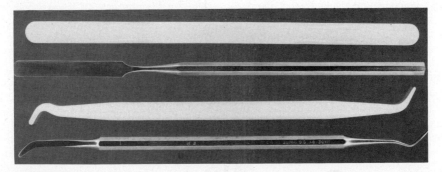

Fig. 5-15. Spatulas and filling instruments. *Top to bottom:* composite spatula, No. 1 324SSW cement spatula, composite filling instrument, FP No. 1 filling instrument.

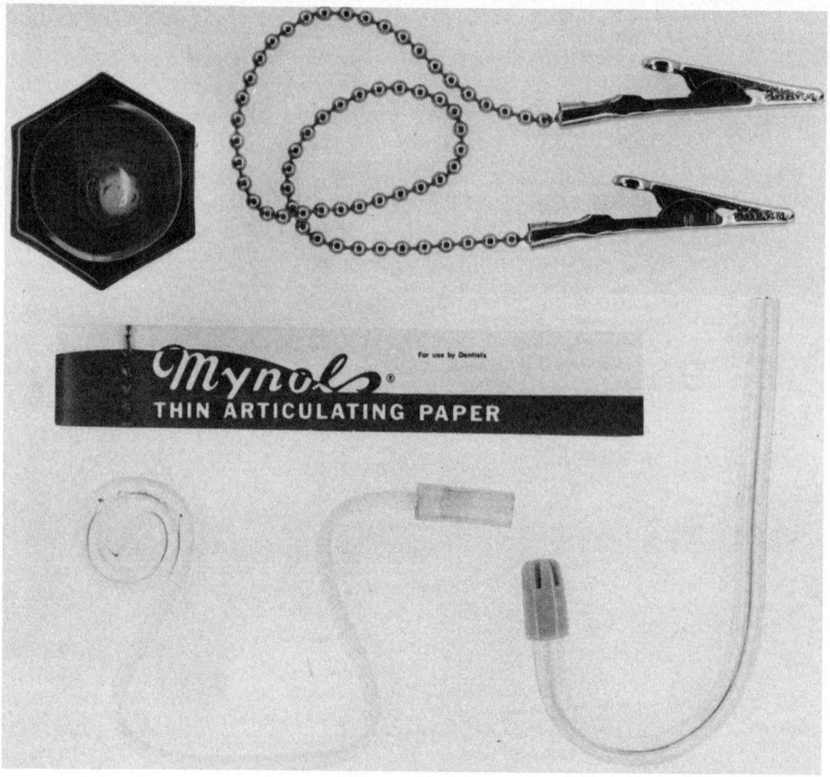

Fig. 5-16. A, Dappen dish. **B,** Napkin holder. **C,** Articulating paper. **D,** Aspirating tongue retractor (Hygoformic). **E,** Saliva ejector.

item available in different styles that is used to secure the dental napkin around the patient's neck. Nonmetal types are often preferable because they are not as cold on the patient's neck as the metal types.

Articulating paper (Fig. 5-16, *C*). Articulating paper is a fairly heavyweight paper that is impregnated with an inklike substance. When the paper is inserted in the patient's mouth and the teeth are closed together, the paper will leave marks indicating where the upper and lower teeth have made contact. In other words, articulating paper is similar to carbon paper that is used in a typewriter.

The marks that are made by the articulating paper aid the dentist in establishing a favorable occlusion for the patient who has excessive contact on a tooth or a restoration.

Articulating paper is available in strips or arch shapes, in red or blue color, and in thick and thin gauges.

Saliva ejector. This item is connected to a low-velocity vacuum hose for purposes of removing saliva from the patient's mouth during a dental procedure. There are various metal styles available that can be sterilized and reused. However, these are all but obsolete in the presence of new disposable types (Fig. 5-16, *E*). Besides their convenience, disposable saliva ejectors have the added attraction of being adaptable to the patient's mouth by being bent into various shapes.

The Hygoformic and Svedopter are saliva ejectors that also provide retraction of the tongue (Fig. 5-16, *D*, Hygoformic and Fig. 5-17, *A*, Svedopter).

Crown and collar scissors (Fig. 5-18). These short-beaked pairs of scissors are used to trim metal matrix bands, temporary crowns, and copper bands. Their husky, "duck-bill" design makes them handy instruments to contour the cervical areas of these devices. The assistant will find these scissors useful in

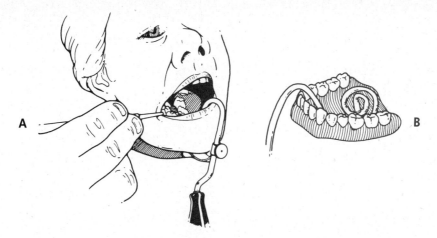

Fig. 5-17. Tongue retraction style saliva ejectors. **A,** Svedopter. **B,** Hygoformic.

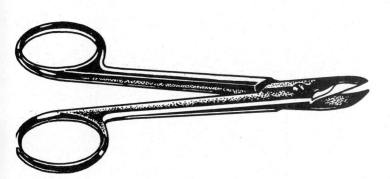

Fig. 5-18. Crown and collar scissors.

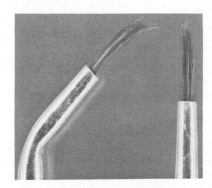

Fig. 5-19. Sable brushes.

cutting the various cotton products for use in the oral cavity.

Sable brushes (Fig. 5-19). The sable brush is a small artist's paintbrush that is used to apply acrylic restorative materials to teeth and existing restorations. The brush is dipped in the liquid (monomer) and then in the acrylic powder (polymer). Next, the wetted powder is painted on the area to be restored. This is often referred to as the brush-in technique.

The sable brush is available in varous sizes and in straight and bent styles.

Cotton pellets (Fig. 5-20). Cotton pellets are one of the most common cotton products used in dentistry and are usually a part of every operative and restorative setup. They are small balls of plain cotton that are used to clean cavity preparations, apply intraoral

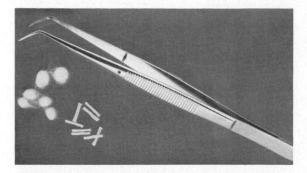

Fig. 5-20. Cotton pellets and pledgets, which are handled with cotton pliers.

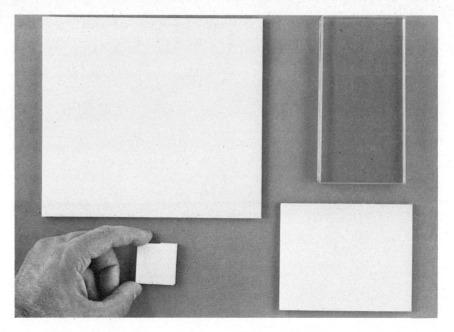

Fig. 5-21. Various sizes of paper mixing pads and a glass mixing slab.

medications, and control small areas of hemorrhage. They are available in various sizes and are usually handled in the mouth with cotton pliers.

Cotton pledgets (Fig. 5-20). Cotton pledgets are small sticks of stiffened cotton that are used to clean cavity preparations and apply cavity varnish. They are usually handled with cotton pliers.

Mixing slabs and pads (Fig. 5-21). Various dental materials are prepared at chairside by the dental assistant. These materials include cavity liners, dental cements, surgical dressings, and various impression materials. Some of these materials are mixed on a paper pad, but others must be prepared on a glass mixing slab.

Paper pads are convenient because clean-up is simply done by tearing off and disposing of the top sheet of the pad after use. Paper pads are available in various sizes. The size of the pad to be used is dictated by the amount of material that has to be prepared on it. The type of paper used in paper pads varies, and the one to use should be chosen according to what materials are going to be mixed on it. Generally speaking, materials of a paste consistency can be mixed on a plain paper pad. On the other hand, materials that involve the mixing of powder and a thin liquid should

be mixed on a parchment or a waxed paper pad. Parchment paper will prevent the absorption of the liquid into the paper, which would alter the proportions of the mix.

Some materials such as zinc phosphate cements are preferably mixed on a cool, dry glass slab. These materials produce heat during the mixing procedure, which must be absorbed by the cool glass slab. Otherwise, the material will set before the dentist can use it.

Cavity liner applicators (Fig. 5-22). These tiny-tipped instruments are handy devices to apply cavity liners in cavity preparations. They are especially useful in the conservative Classes III, IV, and V cavity preparations.

Some dentists prefer to use a small, hand-type ball burnisher or a spoon excavator for this purpose rather than add another instrument to the preset tray.

Isolation devices. The instruments and devices used for isolation of various teeth will be presented in Chapter 8 along with a discussion of their use.

COMMON HAND CUTTING INSTRUMENTS

Hand cutting instruments are those instruments that are operated by hand to remove unwanted tooth struc-

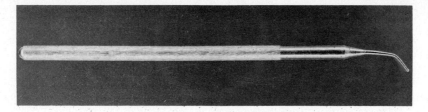

Fig. 5-22. Cavity liner applicator.

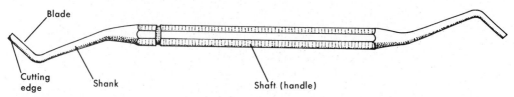

Fig. 5-23. Parts of a hand cutting instrument.

ture. The hand cutting instruments were formerly the major means by which a cavity was prepared. Today, with the use of both the high-speed and conventional-speed handpieces, the hand cutting instruments are used primarily to refine the fine details of the cavity preparation. Fig. 5-23 shows the basic parts of these instruments.

Classes of hand cutting instruments

There are a wide variety of hand cutting instruments available. For the most part, each instrument can be grouped into one of five classes: hatchet, chisel, hoe, margin trimmer, and angle former. Each class has basic design features intended to accomplish a specific task. However, with the changes in cavity preparation design and the desire of dentists to minimize the number of instruments needed for a given procedure, many of the hand instruments are used for more purposes than their intended one. It is not at all uncommon to find that the armamentarium of an experienced dentist contains far fewer hand instruments than that of a recent graduate. One of the ways to increase chairside efficiency is to get maximum use of an instrument during any given procedure.

Hatchets. Hatchets are given the name because of their similarity in design to the woodsman's tool (Fig. 5-24). The cutting edge is in the same plane as the handle of the instrument, and it contains at least one bend in the shank at the point of attachment to the blade.

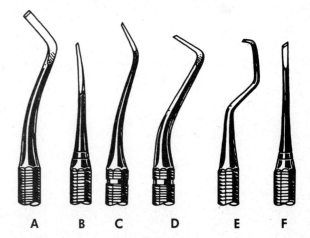

Fig. 5-24. Hand cutting instruments. **A,** Hatchet. **B,** Straight chisel. **C,** Monangle chisel. **D,** Binangle hoe. **E,** Triple angle hoe. **F,** Straight angle former.

Although hatchets are available in single-ended, long-handle (LH) styles, they are more commonly purchased in double-ended (DE) styles. DE instruments are far more practical than the LH styles because they reduce the number of instruments that has to be purchased, sterilized, and handled by the operating team.

The DE hatchet has a right and a left end. The right end is the end of the instrument with the bevel of the cutting edge to the operator's right when the instrument is held in operating position for the mandibular teeth. That is, the cutting edge is down and away from the operator's hand. The right end of the instrument is designated by an indented ring around the instrument handle near or on the shank (Fig. 5-24). The opposite end is the left end of the instrument.

The hatchet is used to plane cavity walls and cervical floors to remove any roughness created by burs during cavity preparation. Hatchets are helpful in sharpening line and point angles in the preparation. Before sit-down dentistry became a mode of practice, the hatchet was primarily considered a mandibular instrument because the dentist lacked access to the maxillary arch while standing next to the patient. Sit-down dentistry has expanded the use of this instrument to both the maxillary and mandibular teeth.

Chisels. The chisel is a rather straight instrument with a single-beveled cutting edge. It is used primarily in the maxillary arch with a push motion to plane enamel margins. The Wedelstaedt chisel is one of the most popular in use today (Fig. 5-24). Chisels can be rather straight, have one bend in the shank (monangle), or two bends in the shank (binangle). Chisels have a blade angle of 12.5 centigrades or less to the shaft of the instrument.

Chisels are often conveniently used to trim margins on esthetic restorations in the anterior areas of the mouth.

Hoes. Like the hatchet, the hoe is given its name because of its resemblance to the garden tool. It has a similar shape in that the blade of the instrument orients the cutting edge to be nearly perpendicular to the handle of the instrument (Fig. 5-24).

The hoe is used with a pull motion to plane cavity walls and floors that are conveniently reached by this instrument. Technically speaking, an instrument with a blade angulation of more than 12.5 centigrades to the shaft is considered to be a hoe.

Angle former. The angle former is actually a chisel with the cutting edge at an angle other than a right angle to the blade (Fig. 5-24). The sides of the blade also are sharpened to form cutting edges. DE angle formers are paired right and left instruments. The right end is identified with an indented ring on the instrument handle near the shank. When viewed from the beveled side of the blade, the right end has the cutting edge on the end sloping toward the handle and to the right, and the left end of the instrument slopes to the left.

These instruments are used as their name implies, that is, to form sharp internal line and point angles of cavity preparations. Cohesive gold preparations require the use of these instruments to enhance the retention form.

Gingival margin trimmer. This is a modified hatchet that is used to place a bevel along the cervical cavosurface margin in amalgam and inlay preparations (Fig. 5-25). There are mesial and distal styles of

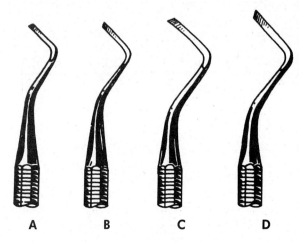

Fig. 5-25. Gingival margin trimmers. **A,** Mesial trimmer (small). **B,** Distal trimmer (small). **C,** Mesial trimmer (large). **D,** Distal trimmer (large).

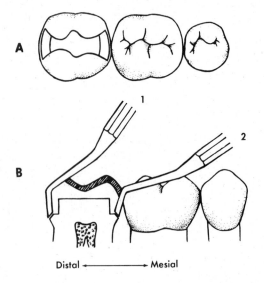

Distal ◄——————► Mesial

Fig. 5-26. A, Occlusal view of cavity preparation. **B,** Lateral view of a longitudinal section of prepared tooth, with gingival margin trimmers in use. *1,* Distal margin trimmer; *2,* mesial margin trimmer.

trimmers available. They are identified by the angle between the cutting edge and the blade of the instrument. When the instrument is held in operating position for the mandibular arch, the cutting edge slopes down and away from the instrument handle in the distal style. The mesial style has the cutting edge sloping down and toward the instrument handle (Fig. 5-26).

The blade of the margin trimmer is curved. This curvature aids in the efficiency of the instrument as it is used in a lateral scraping motion to create the cervical bevel. One end of the instrument curves to the right, the other to the left. It is important to note that the instrument is *not* a combination of a mesial margin trimmer on one end and a distal trimmer on the other. Both ends of one instrument are either for the distal or the mesial.

The gingival margin trimmer is a very common instrument found on amalgam and gold inlay preset trays. It is one instrument that can be used to plane all enamel margins effectively as well as to place cervical bevels. This concept can eliminate the use of some chisels and enamel hatchets on the preset tray that might normally be used for that purpose.

• • •

Within each class of hand cutting instruments further descriptive names are based on the number of angles found in the shank, such as straight—no angles in the shank; monangle—one angle in the shank; binangle—two angles in the shank; and triple angle—three angles in the shank. (The shank is de-

fined as the portion of the instrument connecting the blade to the instrument handle or shaft, Figs. 5-23 and 5-24.)

Today common reference to instruments by name is a combination of the description of the shank and the class of the instrument. For example, a hatchet with two angles in the shank is called a binangled hatchet; a chisel with one angle in the shank is called a monangled chisel.

By and large, these references to instruments should be limited to use among dental personnel out of earshot of the patient. Apprehensive patients may be frightened by the use of such names as hatchets and chisels! Substitutions like ''8E'' for the hatchet and ''Wedelstaedt'' for the chisel are more acceptable.

Instrument formulas

To assist the dentist in purchasing a specific instrument of choice, a universal instrument formula was developed by G.V. Black that is used by instrument manufacturers today. The formula precisely describes an instrument with reference to its shaft, blade, and cutting edge.

If the cutting edge of the instrument forms a right angle with the blade of that instrument, a three-unit formula is used (Fig. 5-27). On the other hand, if the cutting edge forms anything other than a right angle with the blade, a four-unit formula is used (Fig. 5-28).

An instrument with the three-unit instrument formula of 15-8-12 is one with the cutting edge at a right

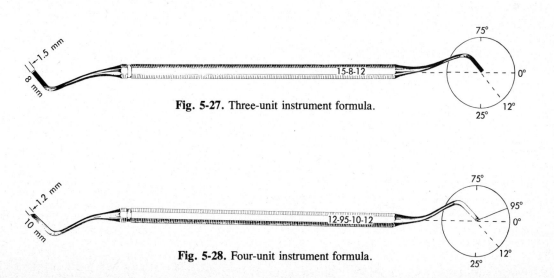

Fig. 5-27. Three-unit instrument formula.

Fig. 5-28. Four-unit instrument formula.

angle to the blade. The formula gives the following information:

15	8	12
First unit indicates width of blade (in tenths of millimeters) = 1.5 mm.	Second unit indicates blade length (in millimeters) = 8 mm.	Third unit indicates angle formed by the blade with instrument shaft (in centigrades) = 12 centigrades.*

An instrument with a four-unit instrument formula is one whose cutting edge is not at a right angle to the blade, and the formula has a slightly different meaning. When the cutting edge is at an angle other than a right angle to the blade, that angle is indicated in the second position of the formula. All other units of the formula retain the same meaning. The formula 12-95-10-12 gives the following information:

12	95	10	12
Width of blade = 1.2 mm.	Cutting edge forms angle of 95 centigrades* to axis of shaft.	Length of blade = 10 mm.	Blade itself forms angle of 12 centigrades* to axis of shaft.

To put instrument formulas into proper perspective, it must be mentioned that they are primarily used in ordering instruments from a manufacturer when a very specific instrument design is desired. In most instances instruments should be indicated by a descriptive name or by a manufacturer's own instrument number. For example, it is much easier in clinical communication to refer to an instrument with a formula of 12-95-10-12 as a distal gingival margin trimmer, which describes its use. After an assistant works with a dentist for a while, even shorter names for instruments will identify the same instrument, such as a ''distal trimmer'' instead of a distal gingival margin trimmer. These abbreviations are unique to the individual dentist and will aid in efficient communication.

SUMMARY

An entire text could be written describing the tremendous variety of instruments and supplies that are available in dentistry today. The volume steadily increases as new dental procedures and techniques are created. Still, some dentists cling to older, traditional methods of treatment, and they may not use every instrument available. Since the dental assistant must adapt to the individual dentist's preferences for instruments, it is recommended that the assistant not attempt to learn every instrument on the market today. Knowledge of basic instruments and supplies will facilitate the adaptation of the assistant to the individual dentist's personal armamentarium.

BIBLIOGRAPHY

Carter, L., Finkbeiner, B., and Yaman, P.: Dental instruments, St. Louis, 1981, The C.V. Mosby Co.
Charbeneau, G.T., et al.: Principles and practice of operative dentistry, ed. 2, Philadelphia, 1981, Lea & Febiger.
Howard, W.W. and Moller, R.C.: Atlas of operative dentistry, ed. 3, St. Louis, 1981, The C.V. Mosby Co.

*Centigrades are one-hundredths of a circle. In other words, a circle is divided into 100 parts instead of the usual 360 degrees.

CHAPTER 6

PROCESSING DENTAL INSTRUMENTS

INSTRUMENT SHARPENING

Hand cutting instruments and scalers become dull as they are used. Dullness results in lack of effectiveness of the instrument. It is the responsibility of the assistant to keep instruments sharpened. The frequency of sharpening an instrument depends on how often it is used and the method used to sterilize the instrument. Steam sterilization techniques tend to dull cutting edges.

The key to maintaining sharp instruments is to learn to recognize when an instrument is dull and when it is sharp. It is not always easy to tell if an instrument is still sharp by using it, unless it is very dull. Many instruments still function when they are slightly dull. However, the operator has to work a lot harder to accomplish the function of the instrument. Since instruments usually become dull gradually, the operator may not notice the loss of effectiveness until the instrument is extremely dull. The objective of good instrument maintenance is to recognize dullness before it reaches this stage.

The sharpness or dullness of any instrument is determined by the shape of the cutting edge that is created by the intersection of two surfaces of the blade of the instrument (Fig. 6-1). Manufacturers design instruments so that a specific angle exists between two blade surfaces to create a sharp cutting edge. This angle must be preserved in sharpening instruments to obtain maximum effectiveness from the cutting edge.

You can examine a cutting edge by looking directly at it while turning the instrument slightly. A dull edge will reflect light along the cutting edge, creating a glare that is visible. The reflection is caused by the rounded intersection of two blade surfaces (Fig. 6-1, A). A sharp edge (Fig. 6-1, B) will not reflect light and will not create a visible glare along the edge. You can inspect instruments rather quickly using this sighting technique.

The goal of instrument sharpening is to eliminate rounded cutting edges while preserving the angle between the two surfaces of the blade that form the cutting edge.

Sharpening devices (Fig. 6-2)

Instruments can be sharpened by hand with a fine-grit Arkansas stone that is held in a stationary position while the instrument is moved over its surface (Fig. 6-3). Mechanical methods involve turning a grinding wheel while the instrument is held in a stationary position against the wheel (Fig. 6-4). Other utensils following this principle are small Arkansas stones that can be mounted in the straight handpiece to sharpen instruments.

Light machine oil is used on the surface of grindstones to prevent them from becoming clogged with metal particles as they grind the instrument. The ro-

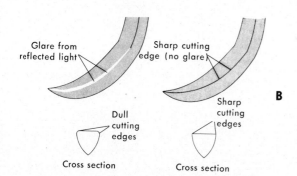

Fig. 6-1. A, Dull sickle scaler. B, Sharp sickle scaler.

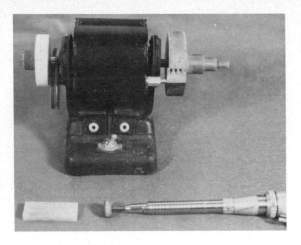

Fig. 6-2. Various instrument sharpening devices.

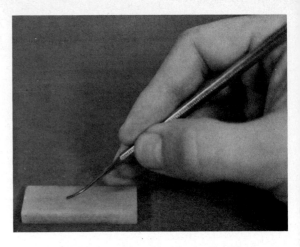

Fig. 6-3. Sharpening chisel by hand method.

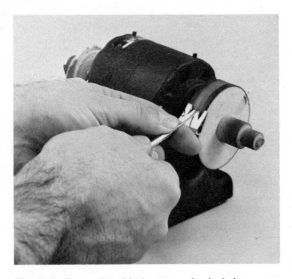

Fig. 6-4. Sharpening chisel on a mechanical sharpener.

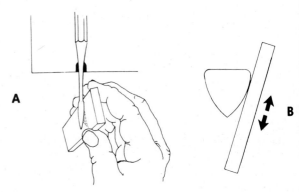

Fig. 6-5. A, Sharpening sickle scaler using small Arkansas stone. **B,** Vertical relationship of sharpening stone to side of scaler while it is being sharpened.

tating grindstones in mechanical sharpeners should be cleaned periodically during sharpening by holding an oil-soaked cotton roll against the turning wheel. Excess oil can be removed by holding a dry cotton roll against the wheel after it has been cleaned. This will prevent spattering of oil.

A common method of sharpening scalers is to use a small rectangular Arkansas stone that is held in the right hand and moved over the surface while the left hand holds the instrument stationary (Fig. 6-5).

Sharpening hand cutting instruments

Hatchets, hoes, chisels, angle formers, and margin trimmers can be sharpened either by hand or on the mechanical sharpener.

Hand sharpening is a slower but more conservative

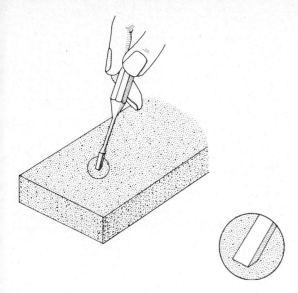

Fig. 6-6. Placing bevel of the instrument flat against stone during sharpening.

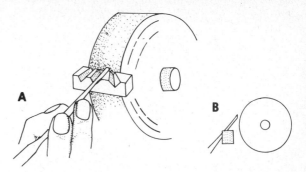

Fig. 6-7. A, Using instrument guide on a mechanical sharpener. **B,** Relationship of bevel of instrument to grinding wheel.

technique of sharpening. There is less chance of ruining the instrument with this technique. The procedure is as follows:

1. Place an Arkansas stone on a flat surface and place a few drops of machine oil on it.
2. Hold the instrument with the pen grasp.
3. Position the instrument on the stone so that the bevel of the blade rests flat on the stone (Fig. 6-6).
4. Hold the instrument firmly and move the entire hand back and forth, rubbing the instrument over the surface of the stone. Strokes about 1 inch in length are used. The last two fingers of the hand should act as guides on the table top to maintain the proper relationship between the surface of the stone and the bevel of the instrument (Fig. 6-3).
5. After several strokes, wipe the instrument clean and inspect the cutting edge. Repeat this procedure until it is sharp.
6. Sometimes a small edge of metal called a bur develops along the edge. This can be removed by gently honing the instrument on the stone with small circular strokes.

Mechanical sharpening is a quicker method of sharpening instruments, but the instrument can be easily damaged if the operator is not careful. These sharpening devices have a guide that holds the instrument in the proper relationship to the grinding wheel. Fig. 6-4 shows that the guide has three dif-

ferent grooves that are designed to hold the various hand cutting instruments. The central groove is used for chisels and hoes, and the two lateral grooves are used for right- and left-angled margin trimmers and angle formers. Following are the steps in the sharpening procedure:

1. Turn the engine on and wipe the stone with an oil-soaked cotton roll.
2. Place the instrument in the appropriate groove on the guide (Fig. 6-7, *A*) and position it so that the entire bevel will contact the surface of the wheel (Fig. 6-7, *B*).
3. Hold the instrument firmly in the guide, using the pen grasp, and lightly press it against the wheel.
4. Remove the instrument from the guide, wipe it clean, and inspect the cutting edge and bevel to see that the edge is sharp and the bevel has its original shape.
5. Use the felt wheel on the opposite end of the engine to remove burs that may develop along the cutting edge. Hold the instrument lightly against the wheel and turn it over a few times to rub away the bur.

Sharpening scalers

It is a matter of opinion, but the hand method is probably a better way for most people to sharpen scalers. Sickle and curette scalers have rather unusual shapes that must be preserved if the instruments are to function properly. Mechanical sharpening methods often grind so quickly that it is difficult to control the amount of metal ground away. This often results in excessive "wear" on the instrument or in extensive alteration of the shape of the working end.

To sharpen a scaler properly, careful attention must be given to the shape of the working end of the instrument before the sharpening procedure is begun.

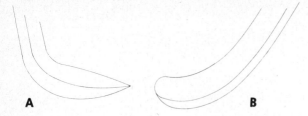

Fig. 6-8. A, Sickle scaler. **B,** Curette scaler.

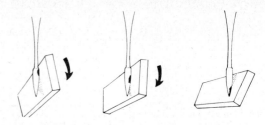

Fig. 6-10. Sharpening sickle scaler from heel to toe of instrument while moving stone up and down in ½-inch strokes. (Top view of scaler.)

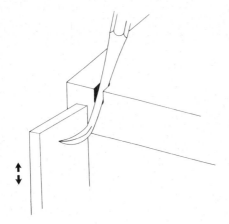

Fig. 6-9. Notched edge of counter top used to stabilize instrument during sharpening.

The original shape of the instrument will serve as a guide during sharpening. Fig. 6-8 demonstrates the shape of sickle and curette scalers. Green and Seyer suggest the following method of sharpening these scalers with a small (1 × 3 inch) lubricated Arkansas stone. A few modifications have been added for convenience.

Sickle scalers. Objectives are to (1) eliminate rounded cutting edges, (2) preserve the angle between the top and the sides of the working end, and (3) preserve the curvature along the cutting edge from the heel to the toe of the instrument.

The procedure is as follows:

1. File a notch on the edge of a counter top or laboratory bench where the instrument will be sharpened. This notch assists in holding the instrument stationary while it is being sharpened (Fig. 6-9).
2. Place the instrument in the notch and hold it firmly with the fingers of the left hand. Hold the rectangular Arkansas stone in the fingers of the right hand.
3. Position the stone at the heel of the working end in the vertical relationship shown in Fig. 6-5, *B*.
4. While maintaining the proper vertical relationship, move the stone up and down, using ½-inch strokes. The entire right hand is moved up and down during the sharpening strokes.
5. The first contact of the stone should be at the heel of the instrument. Rotate the stone toward the toe of the instrument as you continually move the stone up and down along the cutting edge from the heel to the toe (Fig. 6-10). This preserves the curvature along the cutting edge from heel to toe.

   Repeat the same procedure for the cutting edge toward the operator's left hand.
6. Wipe the instrument clean and inspect the cutting edges for sharpness.

Curette scalers. Objectives in sharpening curette scalers are to (1) eliminate rounded cutting edges, (2) preserve the angle between the top and sides of the working end, and (3) round both the end and the undersurface of the working end of the instrument.

The procedure is as follows:

1. Hold the instrument in the notched area on the edge of the bench top as was done with the sickle scaler.
2. Sharpen the cutting edges in the same manner as used for the sickle scaler. Start at the heel and work toward the toe or tip of the working end.
3. After the cutting edges along the sides have been sharpened, the tip should be rounded. Place the stone at approximately 45 degrees to the top surface of the curette. Little by little, rotate the stone around the tip as you continue the up-and-down grinding strokes (Fig. 6-11, *A*).
4. The undersurface of the instrument tends to be lost after repeated sharpening. It is well to recontour this with the stone every time the curette is sharpened to preserve the round shape (Fig. 6-11, *B*).

The operator can tell if the instrument is being sharpened by the accumulation of metal shavings that

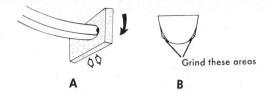

Fig. 6-11. A, Rounding tip of curette scaler. **B,** Cross section of curette scaler. Shaded area is removed during recontouring procedure.

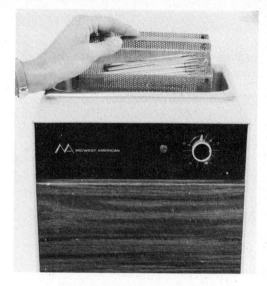

Fig. 6-12. Ultrasonic cleaner.

appears along the cutting edge as the stone is moved up and down against it.

In addition to the visual inspection of the cutting edge for "glare" to determine if an instrument is sharp, there are two other tests that can be used. Both tests involve dragging the cutting edge of the instrument over either the skin or a thumbnail. A sharp instrument will dig into these tissues, but a dull instrument will slide across them rather easily.

DECONTAMINATION PROCEDURES

It has been known for a long time that diseases can be transferred from one person to another by either direct or indirect contact. Contaminated dental instruments and the hands of the operating team are two common sources of indirect transfer of microorganisms from one patient to another. Needless to say, it is the responsibility of the dental team to do everything possible to eliminate this transfer.

There are three basic ways to reduce the transfer of organisms between patients: cleaning, disinfection, and sterilization procedures. Cleaning procedures are nothing more than physical removal of debris and organisms from the surface of an object. Handwashing, instrument scrubbing, and washing oral devices such as dentures and orthodontic appliances fall into the cleaning category. Disinfection is a process of destroying most infectious microorganisms but not necessarily all of them. Some resistant types of bacteria such as those that cause tuberculosis may survive a disinfecting procedure. Hepatitis virus and tetanus spores can also survive disinfection. Sterilization procedures eliminate all infectious microorganisms, including viruses and spores. Therefore the best way to eliminate contamination between patients is to sterilize everything that comes in contact with them. The fact is that this is not possible. Such objects as handpieces, x-ray machines, air-water syringes, and the hands of the operating team cannot be sterilized. Dis-

infection and cleaning procedures must be used on such objects to reduce bacterial transfer.

Cleaning procedures

Handwashing is one of the most frequently employed cleaning procedures used in an office. The operating team must be as thorough as possible when the hands are washed. Disinfectant soaps are available to enhance the elimination of organisms from the skin. Sterile rubber gloves can be used for some dental operations but are awkward to use during procedures that require maximum dexterity.

Swabbing the instruments on the dental unit, counter tops, the operating light handles, and the head of the x-ray machine with a gauze sponge soaked in a disinfecting solution can be viewed as either a cleaning or disinfecting procedure, depending on how thoroughly it is done. Aerosol spray disinfectants are also available.

Cleaning operating instruments of all kinds is a mandatory part of all sterilization and disinfecting methods. Debris on instruments inhibits any attempt to destroy organisms that are harbored in the debris. The first step in preparing instruments for either sterilization of disinfection is to remove debris (blood, plaque, carious tissue, cement, etc.) by either hand scrubbing or use of an ultrasonic cleaner.

Hand scrubbing is merely scrubbing instruments

using a fingernail-style brush under running water. Although several instruments can be cleaned at a time, this can be a laborious task if a lot of instruments need to be processed.

The ultrasonic cleaner is probably the most efficient way to clean instruments (Fig. 6-12). This device is an open bath of cleaning solution that is vibrated at a very high frequency. The action of the vibrating solution shakes debris from the surface of instruments. There are different sizes available to handle various amounts of instruments at one time. The ultrasonic cleaner has a timer that automatically turns the machine off at the end of the cycle. This device can be used for many other purposes besides a step in instrument processing. Different solutions are available for removing cement, gypsum materials, and stains from gold castings and dental appliances.

Disinfection

The most common method used to disinfect instruments is to immerse them in a bath of germicidal solution. Bulky equipment can be disinfected by scrubbing the surface thoroughly with germicide-soaked gauze sponges.

The effectiveness of these solutions depends on the cleanliness of the instrument, the smoothness of the instrument surface, the concentration of the solution, and the time the organisms are exposed to the chemical. This calls for precleaning the instruments, proper mixing of the germicidal solution, and allowing adequate time for instruments to remain in the bath.

Because of the superiority of heat sterilization over chemical disinfection in destroying viruses, spores, and resistant bacteria, only those instruments that cannot be sterilized by heat methods should be chemically disinfected.

Several chemicals can be used as disinfectants. Among these are glutaraldehydes (Cidex*), benzalkonium chloride (Zephiran†), phenols (Staphene‡), and alcohols.

Glutaraldehyde (Cidex). Cidex is a popular agent for obtaining a high level of disinfection of instruments and other items that cannot be sterilized by other means. A 2% solution will provide effective disinfection within 10 minutes without damaging metal instruments or items made of glass, rubber, or plastic.

A fresh solution is a critical factor in the effective-

ness of this agent (Fig. 6-13). Therefore an activator is mixed with the solution when a fresh batch is needed. This avoids the possibility of the solution losing its effectiveness during shipment and storage.

The activity of Cidex is not altered by the presence of small amounts of soap or organic matter. The solution is irritating to the skin and eyes, so care must be taken to avoid contact with the solution.

Benzalkonium chloride (Zephiran). Zephiran has been a common disinfectant used in dentistry for years. Immersion in a 2% solution for 10 to 15 minutes destroys many bacteria and fungi but not viruses, spores, and tubercle bacilli.

Zephiran deteriorates rapidly under heavy use and should be replaced frequently according to manufacturer's recommendations. This agent is also deactivated by soap and by cotton materials. Instruments that are scrubbed with soap must be rinsed thoroughly before placement in Zephiran solution. Swabbing equipment with a Zephiran-saturated cloth or gauze sponge is not recommended.

Because of the irritating nature of this solution to the skin, use of forceps to retrieve instruments from the solution is recommended.

Phenols (Staphene). Staphene is a good disinfectant to use to swab air-water syringes, handpieces, operating light handles, and other parts of dental

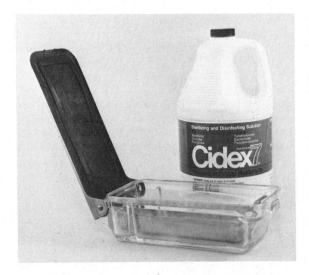

Fig. 6-13. Disinfecting bath that can be used with a variety of disinfecting solutions such as benzalkonium chloride (Zephiran Chloride) or the glutaraldehyde shown.

*Surgikos, Inc., Arlington, Tex.
†Winthrop Laboratories, New York.
‡Vestal, Inc., St. Louis.

equipment that are touched by the operating team during a treatment procedure. Staphene dries slowly and is somewhat effective in destroying tuberculosis-causing organisms. After equipment is swabbed, the Staphene should be allowed to remain for approximately 10 minutes for maximum effectiveness. These equipment items must be dried with sterile gauze before use if air drying has not taken place.

Phenolic substances are very irritating to soft tissue. Care should be taken during the swabbing procedure to either protect the hands with rubber gloves or apply with an aerosol can.

A 2.0% Staphene solution can also be used to disinfect instruments by immersion for 15 minutes in a bath. Leaving instruments in a phenolic bath for several hours can lead to corrosion problems. Instruments should be rinsed and dried with a sterile towel following the disinfection procedure.

Alcohols (isopropyl and ethyl). Alcohols in the concentration of 80% are rather effective agents to use to swab dental equipment. Ethyl alcohol seems to be the more effective of the two alcohols. However, Staphene is even more effective as a swabbing agent because of its effectiveness against tubercle bacilli.

Some dental units in use today draw contaminants from the end of the handpiece up into the water spray line when the handpiece is turned off. The assistant should run the handpiece for a moment after swabbing the working end to help flush out the contaminated water and then swab the handpiece again.

Because these chemicals are not capable of destroying all viruses and spores, they should be referred to as germicides or disinfectants. The term "cold sterilization" has been applied to the process of immersing instruments into such chemicals at room temperature. This is a misnomer because only disinfection, and *not* sterilization, occurs.

Sterilization

The most practical method to achieve true sterilization of dental instruments is by heat. Microorganisms all have an upper limit to the temperature range that is acceptable to their survival. When this upper limit is exceeded, sterilization occurs. Three common ways of achieving sterilization by the use of high temperatures are autoclaving (moist-heat), dry-heat sterilization, and vapor sterilization. There are also some auxiliary methods of sterilizing small numbers of instruments. These methods do not replace autoclaving and dry heat, but they can be helpful for special purposes.

Autoclaving. Autoclaving, or moist-heat sterilization, is one of the most effective and efficient methods of achieving true sterilization. Depending on the size of the autoclave, large quantities of instruments can be sterilized in a relatively short period of time (Fig. 6-14).

The autoclave is a steam chamber into which the instruments to be sterilized are placed. During the sterilization cycle, water flows into the chamber and is heated to the boiling point to create steam (212° F [100° C]). Since the chamber is sealed, pressure increases to approximately 15 pounds per square inch. This increase in pressure allows the heat of the steam to rise from 212° to approximately 250° F (100° to 121° C). When instruments are exposed to this superheated steam, sterilization occurs. Usually this requires about 15 minutes for the more resistant bacterial spores and viruses. Porous materials such as cotton goods and surgical sponges may require as much as 30 minutes for sterilization to occur.

Unfortunately, steam has a corrosive effect on metal instruments. Instruments rust rather quickly when exposed to the steam, and the cutting edges of sharp instruments are dulled by this corrosive process. An oil emulsion has been developed to coat instruments prior to sterilization to prevent these harmful effects (Fig. 6-15). After the instruments are cleaned, they are dipped into the oil emulsion and the excess is drained off before insertion into the autoclave.

If instruments are to be packaged before sterilization, the oil coating is applied just before packaging. When covered metal preset trays are used, the coated

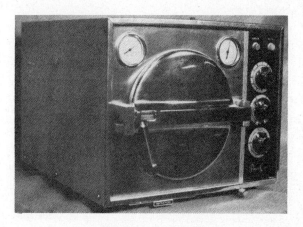

Fig. 6-14. Autoclave.

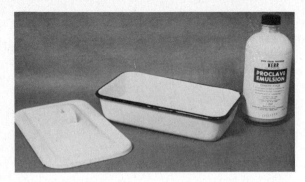

Fig. 6-15. Protective oil emulsion used to prevent corrosion during steam sterilization.

instruments are returned to the tray before insertion into the autoclave.

A general guideline for autoclaving is to sterilize a light, well-spaced load of instruments for 15 minutes at 250° F (121° C) and 15 pounds of pressure. Other factors that may alter the time required for sterilization are the size of the load, the type of instruments or materials, and the method of packaging of the items to be sterilized. If the autoclave is started from a cold condition, an extra 5 minutes must be added to the cycle time to allow for a warm-up period.

The steam must penetrate through the entire load to achieve sterilization. Therefore it is important to avoid overloading the steam chamber with instruments and wrapping instruments too tightly, which would reduce the penetration of the steam.

After the sterilization cycle is complete, the pressure is released from the steam chamber through a vent, and the door can be opened to allow the instruments to dry.

Manufacturer's instructions should be followed closely for the operation of the specific autoclave to be used.

Dry-heat sterilization. This is a popular method of destroying microorganisms on dental instruments. It is essentially a process of "baking" instruments in an oven at temperatures of 320° to 347° F (160° to 175° C). Because the heat used to destroy organisms is dry, there is no danger of corrosion on instruments.

The choice of which heat method to use for sterilization may be based on either personal preference or the type of item to be sterilized. For example, some items made of paper, cloth, plastic, or some metal impression trays with solder joints may be destroyed at the extreme temperatures used in the dry-heat

method. On the other hand, instruments such as endodontic files and reamers are so vulnerable to corrosion that they should be sterilized by dry heat to preserve their usefulness.

Instruments to be processed by dry-heat methods must be cleaned and dried before being placed in the oven. Covered metal preset trays can be used in the dry heat oven, so that tray setups can be sterilized and stored without handling the contents until the tray is actually being used. No oil coating is required for the instruments when the dry-heat method is used.

The dry-heat oven can be a counter-top style sterilizer made by various medical equipment manufacturers. These have a built-in timer and a thermostat to control the temperature. Many dentists use an ordinary kitchen broiler for the same purpose. In fact, regular kitchen ovens are frequently used in offices that sterilize large quantities of instruments by dry heat. The autoclave shown in Fig. 6-14 is a combination moist- and dry-heat sterilizer. A special door is inserted in the sterilizing chamber when it is used as a dry-heat unit.

Sterilization in a dry-heat oven is a little more time-consuming than in the autoclave. Dry-heat sterilization requires the instruments to be heated to 320° to 347° F (160° to 175° C) for approximately 30 minutes. The dry-heat ovens require a warm-up time of approximately 15 minutes to heat the instruments to 320° F (160° C). Thus to be sure sterilization has occurred, a total time of 45 minutes is required for a light load and even an hour for larger loads.

Chemical vapor sterilization. Another method of achieving sterilization of instruments and some supply items is through the use of a combination of heat and chemical vapor. A special sterilizer (Fig. 6-16) is used with a special solution containing alcohol, acetone, ketone, formaldehyde, and distilled water (9.25%).

It has been demonstrated that corrosion and dulling of metal items has been eliminated using this method of sterilization since the water content of the sterilization solution is below 15%.

Instruments must be scrubbed thoroughly or cleaned in an ultrasonic cleaner, rinsed with cold water, and dried with a towel before placement in the sterilizer. Failure to prepare the instruments properly can result in incomplete sterilization, damage to the instruments, or both.

Clean items to be sterilized are packaged loosely in the usual sterilization containers and placed in the sterilizer. The sterilization cycle is run according to

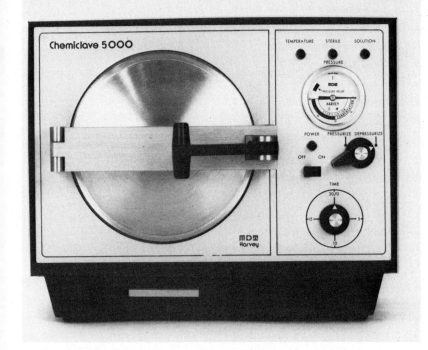

Fig. 6-16. Chemical vapor sterilizer. (Courtesy MDT Corp., Gardena, Calif.)

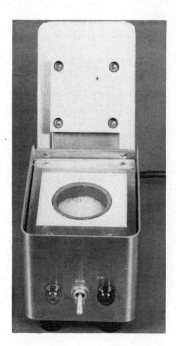

Fig. 6-17. Bead sterilizer.

the manufacturer's instructions which is usually approximately 30 minutes at a temperature of 270° F (132° C) and at a pressure of 20 pounds per square inch.

If heavy loads of soft goods such as cotton rolls, surgical towels, and surgical sponges are sterilized using this method, then biological spore indicators should be used to indicate that sterilization of these items has occurred.

Another advantage of the system is that because of the low water content in the sterilization solution, the instruments are dry at the completion of the cycle.

A well-ventilated sterilization area is recommended to reduce the odor produced by the sterilization solution.

Generally any items that can be sterilized in an autoclave can also be safely sterilized in the chemical vapor sterilizer.

Bead sterilization. Bead sterilization is only used in endodontic therapy. During a root canal procedure it is helpful to resterilize files, reamers, and broaches as they are used. The bead sterilizer is a heating device containing a small pot of tiny glass beads that are

heated to a temperature of 450° F (232°C) (Fig. 6-17). Endodontic instruments are very small and can be heated readily. They are inserted in the pot of beads for 15 to 20 seconds to sterilize them. Heavier metal instruments will require approximately 30 seconds for sterilization.

Open flame sterilization. This has limited use in dentistry. During the culturing sequence (Chapter 22) it is helpful to insert the beaks of the cotton pliers into the flame of the alcohol lamp prior to grasping sterile paper points. This procedure helps to ensure an accurate test of the sterility of a root canal under treatment. Flaming instruments to sterilize them results in damage to the finish of the instrument. It is advisable to use the same instrument for flaming each time to limit this damage to just a few instruments.

• • •

Various instruments and devices used in dentistry will require different methods to sterilize or disinfect them. The choice is based on the nature of the instrument itself. A guideline that can be used in selecting the appropriate method is to select the most effective and efficient method that will not damage the instrument. It is unreasonable to ruin expensive endodontic files in an autoclave when dry heat will serve to accomplish the same task with minimal damage to the instruments. Plastic devices that would melt in high-temperature sterilization must be disinfected in chemical germicides at room temperature. Every dental office will use a variety of the decontamination methods described to process instruments for use in the operatory.

Packaging dental instruments

The best way to maintain sterility of instruments is to sterilize them in some sort of container. The instruments can remain in the containers until they are ready for use. Containers commonly used are paper and cellophane autoclave bags, covered metal trays, and cloth towel wraps.

Paper autoclave bags (Fig. 6-18, *B*) are one of the mose popular containers in use. Instruments are placed in the bags after cleaning and coating with oil emulsion. The bags are folded on top and stapled. The number of the instrument is recorded on the outside of the bag to identify the contents. There is usually a mark on the bag that will darken during the autoclaving process to indicate that the contents have been sterilized.

Preset covered metal trays make good sense from the standpoint of efficiency and maintaining sterility. The instruments are properly arranged in the tray before sterilization and need not be handled again until they are used (Fig. 6-18, *A*).

Towel wraps are useful particularly for surgical instrument setups. An entire setup of heavy surgical instruments can be placed in a towel wrap (Fig. 6-18, *C*). The wraps are secured with autoclave tape. The tape has stripes on it that will change color during autoclaving to indicate that the contents have been sterilized. The towel wrap also serves as a sterile surface during the procedure when the instruments are used.

PRESET TRAY SYSTEM*

An important part of instrument processing is the maintenance on a preset tray system. A preset tray is a well organized group of instruments and supplies needed for a given dental procedure. They are stored on a metal or plastic tray for use when that procedure is performed (Fig. 6-19, *A* and *B*).

Advantages

Reduced downtime. The use of preset trays can substantially reduce the downtime, or time required to

*Adapted from Chasteen, J.E.: Four-handed dentistry in clinical practice, St. Louis, 1978, The C.V. Mosby Co.

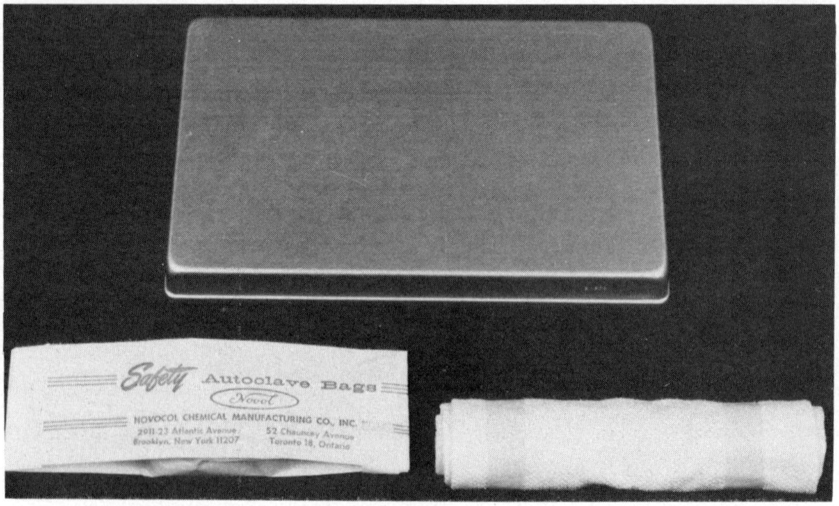

Fig. 6-18. A, Preset covered metal tray. **B,** Paper autoclave bag. **C,** Towel wrap.

prepare an operatory between patients. The armamentarium for a procedure can be readied more easily and quickly by pulling out a tray containing most of the needed instruments and materials rather than searching through several drawers and cabinets for these items. There is less chance of leaving out an item when the instruments and materials for a procedure are handled as a group on a tray.

Improved instrument inventory. The inventory of broken, lost, or dull instruments is easier when the equipment is handled as a group during the procedure and during sterilization.

Improved procedural flow. Organized preset trays help promote the orderly flow of a treatment procedure. The assurance that all items are accounted for on a preset tray (excluding a few add-on items) helps to prevent unnecessary delays. In addition, instruments can be arranged from left to right in the order of their use in a procedure. The tray is used at chairside in a horizontal orientation in front of the assistant, as shown in Fig. 6-19, *A,* when this arrangement is used. However, some assistants prefer to place the tray in a vertical orientation in front of them at chairside, as shown in Fig. 6-19, *B.* In this case, instruments are arranged from bottom to top in the order of their use.

Instruments on preset trays should be arranged in the same sequence that has been established by the dental team for each procedure. The most frequently used items, such as the mirror, explorer, and cotton pliers, should be placed nearest to the patient (Fig. 6-19, *B*). After an instrument is used, it should be returned to the same location on the tray, in case it is needed again. The maintenance of a neat, orderly tray permits the chairside assistant to retrieve instruments quickly as they are needed, without the delay involved in searching through all the instruments for the desired one. Chairside assistants who become familiar with an orderly arrangement of instruments on a tray can substantially reduce the scanning time required to find any instrument in the setup. New employees can learn to work with an operator more quickly if a specific treatment sequence is followed and the instruments are arranged on the tray to match that sequence.

Improved cleaning technique. The use of preset trays can reduce the handling of instruments after sterilization. Depending on the system used, instru-

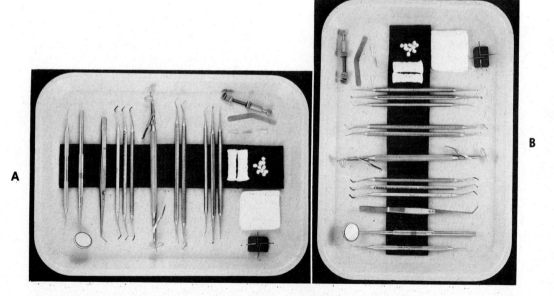

Fig. 6-19. A, Preset tray in horizontal orientation with instruments arranged from left to right in sequence in which they will be used. **B,** Preset tray in vertical orientation with instruments arranged from bottom to top in sequence in which they will be used.

ments can be maintained in a sterile state until they are used at chairside.

Disadvantages

The initial cost of establishing a preset tray system is probably the only real disadvantage. Considerably more instruments are needed for this system, in place of fewer instruments that are sterilized more often. The trays themselves can be rather costly, particularly some of the more elaborate metal ones. However, the longevity of the instruments and the trays should be considered. Preset trays will provide years of convenient service in the office.

General considerations

Preset trays should be kept as simple as possible and stocked only with items that are usually needed in a given procedure. Overstocking trays with instruments that may be used only occasionally creates congestion and tends to defeat the efficiency of the tray system during the procedure. Items that are generally placed on preset trays include the following:

Hand instruments
Burs
Cotton products
Interproximal wedges
Matrix bands
Evacuator tips
Articulating paper

One of the functions of the preset tray is to reduce the time required to set up for a procedure. Thus the inclusion of accessory items at the time the setup is sterilized and assembled reduces the time required for operatory preparation. Items that are impractical to place on a preset tray are considered to be "add-ons" and should be kept in the assistant's mobile cabinet. These include items such as the following:

Restorative materials
Cements
Cavity liners
Impression materials
Interim dressings
Anesthetic syringes and cartridges

The final choice of which items to include on a given tray has to be made by the dentist according to individual technique.

The whole issue of organization of instruments and materials in the dental operatory has to extend beyond consideration of the arrangement of only the preset tray system. This system has to be coordinated with instruments and materials contained in the mobile cabinet and in fixed cabinets. The choice of which items to include on a preset tray is really a matter of priorities established by the individual dentist. Priorities should be based on the frequency with which a service is provided in the daily schedule and convenience to the operating team.

As stated previously, the most frequently used items in a procedure are placed in an orderly sequence on a tray whenever possible. These items represent a primary priority. Add-ons are secondary priority items and are not placed on trays. These should be stored in the most convenient place possible in the assistant's mobile cabinet for favorable access at chairside. Items that are part of operatory preparation or less frequently used items should be located either in the less accessible lower drawers of the mobile cabinet or in nearby fixed cabinets (Fig. 6-20).

The preset tray represents the principal items used in a procedure. From a seated position at chairside, add-on items can quickly be added to an instrument setup from the storage well and upper drawers of the mobile cabinet. Operatory preparation items, such as paper goods, and special-use items, such as the vitalometer, pin kits, and impression trays, may be stored in places that can be reached easily before the assistant is seated in the working position at chairside. An analysis of the individual's practice style is required so that the priorities can be established for each instrument or material.

There are two basic kinds of preset tray systems: the specific procedure tray system and the multipurpose tray system.

Specific procedure tray system. The specific procedure tray system is generally preferable because preset trays are established for rather specific procedures, such as amalgam restorations, composite restorations, cast gold preparations, and cementation of cast restorations. Thus the tray setups are generally less congested, and the instruments can be organized on the tray to match the sequence of the procedure. Each tray can be color coded to identify the purpose for which the tray will be used.

Multipurpose tray system. Although the multipurpose tray system is somewhat less convenient, it is in common use. Trays are established for general categories of procedures, such as operative and crown and bridge. This method can generate preset trays that are more congested and not necessarily organized to match the specific procedural sequence at hand. If a multipurpose preset tray becomes too crowded, the specific procedure tray method should be considered.

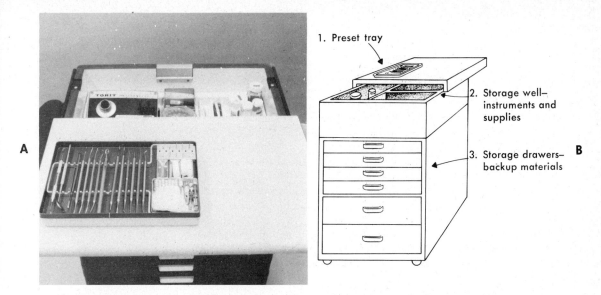

1. Preset tray

2. Storage well—
instruments and
supplies

3. Storage drawers—
backup materials

A

B

Fig. 6-20. A, Preset tray in working position on assistant's mobile cabinet. **B,** Instruments and materials arranged according to their priority in mobile cabinet.

Some dentists use a combination of specific procedure and multipurpose trays in their practices.

Establishing a system

To establish a preset tray system, the dental team has to analyze the requirements of the individual practice and establish priorities for the location of instruments and materials according to the previous discussion. Next, the sterilization method that will be used should be identified, so that appropriately styled trays can be selected. Then, the sterilization area should be arranged to accommodate the mass processing of trays and their contents to prepare them for use in the operatory areas. An identification code is selected for convenient labeling of trays according to their intended use. Color coding is a popular labeling method.

Tray selection. The two basic styles of trays available for use in a preset tray system are the open style and the covered style. Various modifications of these two basic tray styles are available.

Open-style trays (Fig. 6-21). Open-style trays are available in either stainless steel or plastic. Stainless steel trays are durable and can be autoclaved. They are more expensive than plastic trays and have no color that can be used in a coding system. Plastic open-style trays are the least expensive trays avail-

able. They are rather durable, but many of them cannot be autoclaved and they must be washed after every use. Plastic trays are available in an assortment of colors that is useful in a color-coding system. Molded plastic trays that provide compartments for materials and an instrument mat or holder for hand instruments are available (Fig. 6-21, *C*). Also useful are paper tray covers for use with unmolded types of open-style trays (Fig. 6-22).

Instrument mats are also available commercially for use on open-style trays. Instrument mats are devices that hold hand instruments in place on the preset tray. They allow instruments to be positioned for easy identification and retrieval by the chairside assistant. The mat elevates hand instruments so that the assistant can pick up instruments with the thumb and index finger (Fig. 6-23).

Custom-made instrument mats can be fabricated from grooved-style automobile floor mats. They can be cut to any desired length, but the width should be approximately 2 inches for best results (Fig. 6-24). These floor mats are available at many auto supply stores and discount department stores. They can be autoclaved and are durable, considering the rather low cost.

Tray racks can be made to hold trays in a cupboard-style cabinet in each operatory (Fig. 6-25). Trays

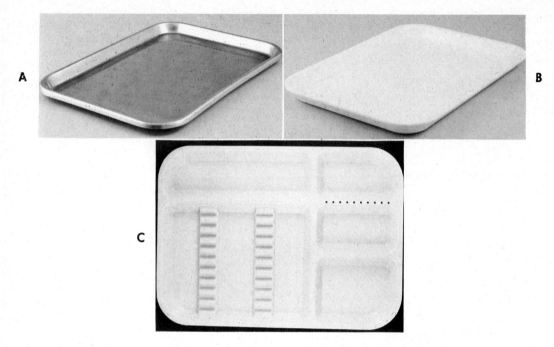

Fig. 6-21. Open-style instrument trays. **A,** Stainless steel. **B,** Plastic. **C,** Molded version of plastic open-style tray.

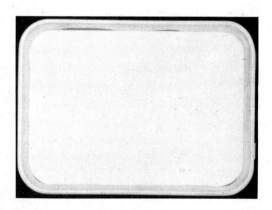

Fig. 6-22. Paper covers for open-style trays are available commercially.

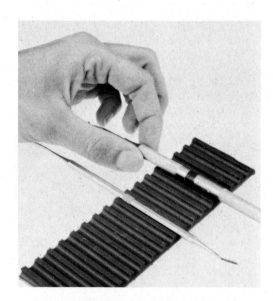

Fig. 6-23. Instrument mat.

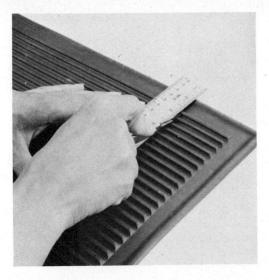

Fig. 6-24. Instrument mats can be fabricated from grooved automobile floor mats.

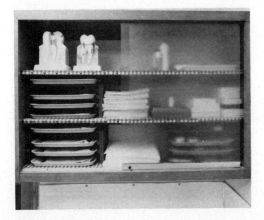

Fig. 6-25. Storage cupboard for preset trays and preparation items for the operatory.

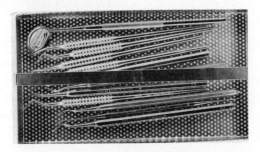

Fig. 6-26. Sterilizing basket.

should be placed so that any tray identification (color coding) is visible when the cupboard is opened.

The technique used to sterilize instruments for the open-style tray depends on the type of tray used, the method of decontamination that the operator prefers, and the capacity of the equipment available in the sterilization area. If stainless steel trays are used, instruments can be debrided, dipped in emulsion, set on the instrument mat on the tray, and placed as an entire unit in the autoclave if its chamber is large enough to accommodate the trays.

If the autoclave chamber is too small or if plastic trays are used, instruments are processed together as a setup in sterilizing baskets (Fig. 6-26), with each basket containing a separate tray setup of instruments. These can be debrided in an ultrasonic cleaner (Fig. 6-12), dipped in protective emulsion, drained, and then placed in the autoclave. The trays are washed, and the instruments that have been autoclaved are returned to the clean trays or a clean paper tray cover.

One disadvantage of this method is that the instruments have to be handled after they have been sterilized to return them to the trays for use in the operatories.

Covered-style trays. Covered-style trays are available in either aluminum or stainless steel (Fig. 6-27). These trays are compact and can be sterilized in the autoclave or a dry-heat oven. Complete instrument setups can be sterilized as units and preserved in a sterile condition until the instruments are used. The lid that covers the tray helps to prolong the sterile state of the instruments. This is a feature not found with many brands of open-style trays.

Covered trays usually contain a metal instrument

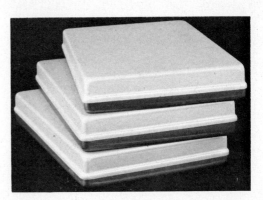

Fig. 6-27. Aluminum covered-style trays available in assorted colors for convenient coding.

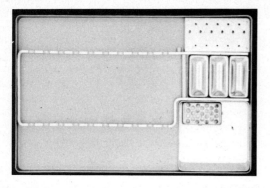

Fig. 6-28. Interior of covered-style tray, containing instrument rack, cotton pellet dispenser, metal dappen dishes, and bur holder.

mat, and some provide small compartments for bur holders, cotton pellets, and other miscellaneous materials (Fig. 6-28). One potential disadvantage is a slight limitation on the arrangement of instruments on the tray. The only major disadvantage is the initial cost of this tray system; however, the investment is a good one, since the trays provide years of service. Some manufacturers provide a variety of colors that are helpful in establishing a color code for easy tray identification.

Dental practices that use a large number of preset trays each day should consider using a covered metal tray system and a dry-heat oven that will accommodate several trays at one time. This method is one of the most efficient ways to process instruments en

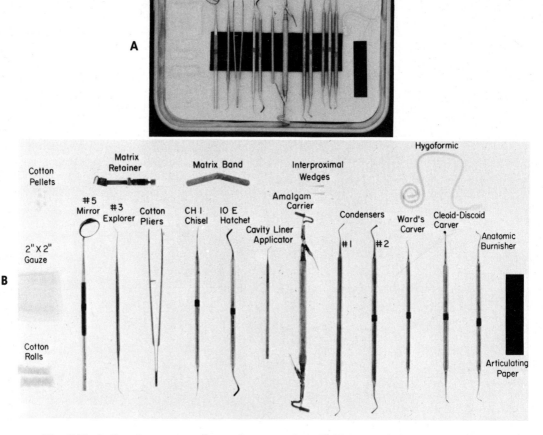

Fig. 6-29. A, Sample preset tray for amalgam procedure. **B,** Tray map for amalgam preset tray.

masse with the least amount of effort by sterilization personnel.

If covered metal trays are sterilized in an autoclave, it is suggested that a paper towel be placed under the instrument mat before sterilization to absorb emulsion and water from the autoclave.

Tray organization

Tray maps. A key requirement of any system is coordination among personnel who use it. To assure uniformity in the preparation of preset trays, it is helpful to develop guides for sterilization personnel to use in setting up instrument trays. The tray map is an example of such a guide (Fig. 6-29).

A tray map is a pictorial display of the contents and arrangement of instruments on a given preset tray. All personnel who work in the sterilization area can use these maps as a guide to be sure all items on a preset tray are accounted for and arranged in the proper configuration. Tray maps are particularly helpful for new employees or employees who are assigned to sterilization only on an occasional basis.

Elaborate tray maps can be made by photographing each instrument setup and labeling each instrument as shown in Fig. 6-29, *B*. Photographs can be dry mounted on poster board (8 × 10 inch size) and stored in the sterilization area for quick reference as they are needed. A less sophisticated method is to use a copying machine (Xerox) to photograph a preset tray.

Instruments are simply placed on the copy machine in the desired arrangement, and the copy is made. The paper copy can then be labeled with a typewriter. There are many instant-copy stores that could provide this service. The finished copy can be placed in a transparent plastic cover available through office supply stores (Fig. 6-30).

The V arrangement. Still another method of organizing instruments on trays is to carefully place color coding identification tape on the handles of the instruments so that they form a distinct V pattern (Fig. 6-31, *A*). The assistant can tell at a glance if the instruments are properly arranged on the tray. Figure 6-31, *B* is the same instrument setup but placed out of sequence on the tray.

Color-coding systems

Color-coding preset trays. Color coding is probably one of the most convenient ways to identify the intended use of any preset tray. Colors can be arbitrarily assigned to the various procedures. For example, blue might be assigned to amalgam restorations; gold to cast-gold restorations, and pink to composite restorations.

Coding of this kind permits rapid visual identification. Some tray manufacturers provide various colors of trays for use in a color-coded system. Stainless steel trays can be coded by using color-coding tape on

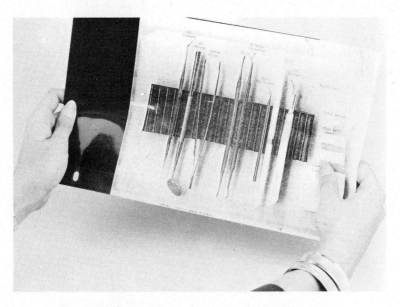

Fig. 6-30. Xerox picture of tray setup in protective cover.

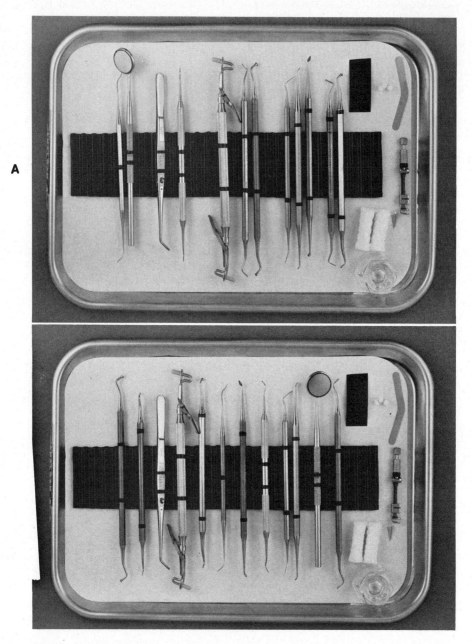

Fig. 6-31. A, V pattern indicates instruments are in proper order. **B,** Same preset tray but the instruments are out of order.

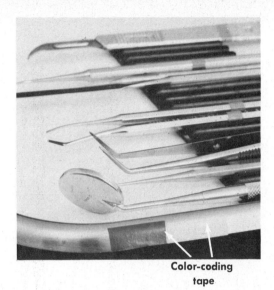

Color-coding
tape

Fig. 6-32. Stainless steel open-style tray with color-coding tape on edge.

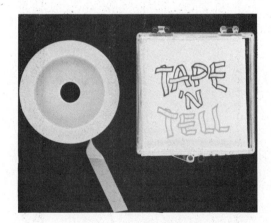

Fig. 6-33. Color-coding tape.

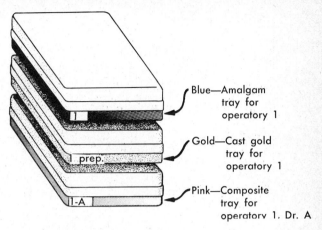

Blue—Amalgam
tray for
operatory 1

Gold—Cast gold
tray for
operatory 1

Pink—Composite
tray for
operatory 1. Dr. A

Fig. 6-34. Color-coded covered metal trays.

the edge of the tray (Fig. 6-32). The tape is available in rolls of assorted colors and will withstand steam sterilization (Fig. 6-33).

Practitioners have elaborated on the basic color-code system, refining it to suit their individual practice needs. Various combinations of colored trays, identification tape, and letters and numbers are used to designate not only the use of the tray but also the operatory in which it belongs and, in group practices, which operator will use it.

Some offices employ a system that codes trays for both the purpose of the tray and the operatory in which the tray belongs. Fig. 6-34 shows that the blue tray is coded for amalgam and is to be stored in operatory 1. This color and number coding is helpful to sterilization personnel and ensures that each operatory is supplied with the appropriate number of trays. If special designations are needed, abbreviations can be placed on the tray. For example, the gold tray in Fig. 6-34 is to be stored in operatory 1 and is a cast-gold preparation tray. The abbreviation *prep* is used to designate its special use. A gold tray with the designation *No. 1 Seat* could indicate that it is a tray for cast gold containing instruments used to seat a cast restoration. Some dentists prefer to use double colors to indicate the purpose and the operatory. One color indicates the purpose, and the other designates the operatory in which the tray belongs. The color that designates the operatory usually matches its predominant color scheme, to simplify the code.

Group practices in which various dentists use different operatories and want their own special preset trays might use a three-part designation on the trays. The pink tray in Fig. 6-34 indicates that the tray contains the equipment for a composite restoration, is to be stored in operatory 1, and is Dr. A's special setup for the procedure.

Some dental offices have a central dispensing area in which all preset trays are stored. In these offices, operatory designations are not needed on the trays, since sterilization personnel can conveniently monitor the supply of trays in the central dispensing area.

Color-coding instruments. Colored identification

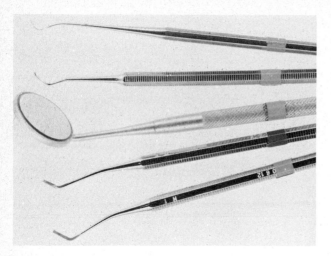

Fig. 6-35. Color-coded instruments with colored identification tape on handles.

tape can be placed on the handles of instruments to match the color code on the tray (Fig. 6-35). Although this may be helpful for quickly locating the tray on which a stray instrument may belong, it is not absolutely necessary if the contents of each preset tray are processed together and tray maps are used. Color-coding instruments with identification tape requires continuous maintenance, since the tape becomes dingy after repeated sterilization and sometimes separates from the instruments during processing. The choice of whether to code individual instruments is left to the operatory team.

In large clinical facilities, such as hospitals, dental schools, and military clinics, this type of coding is often found helpful in maintaining an orderly preset tray system.

SUMMARY

Instrument processing is an integral part of an efficient dental practice. All the dental auxiliaries in the office, not just the dental assistant, should be able to perform the tasks associated with instrument processing. The ability to delegate instrument processing to an assistant, hygienist, or receptionist adds valuable flexibility to office procedure, which contributes to greater efficiency in the dental practice.

BIBLIOGRAPHY

Barton, R.E., et al.: The dental assistant, ed. 5, New York, 1978, McGraw-Hill Book Co.

Chasteen, J.E.: Four-handed dentistry in clinical practice, St. Louis, 1978, The C.V. Mosby Co.

Coughlin, J.W., et al.: Comparison of dry heat, autoclave and vapor sterilizers, J. Ont. Dent. Soc. **45:**137, April 1968.

Green, E., and Seyer, P.C.: Sharpening curets and sickle scalers, San Francisco, 1972, Praxis Publishing Co.

Lawrence, C.A., and Block, S.S.: Disinfection, sterilization, and preservation, Philadelphia, 1968, Lea & Febiger.

CHAPTER 7

LOCAL ANESTHESIA AND
PREMEDICATION

LOCAL ANESTHESIA

Many dental procedures involve the cutting or painful manipulation of living tissue. The painful stimulus of these procedures to the patient has determined the need for use of anesthesia in dentistry. Anesthesia is the loss of sensation or feeling in a body part. There are various drugs available that will produce temporary anesthesia in the body. These drugs are classified as either general anesthetics or local anesthetics.

A general anesthetic temporarily alters the central nervous system so that sensation is lost throughout the entire body. The patient is unconscious under the influence of general anesthetics.

Local anesthetics temporarily prevent the conduction of sensory impulses such as pain, touch, and thermal change from a body part along nerve pathways to the brain. Thus only certain selected regions of the body lose sensation under local anesthesia. Patients remain conscious under the influence of local anesthetic agents. With the exception of certain surgical and operative procedures, local anesthesia is more commonly used than general anesthesia in dentistry.

For local anesthetics to work, they must come in direct contact with either the nerve fibers carrying the sensory impulse to the brain or the tiny nerve endings that pick up sensations in the tissues.

A special type of local anesthetic that acts only on tiny nerve endings located in the surface of skin and mucosa is called a topical anesthetic. Topical anesthetics eliminate some sensation on surface tissues such as skin and especially mucosa. Sunburn lotion usually contains a topical anesthetic that temporarily eliminates the discomfort of sunburn. Oral mucosa can be anesthetized by wiping a topical anesthetic on the tissue surface. This is helpful in reducing the dis-

comfort of dental injections and eliminating the gag reflex during impression-making and radiographic procedures. These agents are available in liquid, paste, and cream forms (Fig. 7-1).

Local anesthetics used for operative and surgical procedures must be injected into the soft tissue so that the anesthetic agent can come in contact with sensory nerve fibers. Once an anesthetic solution surrounds a nerve, sensations cannot pass through the nerve at that point. As a result, the structure that receives its innervation from the surrounded nerve can be operated on without pain. Local anesthetic agents that are

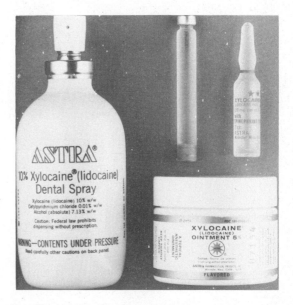

Fig. 7-1. Anesthetic agents. *Left* and *bottom right,* Topical agents. *Top right,* Injectable agents.

used for injection purposes are supplied in liquid form in premeasured cartridges and ampules (Fig. 7-1).

Methods of injection

The three principal injection methods used in dentistry are (1) infiltration, (2) field block, and (3) nerve block.

The term *infiltration anesthesia* is often misused. Specifically, infiltration is an injection method used to deposit anesthetic solution so that it will prevent the sensation of pain from being picked up by tiny terminal nerve branches that are located throughout living tissue. It is a fairly common procedure to infiltrate an area of soft tissue so that an incision can be made in the tissue without producing pain. This method of administration of anesthesia is used in procedures such as biopsy, gingivectomy, frenectomy, and the excision of abnormal tissue.

The term *infiltration anesthesia* is often interchangeably with *field block anesthesia*. The methods of injection appear to be similar to both. The difference between infiltration and field block anesthesia centers on which branches of the nerve are the targets of the injection procedure. Infiltration procedures are directed toward the *tiny* terminal branches of the nerve. Field block procedures are directed toward larger terminal branches. The intended target is the difference between the two procedures. It is true that in the orodental region field blocks often accomplish infiltration anesthesia at the same time. Anesthetic solutions that are injected into areas near large terminal nerve branches will also eliminate pain impulses from adjacent tiny nerve branches. These solutions are not selective as to which branches they will anesthetize in any given area. Fig. 7-2, *A* and *C*, demonstrates the difference between the two proce-

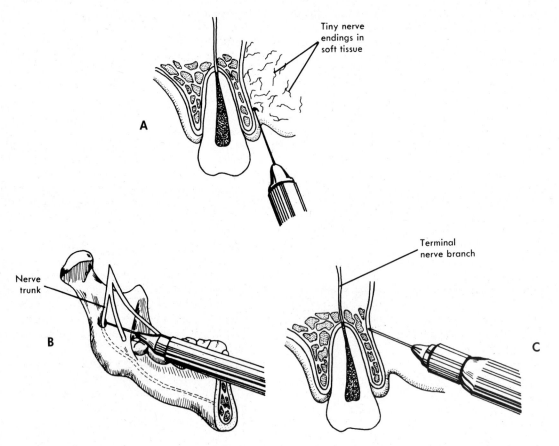

Fig. 7-2. Needle placement. **A,** For infiltration anesthesia. **B,** For nerve block anesthesia. **C,** For field block anesthesia.

dures as far as needle placement is concerned.

Nerve block anesthesia involves the deposition of anesthetic solution near a main nerve trunk. A successful nerve block will prevent passage of any pain impulse past the site of injection to the brain. Therefore any structure that is innervated by the nerve trunk or any of its branches beyond the injection site away from the brain will be anesthetized. Nerve blocks eliminate pain sensation from larger areas than either the field block or infiltration method.

Soft tissue surgery is preceded by infiltration anesthesia procedures everywhere in the oral cavity.

Field block anesthesia is used whenever teeth or bone are going to be operated on in the maxillary or sometimes in the mandibular anterior region. Larger terminal branches of the trigeminal nerve provide innervation to the teeth and bone in these areas. Field block anesthesia cannot be used to successfully anesthetize the posterior mandibular teeth. These teeth are surrounded by very dense bone that does not allow penetration of the anesthetic solution through it to reach the terminal branches that innervate the teeth. Field block procedures are successful throughout the entire maxilla and in the mandibular anterior area because the bone surrounding the teeth is thinner and less dense. Hence the anesthetic solution can penetrate this bone and contact the terminal nerve branches that innervate these teeth. Some patients can be anesthetized in the mandibular premolar region by a field block injection; however, this varies with the anatomic features of the individual patient.

The most common nerve block that is used in dentistry is the mandibular nerve block. The inferior alveolar nerve supplies all the mandibular teeth and surrounding bone. To anesthetize these structures, a needle is placed near the mandibular foramen on the medial aspect of the ramus (Fig. 7-2, *B*). The solution is deposited near this main nerve trunk where it enters the mandible. All the mandibular teeth and bone will be anesthetized beyond this point to the patient's midline.

Following is a summary of which injection procedures are used to anesthetize specific structures for dental procedures.

Structure	Injection method
Oral soft tissue	Infiltration
Maxillary teeth and bone	Field block
Mandibular anterior teeth and bone	Field block
All mandibular teeth and bone	Mandibular nerve block

The trigeminal nerve is the fifth cranial nerve, and it provides sensory innervation to the orofacial region of the body.

Anesthetic agents

Although there are approximately 15 different anesthetics available for dental use, 2% lidocaine (Xylocaine) and 2% mepivacaine (Carbocaine) are probably the most commonly used. These two agents are similar in that they have a rapid onset of action, last approximately 90 to 180 minutes, and provide profound local anesthesia.

The trend in dental practice is to do more dental procedures during longer appointments. When these agents are used with vasoconstrictors, they provide a favorable working time for this type of practice.

If a short procedure is anticipated, anesthesia with a short duration can be accomplished with a 3% mepivacaine (Carbocaine) solution without a vasoconstrictor. A short duration is considered to be 45 to 75 minutes.

Vasoconstrictors

Vasoconstrictors are drugs that cause blood vessels to constrict so that blood flow through these vessels is reduced. The drugs accomplish this by stimulating certain receptors in the arterial system. When vasoconstrictors are used in combination with local anesthetic agents, they reduce blood flow at the site of the injected solution. The effect is to retard absorption of the anesthetic solution into the bloodstream. This is desirable because the anesthetic solution is kept in the injection site for a longer period of time rather than being carried away into the bloodstream. Thus the profoundness and duration of the anesthesia are increased.

Since most anesthetics are somewhat toxic to the central nervous system, vasoconstrictors increase the safety margin because smaller quantities of anesthetic can be used to obtain adequate anesthesia. In addition, the amount of anesthetic that is used cannot enter the bloodstream rapidly and be carried to the brain in great enough quantity to produce a toxic effect.

The most common vasoconstrictors used are epinephrine (used with lidocaine), and Neo-Cobefrin (used with mepivacaine). Lidocaine, 2%, is available in two forms: (1) without any vasoconstrictor or (2) with epinephrine in either a 1:100,000 or a 1:50,000 concentration. A concentration of 1:50,000 means that 1 part of vasoconstrictor is diluted by 50,000 parts of nonvasoconstrictor. The 1:100,000 concentration seems to be the most favorable. Mepivacaine is available in a 3% solution without a vasoconstrictor or in a 2% solution with a 1:20,000 concentration of Neo-Cobefrin. The anesthetic solutions without vasoconstrictors are a convenient choice for short-acting anesthetics.

Armamentarium

The armamentarium needed to administer local anesthesia in the oral cavity is shown in Fig. 7-3.

Syringes. Dental injection syringes vary in design. The choice of syringe design is a matter of personal preference of the dentist.

Probably the most widely used aspirating syringe is the metal breech-loading style with a harpoon-type plunger (Fig. 7-4). This type of syringe is available with a thumb ring, which helps the dentist apply back pressure on the plunger after needle placement in the tissue.

As was mentioned previously, all local anesthetics are potentially toxic to the central nervous system if injected in sufficient quantities into the bloodstream. This can occur if a needle is inadvertently placed in a blood vessel and the solution is injected directly into the bloodstream. To prevent this from occurring, the dentist must apply back pressure on the plunger after needle placement. If the needle is in a vessel, blood will be drawn into the anesthetic cartridge, which is called *aspiration*. If blood does enter the cartridge, it is recommended that the needle be removed and the injection started again in a different position. This procedure is a safety measure designed to protect the patient. Aspiration is not as important in field block and infiltration injections as it is in nerve blocks, since the larger vessels are located deep in the tissues near main nerve trunks.

When the syringe is loaded, it is important to drive the small harpoon on the end of the plunger into the rubber stopper in the anesthetic cartridge. The harpoon will engage the rubber stopper when back pressure is applied to the plunger, allowing the aspiration to occur.

Injection needles. One of the best developments in medicine and dentistry in recent years has been the advent of the disposable injection needle. These needles are packaged under sterile conditions in individual protective plastic containers. They are ready to use with no further preparation necessary.

The disposable needle has the following advantages:

1. It is convenient, since no further sterilization is required.
2. There is no danger of cross contamination from one patient to another, since the needle is thrown away after use.
3. The needle is sharper, since it is not used repeatedly, as is the nondisposable type.

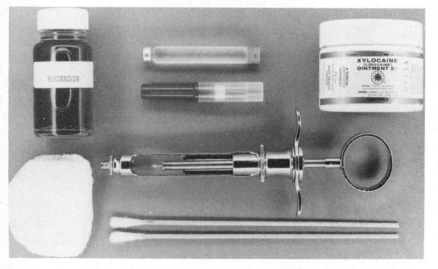

Topical disinfectant (Mecresin or Metaphen)
Anesthetic cartridge
Injection needle
Topical anesthetic (optional)
Gauze sponges, 2 × 2 inch
Syringe
Cotton swabs

Fig. 7-3. Local anesthetic armamentarium.

A common type of disposable needle has two sections to its plastic container. One section covers the hub portion of the needle. The other section covers the shaft and bevel portion of the needle (Fig. 7-5). After the syringe is loaded with an anesthetic cartridge, the hub portion of the needle can be uncovered and screwed onto the end of the syringe. The small portion of the needle extending from the hub will puncture the small rubber seal in the center of the metal end of the cartridge. The section of the plastic container covering the shaft of the needle is left in place until the needle is to be used. This prevents contamination of the needle. After the injection, it is wise to cover the needle again with the plastic container in case the needle is needed for another injection in the same patient. This is also a safety measure to protect the dental assistant.

Needles are available in different lengths and gauges. Length is measured from the hub to the tip of the needle bevel. Two of the more common lengths in use are the 1-inch needle (short needle) and the 1⅝-inch needle (long needle). A fairly common practice is to use a short needle for infiltration and field blocks and a long needle for deep nerve blocks such as the mandibular nerve block. Again, this is determined by the personal preference of the dentist. The gauge of a needle is the measurement of the diameter of the needle shaft. Some of the common gauges used in

dentistry are 23, 25, 27, and 30 gauge. The *lower* gauge number indicates the *larger* diameter of needle shaft.

The selection of needle gauge is dictated somewhat by the depth of the injection and the needle length used. Generally speaking, the longer the needle length, the larger the diameter of needle that should be used. Although small-diameter needles may be less painful, they can be easily deflected in the tissue and miss the intended target. This is especially true when long, thin needles are used for deep injections. Inadequate anesthesia is often the result of needle deviation, since the solution will be deposited away from the nerve target. Fine-gauge needles such as short-length needles of 27 and 30 gauge are recommended for shallow infiltration and field block injections.

Anesthetic cartridges. Without doubt, the premeasured anesthetic cartridge is the most convenient way to purchase a local anesthetic. It eliminates measuring errors, reduces the possibility of bacterial contamination, and ensures uniformity in the concentration of the solution.

The cartridge is essentially a glass tube with one end sealed with a metal cap. The metal cap has a rubber center into which the needle is inserted after the cartridge is loaded into the syringe (Fig. 7-6). The other end of the tube is sealed with a rubber stopper. The small harpoon is driven into this stopper after the cartridge is loaded into the syringe.

Most cartridges contain 1.8 ml of anesthetic solution, which is an adequate dose for most dental procedures.

There are variations in disposable needles, cartridges, and even syringes. Some cartridges are available with the needle already attached, all in one unit. On the other hand, there are plastic syringes available with attached needles that are loaded with a standard anesthetic cartridge. The entire assembly can be dis-

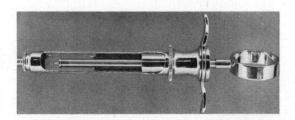

Fig. 7-4. Breech-loading injection syringe.

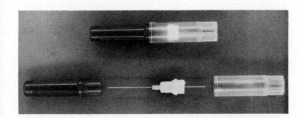

Fig. 7-5. Disposable injection needle. *Top,* Covered. *Bottom,* Uncovered.

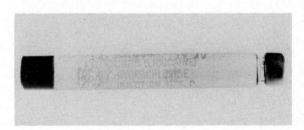

Fig. 7-6. Anesthetic cartridge.

carded after it is used. Items such as these might be given strong consideration because of their convenience.

It has been suggested that anesthetic cartridges be stored with the cartridges on end and the metal-capped end immersed in isopropyl alcohol to prevent contamination of the rubber seal in the center of the cap.

Auxiliary items. The auxiliary items used in the administration of local anesthesia are all used to prepare the injection site before inserting the needle into the tissue.

Gauze sponge, 2 × 2 inch. This is used to dry the mucosa before applications of both the topical anesthetic and the disinfectant. It is also used as a compress after the injection.

Cotton swabs. These are used to apply the topical anesthetic and disinfectant.

Topical anesthetic. Before the injection this is applied to the mucosa to reduce the discomfort of the needle penetration into the tissues.

Topical disinfectant. It is used to clean the injection site before the injection.

Preparation of the injection syringe

Following is a suggested sequence of preparing an injection syringe for use:

1. Load an anesthetic cartridge into a sterile syringe by pulling the plunger mechanism as far back as possible and dropping the cartridge into the large opening on the side of the barrel of the syringe. Place the metal-capped end of the cartridge toward the end of the syringe where the needle will be attached (Fig. 7-7, *A*).
2. After the cartridge is in place, remove the plastic cover from the hub end of the needle. Force the small projection of the needle into the cartridge toward the soft rubber center of the metal cap. Then screw the hub onto the syringe until it is tight. Leave the plastic cover on the shaft portion of the needle (Fig. 7-7, *B*).

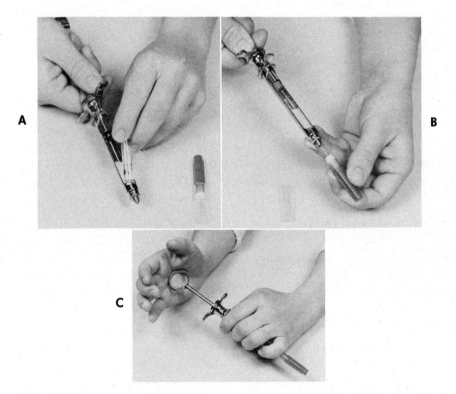

Fig. 7-7. Preparation of anesthetic syringe. **A,** Insertion of anesthetic cartridge. **B,** Attachment of disposable needle. **C,** Setting harpoon-shaped plunger into rubber stopper of cartridge.

3. Grasp the syringe firmly with one hand on the barrel and tap the thumb ring firmly with the open palm of the other hand (Fig. 7-7, *C*). This drives the harpoon of the plunger into the rubber stopper.
4. Remove the needle cover and express a few drops of anesthetic out of the needle to make sure the apparatus is functioning.
5. Place slight back pressure on the thumb ring to check whether the harpoon is properly engaged in the rubber stopper.
6. Cover the needle again with the plastic cap until the syringe is needed.

Preparation of the injection site

An ideal method of preparing an injection site is as follows:

1. Dry the mucosa at the injection site with a 2 × 2 inch gauze sponge.
2. Apply a topical anesthetic with a cotton swab and cover the area with the 2 × 2 inch gauze. Wait 30 to 60 seconds for the topical anesthetic to take effect.
3. Remove the gauze and paint the site with disinfectant (Mecresin).
4. The injection is made immediately after the disinfectant is applied.
5. After the injection, place a fresh 2 × 2 inch gauze over the injection site while waiting for the anesthetic to take effect. This catches any blood or anesthetic solution that may seep out of the needle hole in the tissue.

If the needle is inadvertently touched at any time before the injection, it should be discarded and replaced with a new sterile needle.

Hidden syringe transfer

A technique for transferring the anesthetic syringe to the dentist out of the patient's view is discussed on p. 171.

Standard injection sites (Fig. 7-8)

All field blocks to anesthetize teeth are administered in the mucobuccal and mucolabial fold areas over the roots of the teeth to be anesthetized. Alveolar bone is thinner on the buccal and labial aspects of teeth.

Infiltrations are shallow injections that are placed wherever soft tissues need to be anesthetized. These injections are done right at or very near the surgical site.

Mandibular blocks are administered near the anterior pillar of the soft palate, along the anterior border of the ramus.

PREMEDICATION

Premedication is the administration of a drug before the actual treatment of the patient. Premedication can also be an adjustment of the dosage of a drug that the patient is already taking routinely for a systemic disorder. Premedication is most frequently employed to control apprehension. However, it may be necessary to administer certain drugs to protect the patient from undesirable effects of a procedure or to improve working conditions for the operator. The intent of this section is to discuss some of the most common uses of premedication in general dentistry.

Agents to control apprehension

Despite the fact that dentistry has eliminated pain in most routine procedures, some dental patients are still apprehensive about receiving dental services. If in the opinion of the dentist the patient's apprehension is great enough to interfere significantly with the proposed treatment, premedication of the patient with an antiapprehension agent is indicated.

The decision to premedicate a patient for any purpose must be based on the study of the general health of the patient. Such information is acquired during the recording of the medical-dental history discussed previously. This information, coupled with the dentist's knowledge of the effects of drugs on the vital systems of the body, leads the dentist to a sound decision on the advisability of premedication.

Preoperative sedation through the use of drugs can be achieved with agents such as narcotics, barbiturates, and nitrous oxide analgesia.

Narcotic agents. Narcotic agents are extremely useful drugs for preoperative sedation in the presence of severe preoperative pain. Narcotics are effective as sedatives and even more as analgesics (pain relievers). The fact that they are addictive has caused many dentists to avoid their use. If the drugs are used properly, there is little danger of addiction under normal use. Morphine sulfate and meperidine hydrochloride (Demerol) are examples of such narcotic agents. Obviously the dentist will not select these agents for routine use as a preoperative sedative when other agents are available that accomplish the same task in most patients.

Barbiturates. Barbiturates are principally sedative agents, whereas narcotics are principally analgesics. Barbiturates are superior to narcotic agents in relieving apprehension. Because of this fact and because there is very little tendency toward addiction, the bar-

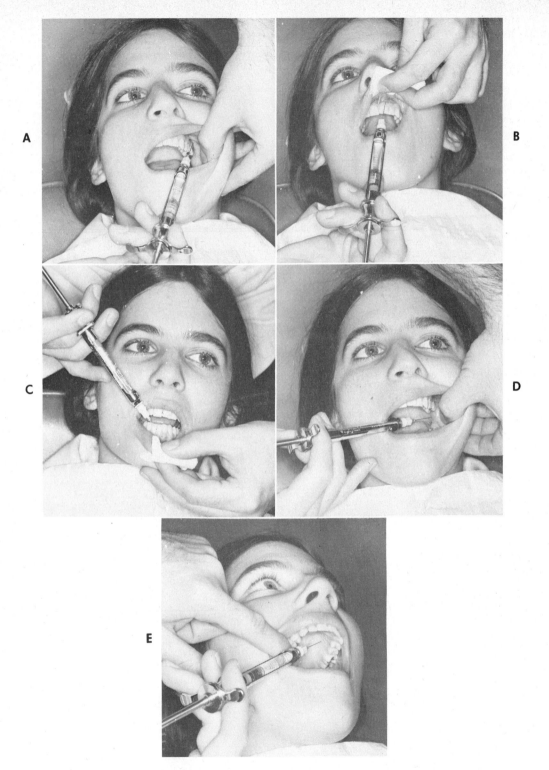

Fig. 7-8. Standard injection sites. **A,** Maxillary posterior teeth. **B,** Maxillary anterior teeth. **C,** Mandibular anterior teeth. **D,** Mandibular posterior teeth. **E,** Palatal soft tissue.

biturates have become popular in dentistry as preoperative sedatives. Short-acting barbiturates such as pentobarbital (Nembutal) and secobarbital (Seconal) are usually the drugs of choice.

These agents are given orally approximately 45 minutes before the appointment time. Caution must be exercised in prescribing either of these drugs because the effects last from 3 to 4 hours. This creates a distinct disadvantage for many patients because they should be escorted to and from the dental office while under the influence of the drug. Another disadvantage is that the effect of the drug lasts longer than it is needed in most instances.

Combinations of various sedatives are sometimes selected to achieve a sedative effect. Demerol compound is such a drug. It is a combination of meperidine (Demerol), promethazine (Phenergan), and chlorpromazine (Thorazine). This agent is effective for use in children through the age of 12 years. The dosage is calculated according to the child's body weight.

Nitrous oxide analgesia. Nitrous oxide analgesia, or ''tranquilizing air'' as it is sometimes called, can be used as a convenient preoperative sedative. Nitrous oxide is actually a general anesthetic that has been available since around 1844. Although the early use of nitrous oxide gas was relatively crude by today's standards, it was the most popular anesthetic in common use by dentists until local anesthesia was developed around 1905. Local anesthesia rapidly gained popularity and virtually eliminated the use of nitrous oxide as an anesthetic in dental practice.

For many years nitrous oxide has been slowly returning to popularity in dental practice, not as an anesthetic but rather as a means of sedating a patient and raising the pain reaction threshold while the patient remains conscious. The general idea of nitrous oxide analgesia is to provide preoperative sedation for the patient just before the dental procedure begins. Other means of achieving sedation by the use of oral agents require that the patient take the medication well in advance of the dental appointment. Although intravenous sedatives eliminate this problem, they require an injection procedure that is often objectionable to the apprehensive patient. Nitrous oxide analgesia can be continually administered to the patient throughout the dental procedure to maintain sedation. After completion of the dental appointment the nitrous oxide can be discontinued, and the patient returns to a normal alert status and can drive home

safely. This is not possible with oral sedatives. In short, sedation with nitrous oxide can be initiated immediately before a dental procedure, maintained throughout the procedure at a constant level, and then terminated quickly at the end of the appointment. This is very convenient for both the dentist and the patient.

Since nitrous oxide is a gaseous substance, it is administered with a gas machine, in which it is mixed with oxygen and delivered to the patient through a nosepiece (Fig. 7-9). The patient inhales this mixture, and sedation results. The mixture commonly used is approximately 15% nitrous oxide and 85% oxygen. The mixture is almost odorless and not unpleasant for the patient. Normal atmospheric air contains approximately 80% nitrogen and 20% oxygen. The patient actually receives more oxygen through the nosepiece (85%) than by breathing normal room air. Thus asphyxiation is not a problem in the use of nitrous oxide analgesia.

After the nitrous oxide enters the lungs, it is absorbed into the bloodstream and depresses the central nervous system. The degree of central nervous system depression is controlled by the mixture of gases delivered to the patient. Patients in the analgetic state

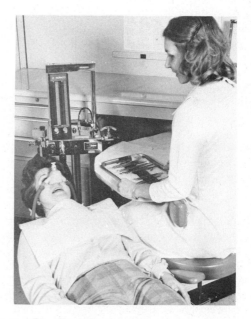

Fig. 7-9. Nitrous oxide analgesia setup.

created by nitrous oxide have the following characteristics:

1. Are still conscious, communicative, and cooperative
2. Are relaxed, breathe normally, and can hold their mouth open voluntarily
3. Have an elevated pain reaction threshold and do not react to a minor pain stimulus such as the injection of a local anesthetic

This state is very safe because the patient remains conscious, whereas protective reflex mechanisms such as the cough reflex and blinking of the eyes remain. The patient will have a feeling of profound relaxation, tingling in fingers, toes, and the tongue, and a general feeling of well-being. It is recommended that all dentists and auxiliary personnel experience nitrous oxide analgesia if it is to be used in the office. This experience will help in reassuring the patient as to what is to be expected under the influence of nitrous oxide.

After completion of the procedure, the flow of nitrous oxide to the patient is discontinued, and for approximately 3 minutes only oxygen mixed with room air is inhaled through the nosepiece to "clear" the patient. When the patient has returned to normal alertness, postoperative instructions can be given. Then the patient can be dismissed.

Premedications to protect the patient

Sometimes patients have a systemic disorder that requires continued use of certain drugs to maintain their health. Examples of such conditions include diabetes, epilepsy, hypothyroidism, hypertension, coronary thrombosis, and rheumatic heart disease. The medical-dental history taken at the diagnostic appointment will reveal these conditions and the medications that are taken to control them. The dentist often works with the patient's physician to regulate dosages of these drugs at the time dental treatment is being done. For example, patients who are taking anticoagulants (blood-thinning agents) must have the dosage carefully regulated to avoid problems of bleeding after oral surgical procedures.

Patients with rheumatic heart disease or various blood diseases that make them extremely vulnerable to severe systemic infections must be premedicated with antibiotics to protect them during transient bacteremias. A transient bacteremia (bacteria in the blood) can occur as a result of the entry of organisms into the bloodstream through ruptured oral soft tissues. Not only do obvious procedures such as oral surgery allow bacteria from the oral cavity to enter the bloodstream, but also a routine cleaning of the teeth can cause a bacteremia. Patients with normal defense mechanisms will destroy these organisms without assistance from antibiotics. However, patients with a depressed defense mechanism need protection from antibiotics to prevent serious systemic infection.

Premedication for operator convenience

Certainly the preoperative sedative agents provide convenience for the dentist, since the apprehensive patient is rendered more cooperative. There are other agents that are helpful to control such problems as excessive salivation, gagging, and muscle spasm, which create technical difficulties for the operating team.

Excessive salivation occurs in patients with extremely active salivary glands and can create difficulty in isolation of the operative field. This is of particular significance in procedures for which a rubber dam cannot be used, such as surgery and impression-taking. Premedication with an agent such as propantheline (Pro-Banthine), atropine, or scopolamine will decrease the secretion from the salivary glands temporarily while the dental procedure is accomplished.

Gagging can be a problem during restorative, surgical, and radiographic procedures. Nitrous oxide analgesia will reduce the gag reflex significantly. Simply applying a topical anesthetic to the mucosa in the posterior regions of the mouth will be of temporary assistance for short procedures. This is especially useful in the taking of radiographs of posterior regions of the mouth, where contact of the film packet with the mucosa triggers the gag reflex.

Sometimes patients present themselves for dental treatment when their muscles of mastication are in a state of constant contraction, or spasm. This is often so profound that the patient cannot open his or her mouth wide enough for the dentist to correct the intraoral cause of the spasm. Other patients experience problems of muscle spasm or cramping during dental procedures because of fatigue as a result of holding the mouth open. The dentist can often overcome this problem by prescribing skeletal muscle relaxants such as methocarbamol (Robaxin), diazepam (Valium), and orphenadrine (Norflex) preoperatively. Nitrous oxide analgesia has also been useful in circumventing this problem.

SUMMARY

The preparation of anesthetic syringes and the administration of local anesthetics are a daily activity in a general dental practice. Dental assistants must be thoroughly familiar with the types of anesthetics to be used as well as the procedure itself.

Handling of patients who require premedication is a responsibility shared by all members of the dental team. The dental assistant is well advised to be aware of the patients who require this service and to be familiar with the specific medications that are used in the office.

BIBLIOGRAPHY

Bennett, C.R.: Monheim's local anesthesia and pain control in dental practice, ed. 7, St. Louis, 1984, The C.V. Mosby Co.

Holroyd, S.V., and Wynn, R.L.: Clinical pharmacology in dental practice, ed. 3, St. Louis, 1983, The C.V. Mosby Co.

Langa, H.: Relative analgesia in dental practice, Philadelphia, 1968, W.B. Saunders Co.

CHAPTER 8

ISOLATION PROCEDURES

Isolation of the operating field is the process of retracting soft tissue out of the way to gain access to and visibility of the area to be treated. Since the oral cavity is a wet environment, an important function of isolation procedures is to control salivary contamination of the operative field. Virtually all restorative materials require a clean, dry environment at the time of their insertion into a prepared cavity if maximum quality is to be achieved. Hence effective isolation should be an integral part of any restorative procedure.

Many devices and methods are available to accomplish adequate isolation. No attempt will be made here to discuss all of them, but rather the discussion will be limited to the two most widely used methods: (1) cotton roll isolation and (2) rubber dam isolation.

COTTON ROLL ISOLATION

One of the oldest and still popular isolation methods is the cotton roll method. It is a simple and rapid way to isolate the operative field. However, it is by no means the most reliable isolation method. The cotton roll method does not prevent the patient from inadvertently contaminating the operative field while swallowing or with a "curious tongue." This method does not prevent debris from the operative procedure from dropping into the throat area and under the tongue. On the other hand, the rubber dam isolation technique does provide ideal isolation in all respects.

A typical cotton roll isolation setup for operating anywhere in the maxillary arch is accomplished by placing an appropriate-sized cotton roll in the mucobuccal or mucolabial area in the region of the teeth to be treated (Fig. 8-1, A and B). There are various sizes of cotton rolls available. Some are wrapped in cotton thread to prevent them from sticking to the mucosa when removed. Dry cotton rolls should be moistened with the water syringe before they are removed. This prevents the cotton roll from pulling off the delicate epithelial covering of the mucosa, which is often referred to as "cotton roll burn."

The mandibular arch requires a little more gadgetry to isolate the posterior teeth because of the presence of the tongue and the pooling of saliva in the floor of the mouth. A time-honored method is to use cotton roll holders that place a cotton roll on both the buccal and lingual aspect of the arch (Fig. 8-1, C). These holding devices are available in different sizes, and they are purchased in right-side and left-side styles. The device is held in place by a metal clamp that is tightened under the patient's chin. Smaller disposable cotton roll holders are now available that are less bulky than the metal styles (Fig. 8-1, D). Saliva is removed by placing a disposable saliva ejector in the sublingual area.

Another more comfortable method of isolating the mandibular posterior area is to place a cotton roll on the buccal aspect of the arch and use an aspirating tongue retractor on the lingual aspect (Fig. 8-1, E). These retractors are available in various styles (Fig. 8-2). The disposable types are preferable because they are adjustable to fit the patient and can be thrown away after use. These devices are connected to the saliva-ejector hose.

An auxiliary device that is helpful in isolating posterior areas is the triangular-shaped absorbent paper disk (Theta Dri-Angle) (Fig. 8-3). The disk aids in the retraction of the buccal mucosa and is a helpful companion device to cotton roll isolation.

The mandibular anterior teeth can usually be isolated with a small cotton roll placed in the mucolabial fold (Fig. 8-1, F).

One small disadvantage of the cotton roll isolation technique is that the cotton rolls must be replaced after they are wetted by the water coolant during the cavity preparation phase. The new dry cotton rolls ensure a dry field during the insertion of the restorative material.

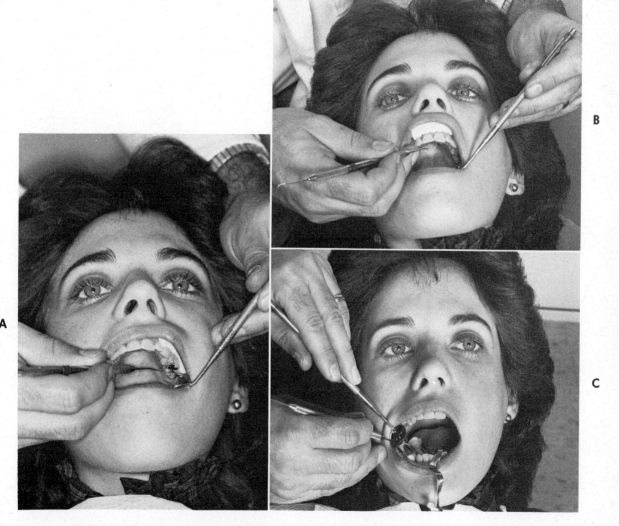

Fig. 8-1. Cotton roll isolation. **A,** Maxillary posterior area. **B,** Maxillary anterior area. **C,** Mandibular posterior area (with traditional cotton roll holder). *Continued.*

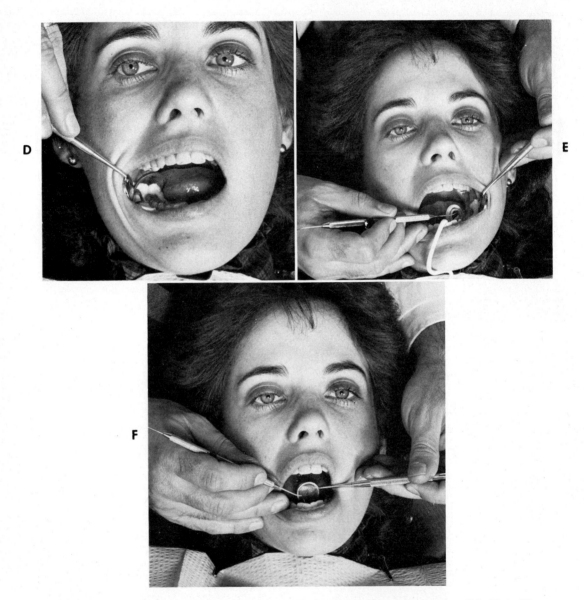

Fig. 8-1, cont'd. D, Mandibular posterior area (with plastic disposable cotton roll holder). **E,** Mandibular posterior area (with Hygoformic tongue retractor). **F,** Mandibular anterior area.

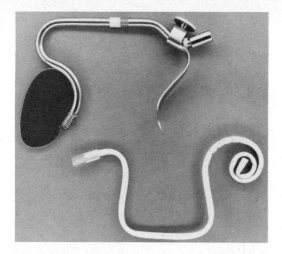

Fig. 8-2. Aspirating tongue retractors. *Top,* Svedopter. *Bottom,* Hygoformic.

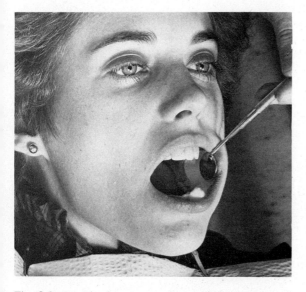

Fig. 8-3. Combination cotton roll and absorbent paper triangle used for isolation.

RUBBER DAM ISOLATION

The rubber dam isolation method is a much more complicated procedure but is extremely worthwhile in terms of quality of isolation. There is no doubt that the use of the rubber dam is the best isolation method available in dentistry. It does require a little more time to apply than the cotton roll method, but its dividends in time saving and convenience during the restorative procedure make up for the additional effort required in the application.

The concept of the rubber dam procedure is to place a sheet of latex rubber over the lower face so that only those teeth to be treated, plus a few adjacent teeth, project through the rubber sheet. The rubber dam is held in place by clamps and a ligature. All other structures and saliva are located under the rubber dam (Fig. 8-8, *K*). Once the dam is in place, all phases of the restorative procedure can be accomplished with easy access and good visibility, and the environment will be absolutely dry during the insertion of the restorative material. All debris from the restorative procedure is kept out of the throat area and can be easily removed with the oral evacuator.

Armamentarium

The rubber dam procedure requires a separate tray setup for convenience (Fig. 8-4).

Rubber dam clamps. The use of a rubber dam clamp is a convenient way to hold the rubber dam in place. Various clamps are available to meet the particular needs of the individual restorative procedure. The clamps shown in Fig. 8-5 are some of the most common types used. The beaks of the clamp engage the cervical portion of the tooth to hold it in place.

Rubber dam punch. The rubber dam punch is used to punch holes in the dam so that the dam can be placed over the teeth. The punch has an adjustment wheel on it so that holes of the proper size can be made (Fig. 8-6).

Rubber dam stamp. The rubber dam stamp (Fig. 8-7) is helpful to the assistant in positioning the holes properly on the dam. Although the arrangement of hole markers on the stamp does not fit every case, its use as a guide is a valuable aid. The rubber dam can be stamped well in advance of the procedure.

In situations involving malposed or missing teeth in the area to be isolated, the positions of the holes must be altered to accommodate the changes. For example, if a tooth is located more buccally than normal, the hole that will be punched for it will have to be punched in a more buccal position. Holes are not punched in areas where teeth are missing.

It is helpful to attach the dam to the frame while it is being punched. This makes it easier to visualize the desired position of the holes.

Rubber dam forceps. The rubber dam forceps are used to spread the beaks of the rubber dam clamp

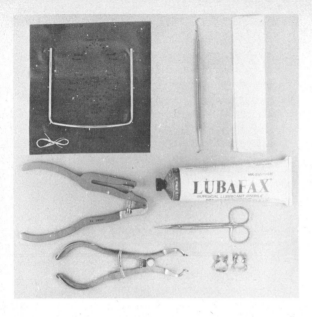

Heavy rubber dam (prestamped)
Young frame
Dental floss
Spoon excavator
Gauze napkin
Rubber dam punch
Water-soluble lubricant
Rubber dam forceps
Scissors
Clamps

Fig. 8-4. Rubber dam armamentarium.

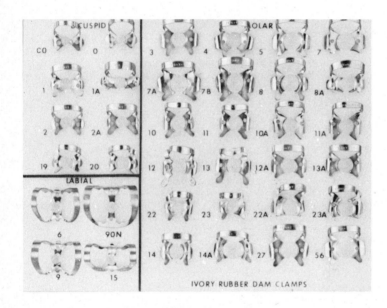

Fig. 8-5. Rubber dam clamp assortment. (Courtesy The Ivory Co, Inc., Philadelphia.)

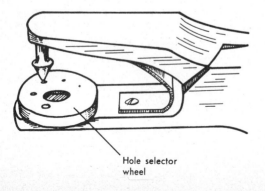

Hole selector wheel

Fig. 8-6. Rubber dam punch, showing various sizes of holes that can be punched in dam.

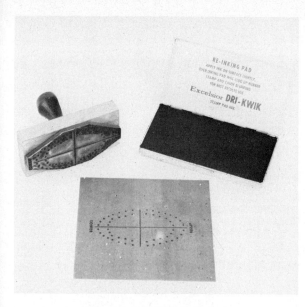

Fig. 8-7. Rubber dam stamp.

while it is used to both place and remove the clamp from the anchor tooth (Fig. 8-8, *D*). The tips of the forceps are inserted into the two holes located on the beaks of the clamp. The clamp beaks are spread open by the forceps and locked in this position by a locking device on the forceps. After the clamp is placed over the anchor tooth, the locking mechanism is released and the clamp closes around the cervical area of the tooth.

Rubber dam. Rubber dam material is available in light and heavy weights, in light or dark colors, and in either sheet or roll form. Most dentists prefer 6- or 8-inch–square, dark-colored sheet forms. Heavy-weight dam material is preferred because it resists tearing and provides better soft tissue retraction. The dark color gives a better background to contrast with the white teeth. Precut sheets are convenient for the assistant to handle. The sheets can be stamped with the rubber dam stamp (Fig. 8-7) at the convenience of the assistant before they are needed.

Rubber dam napkins. Rubber dam napkins are flannel cloth sheets that are placed under the rubber dam after it is in place. These napkins provide for patient comfort during the procedure. They can be purchased ready made, or they can easily be made from flannel material or large gauze rectangles.

Rubber dam (Young) frame. The rubber dam frame is used to support the dam on a patient's face. It maintains the isolation effect by holding the dam out of the way.

• • •

Use of the other items in the rubber dam setup will be described in the discussion on how the dam is applied and removed.

Rubber dam procedure

The detailed explanation of the rubber dam procedure that follows is intended to give the assistant a thorough understanding of the technique. Thus greater assistance can be offered the dentist to increase the efficiency of the rubber dam technique. In addition, many dentists are using dental assistants to apply the dam by themselves as a part of patient preparation.

Applying the rubber dam. Following is a step-by-step procedure of applying the rubber dam. It is by no means the only method that can be used, but rather it is one of the most common techniques. Isolation of the mandibular left quadrant will be used as an example (Fig. 8-8).

1. Attach the prestamped rubber dam to the rubber dam frame (Young frame) by stretching the material over the metal pegs along the sides and bottom of the frame. The dam is oriented so that the top of the frame is the open end that will rest under the patient's nose. The curved lower portion of the frame will rest over the patient's chin area, with the frame curving toward the patient's face (Fig. 8-8, *A*).
2. Punch holes in the dam in the area to be isolated using the rubber dam punch at the hole marks made by the stamp. The largest hole is generally used for molars, a medium-sized hole for premolars and canines, and the smaller holes are used for incisors (Fig. 8-8, *B*).
3. Tie a 12-inch strand of dental floss around the bow of a wing-style clamp before testing the fit on the patient's tooth. This is a safety precaution in the event that the clamp becomes dislodged and is either swallowed or aspirated by the patient (Fig. 8-8, *C*).
4. Using the rubber dam forceps, place the clamp on the selected anchor tooth. Usually the second molar is used as the anchor tooth if an entire quadrant is to be isolated. A proper fit is indicated when the beaks contact the anchor tooth at four different points around the cervical area and the clamp does not rock when finger pressure is applied (Fig. 8-8, *D*).
5. Once the proper clamp is selected and tested for fit, it is removed from the patient's mouth and placed in the most posterior hole in the punched rubber dam. The clamp should be oriented so that the bow is on top for lower teeth and on bottom for upper teeth. The wings

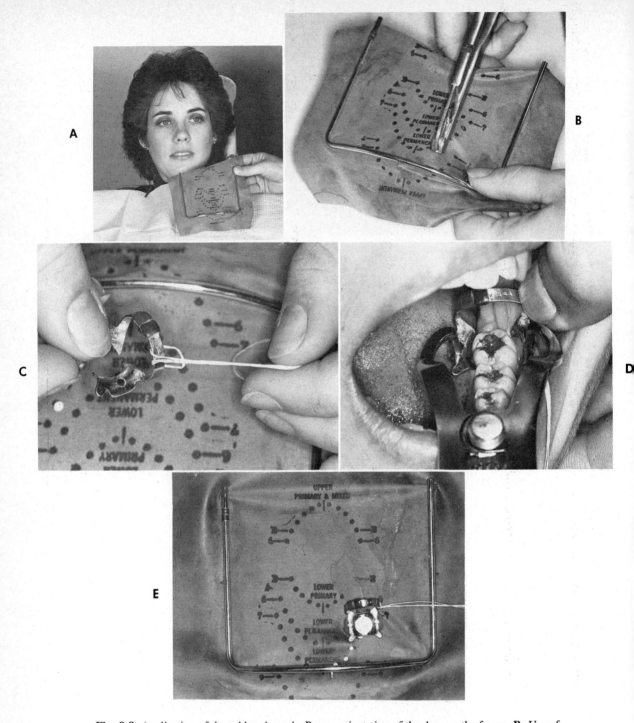

Fig. 8-8. Application of the rubber dam. **A,** Proper orientation of the dam on the frame. **B,** Use of the rubber dam punch. **C,** Placing safety floss on clamp. **D,** Testing clamp for fit. **E,** Placement of clamp in dam. **F,** Placement of clamp on anchor tooth. **G,** Placement of anterior ligature. **H,** Pulling dam between the teeth using dental floss. **I,** Tucking (everting) dam around the teeth. **J,** Placing gauze napkin. **K,** Rubber dam assembly in place.

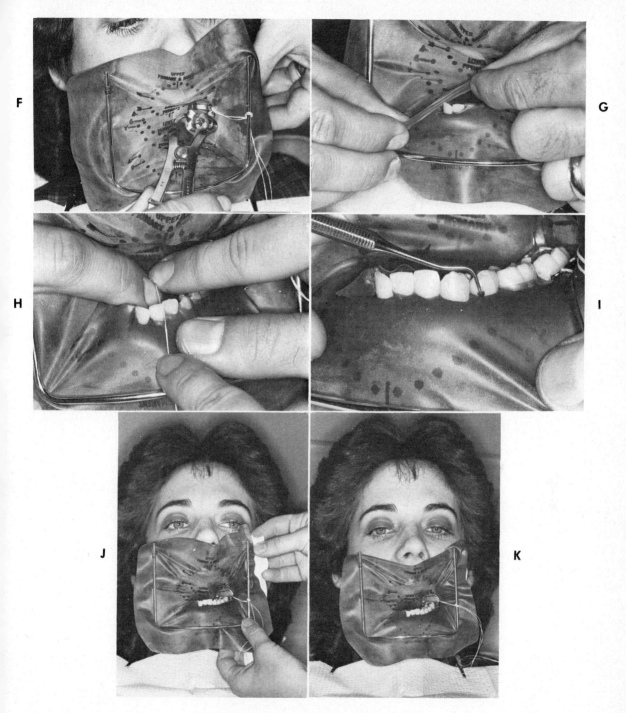

Fig. 8-8, cont'd. For legend see opposite page.

on the clamp serve as holding points to secure the clamp in the dam (Fig. 8-8, *E*).

6. The dam is lubricated lightly with a water-soluble lubricant around the punched holes. Only the tissue surface of the rubber dam is lubricated. This aids in passing the rubber dam between the teeth during application.

7. Floss the interproximal areas of the teeth to be isolated. This removes debris from between the teeth which may interfere with the passage of rubber dam material past the contact areas.

8. Place the tips of the forceps in the holes located on the beaks of the clamp. Spread the clamp beaks and lock the forceps open.

9. Place the open clamp on the anchor tooth. The lingual beak is seated first followed by the buccal beak. Slowly close the clamp on the tooth by releasing the lock on the forceps (Fig. 8-8, *F*).

10. Center the most anterior hole over the lateral incisor and pass the dam through the interproximal areas mesial and distal to the incisor. This can be done by pulling the border of the rubber between the teeth with dental floss. Once the rubber is between the teeth, it can be held in place by stretching a 1 × ¼ inch strip of rubber dam material and pulling it through the mesial contact of the lateral incisor (Fig. 8-8, *G*). This serves as a ligature.

11. Now center the remaining holes over the corresponding teeth between the first molar and lateral incisor and pass the rubber between the holes through interproximal contacts, using dental floss. This is more easily accomplished if one member of the operating team stretches the dam over the teeth while the other passes the floss between the teeth to pull the rubber dam through the contacts (Fig. 8-8, *H*).

12. Once the dam is over the teeth, form a seal around each tooth to prevent salivary leakage by tucking the dam toward the gingiva around each tooth. This is accomplished with a spoon excavator to invert the dam while the assistant dries the dam with the air syringe (Fig. 8-8, *I*). The dam is lifted off the wings of the clamp to allow a seal to form around the anchor tooth.

13. With the dam in place, apply the gauze napkin for patient comfort by gently sliding the napkin between the face and the dam (Fig. 8-8, *J*).

14. Wrinkles can be eliminated by reorienting the rubber dam on the frame as needed.

15. The upper border of the dam should not cover the patient's nasal passages. If necessary, cut away the upper portion of the dam to open the airway (Fig. 8-8, *K*).

Problem solving. In any technique for applying the rubber dam, some common problems may be encountered during the application and use of the dam. Listed are some of these problems and some suggested solutions:

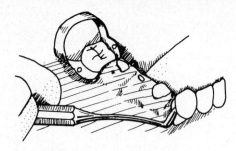

Fig. 8-9. Separating the teeth with a plastic filling instrument.

Problem: Clamp slipping off the anchor tooth

1. Try a different style clamp or grind the beaks of the clamp in use to improve the fit of the clamp.
2. Allow a little slack in the dam by loosening it on the Young frame to lessen the tension on the clamp.
3. Stabilize the clamp by drying the anchor tooth and adding dental compound around the tooth to hold the clamp in place.

Problem: Difficulty in pulling the dam through contact areas

1. Separate the teeth slightly by forcing a plastic instrument upward toward the contact area (Fig. 8-9).
2. Sometimes you will have to polish rough margins of old restorations before dam application to allow the rubber to slip between the teeth.
3. In extremely difficult situations, the preparations can be roughed-in without the dam. Then apply it after the contacts are opened.

Problem: Difficulty in tucking or everting the dam around the teeth

1. Pull the rubber dam away from the teeth so that the hole around the tooth is enlarged. Using the air-water syringe, dry the under surface of the dam and the cervical area of the tooth. Relax the dam and proceed with the eversion process.
2. Some patients who salivate excessively may require the use of an unfolded 2 × 2 inch gauze sponge placed in the mucobuccal fold under the dam to keep the teeth dry until the eversion procedure is complete.

Problem: Wrinkling or creasing of the dam

1. Punch the holes closer together.
2. Reorient the dam on the frame.

Problem: Spaces between the dam and the teeth

1. The holes have been punched too close together. Remove the dam and apply a new dam in which the holes are farther apart.

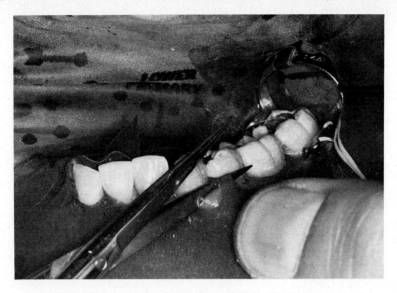

Fig. 8-10. Cutting interproximal rubber dam material before removal.

Problem: Rotary instruments catching interproximal rubber

1. Place a wooden wedge between the teeth to force the dam cervically. The bur may cut into the wedge during the preparation of Class II cavities, but it will not tangle in the dam.

Problem: Saliva accumulation in the patient's mouth

1. Since the patient's saliva is free of contamination when the dam is in place, instruct the patient to swallow in a normal manner.
2. If the patient is still reluctant to swallow, cut a hole in the lingual area of the dam and insert a disposable saliva ejector through the dam.

Removal of the rubber dam. After the restorations have been placed, the dam must be removed to check the patient's occlusion, or biting relationship, on the new restorations. The removal sequence is as follows:

1. Pull the dam in a buccal direction so that the interproximal rubber can be cut with the scissors (Fig. 8-10). This prevents fracture of newly placed restorations such as temporary dressings and amalgam.
2. Remove the anterior rubber dam retention strip (ligature) mesial to the lateral incisor.

3. Remove the clamp with the rubber dam forceps.
4. Remove the entire dam and napkin assembly. Check the interproximal areas to be sure no rubber has been torn and trapped between the teeth. Also, inspect the rubber dam itself for pieces of rubber that may be missing between the holes.
5. Rinse and evacuate the mouth.

SUMMARY

The rubber dam procedure was presented in detail since several states now permit dental auxiliaries to perform this task alone. However, because of the nature of the procedure, it can be accomplished far more efficiently by two people. When the dentist and assistant work together as a team, an extra pair of hands is available to assist with the passage of rubber dam material through the contact areas. This is usually the most difficult step in the procedure when the dam is applied by one person.

It should be emphasized that the technique described in this chapter is only one of several methods in common use today.

BIBLIOGRAPHY

Howard, W.W., and Moller, R.C.: Atlas of operative dentistry, ed. 3, St. Louis, 1981, The C.V. Mosby Co.

CHAPTER 9

MEDICAL EMERGENCIES IN THE DENTAL OFFICE

Life-threatening emergencies can and do occur occasionally in the dental office. The dental team has the responsibility of providing emergency treatment to safeguard the life and welfare of the patient until a physician can attend to the patient. In many emergencies the initial treatment is most important in the prevention of a tragedy.

The dental team should be well prepared to handle such emergencies if they should arise. Preparation includes a basic knowledge of emergency care, emergency equipment and supplies, a knowledge of the patient's medical history, and a preplanned approach to handling unexpected emergencies.

MEDICAL HISTORY

The old saying ''Know your patient'' certainly applies to emergency care. This knowledge can be gained by taking a thorough medical history when the patient is first seen and updating it periodically. The medical history is a useful tool for the operating team in handling emergencies. It should reveal known systemic conditions that would make a patient a more likely candidate for an emergency situation. Probably the greatest problem to overcome in a medical crisis is panic. If the dentist and the assistant lose control in a medical crisis, this only enhances the crisis further. Panic is usually a product of surprise and unpreparedness. There is no excuse for being unprepared for medical emergencies. The element of surprise can often be reduced by knowing the medical history of the patient. This knowledge should create some degree of anticipation of a possible emergency in the mind of the operating team. If a patient has a history of epilepsy, the operating team should anticipate the possibility of a convulsive episode while the patient is in the dental office. The truly prepared operating team should be even better prepared to handle the emer-

gency should it occur. Enough patients with a favorable medical history can surprise the operating team with an unexpected emergency without overlooking those patients with unfavorable histories.

The medical history also assists the dentist in selecting the proper treatment as quickly as possible. If a patient with a history of a heart condition such as angina pectoris complains of chest pains, there should be little doubt as to what treatment to administer immediately. Time is of utmost value in many serious emergencies. Proper diagnosis and prompt treatment can save valuable time and prevent unnecessary harm to the patient.

The history can also reveal allergies and medications that the patient is already taking. These would also influence the dentist's choice of drugs for emergency treatment.

STANDARD EMERGENCY EQUIPMENT

A recommended emergency armamentarium includes the following items (Fig. 9-1):
1. Oxygen supply
2. Emergency drug kit
3. Blood pressure cuff
4. Stethoscope

Oxygen supply

An oxygen supply is an essential part of any emergency setup. Any emergency that could deprive the brain of oxygen for even the shortest period of time will require the use of an oxygen supply. Most oxygen systems are easy to use. They consist of a storage tank, a regulator to control the flow of oxygen, and a hose and mask to deliver the oxygen to the patient. If the patient collapses and breathing is reduced, oxygen is indicated. The mask is placed over the patient's nose, and the regulator is turned on. The patient breathes a higher concentration of oxygen than would be received by breathing room air. This compensates for the decreased oxygen intake that results from the suppressed respiration during the emergency. Oxygen therapy should be continued until the patient recovers completely.

Emergency drug kit

The emergency drug kit is a backup support system designed to provide a variety of drugs in convenient dosage forms for easy administration to the patient. These kits include the syringes and needles needed to administer the drugs and a reference chart to quickly determine the proper dosage and route of administration for each drug in the kit. The drugs should be checked periodically to be sure that they have not passed their expiration date. Any drugs that are used from the kit should be replaced immediately. It would be a tragedy to discover during an emergency that a badly needed drug was missing from the kit or had passed the expiration date when it could have been used to save the patient's life.

Stethoscope and blood pressure cuff

The stethoscope and blood pressure cuff (sphygmomanometer) are of value after the crisis has passed. The patient's blood pressure can be monitored after the individual is on the road to recovery. It is a waste of time to take the blood pressure of an obviously collapsed patient when the time could be better spent on supporting respiration and circulation.

The telephone number of a reliable ambulance service should be attached to every telephone in the office. The ambulance service should be called after initial treatment has been started if the dentist needs this additional support.

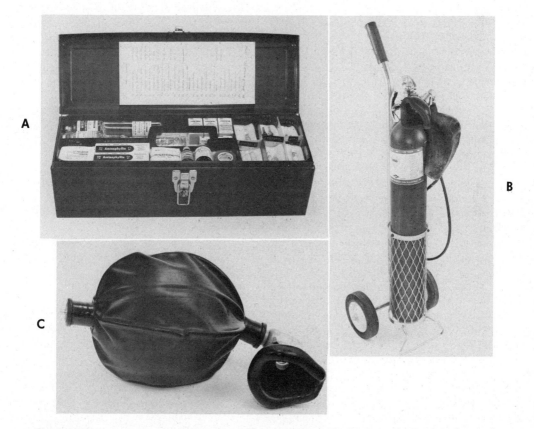

Fig. 9-1. Emergency armamentarium. **A,** Emergency drug kit. **B,** Oxygen unit. **C,** Manual resuscitator (optional).

COMMON MEDICAL EMERGENCIES

A great number of medical emergencies can occur while the patient is in the dental office. Some emergencies are more common than others. It certainly is a great assistance for the dentist to be able to diagnose the specific condition causing the emergency. However, it is not absolutely necessary that the specific cause of the emergency be determined before treatment is started. It is far more important to diagnose the patient's present physical status than to determine the cause of the emergency. If a patient stops breathing, it is more important to begin respiration support than to sit idle trying to determine why breathing has stopped.

Some of the most common emergency conditions will be discussed here either because of their frequency of occurrence or because of their life-threatening consequences.

Airway obstruction

The two most common causes of airway obstruction in a dental office are a relaxed tongue in an unconscious patient and foreign objects inadvertently dropped into the throat during dental treatment. Both are extremely serious life-threatening conditions and must be attended to immediately.

First, consider the situation when a patient loses consciousness. Loss of consciousness results in a generalized decrease in muscle tone throughout the body. Since the tongue is predominantly a muscle, it relaxes and sags into the pharynx (throat) of the victim. The tongue comes to rest against the posterior wall of the pharynx and obstructs the airway to the lungs (Fig. 9-2). The following steps are recommended for recognition and treatment of this situation:

1. Shake the patient's shoulders and shout, "Are you all right?" in an attempt to arouse the patient. If this fails, pinch the skin just above the shoulder blade firmly to elicit a response. If the patient does not awaken, proceed to the following life-support procedures.
2. Place the patient in a slightly lower than supine position with the feet elevated slightly above the head (Trendelenburg's position). Women in the third trimester of pregnancy should be placed on their sides while in this position. Remove the head support if a contour chair is used (Fig. 9-3).
3. Tilt the patient's head back by placing a hand on the patient's forehead and lifting the patient's neck upward with the other hand (Fig. 9-4). Maintain this position until consciousness returns.

This maneuver lifts the relaxed tongue away from the posterior wall of the pharynx and opens the airway in approximately 80% of unconscious patients (Fig. 9-5). Success can be determined immediately by placing one ear close to the patient's mouth or nose to feel and listen for air flow. The rescuer can also simultaneously watch for chest or abdominal movement that may indicate that the patient is breathing or attempting to breathe (Fig. 9-6). If no air flow is detected, reposition the head in a greater tilt backward to lift the tongue forward. If this fails, pull the patient's mandible forward firmly while supporting the neck with one hand.

If an obstruction of the airway is caused by some foreign material lodged in the patient's airway, an abdominal thrust maneuver is recommended. Basically this maneuver is designed to sharply increase the pressure inside the chest cavity to use the air in the lungs to blow the obstruction out of the patient's trachea (windpipe).

If the patient is still conscious, upright, and choking, the following procedure is recommended:

1. Stand behind the patient and wrap both arms around the patient's wrist.
2. Place the thumb of one fist into the soft tissue between the navel and the rib cage. Grasp the fist with the other hand (Fig. 9-7).
3. Pull the fist quickly into the patient's abdomen with a firm upward movement. Repeat as necessary.

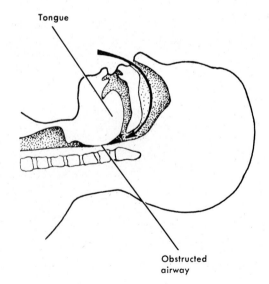

Tongue

Obstructed airway

Fig. 9-2. Obstructed airway caused by tongue resting against posterior wall of the pharynx.

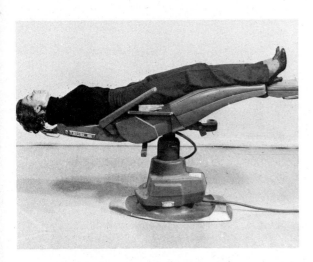

Fig. 9-3. Trendelenburg's position.

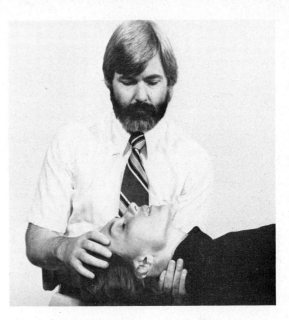

Fig. 9-4. Head-tilt maneuver to maintain open airway.

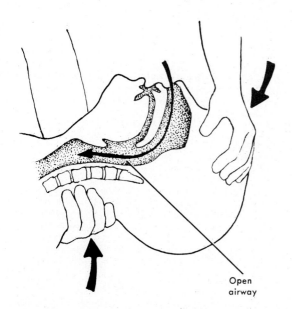

Open
airway

Fig. 9-5. The head-tilt maneuver lifts tongue away from posterior wall of pharynx to open airway.

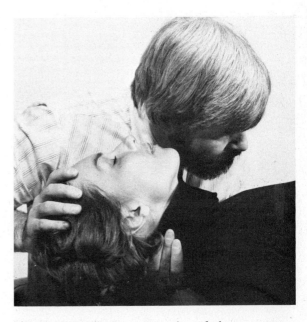

Fig. 9-6. Simultaneous observation of chest movement while listening for flow of air through patient's nose or mouth.

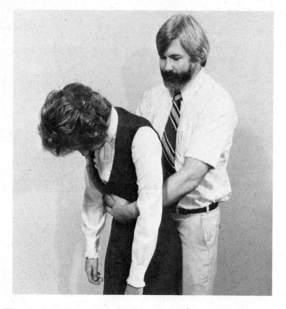

Fig. 9-7. Standing abdominal thrust (Heimlich maneuver).

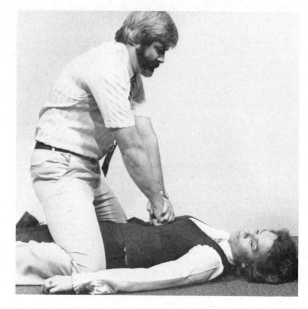

Fig. 9-8. Reclined abdominal thrust.

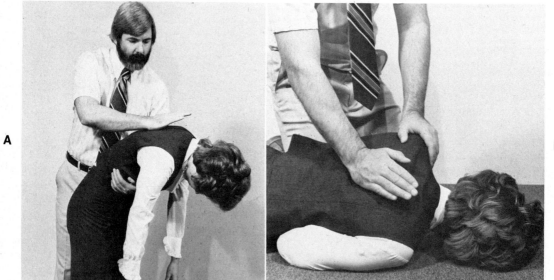

Fig. 9-9. Back-blow technique for dislodging foreign objects in trachea. **A,** Standing position. **B,** Reclining position.

If the patient is already in the dental chair and is unconscious while lying down, the following actions should be taken:

1. Place the patient in the supine position and remove all articles from the patient's mouth.
2. Sit astride the patient.
3. Form a fist with one hand and place it on soft tissue between the patient's navel and rib cage. Use the other hand to support the wrist (Fig. 9-8).
4. Press the fist into the patient's abdomen with a rapid, upward thrust. Repeat as necessary.

These rescue techniques are patterned after the recommendations made by Dr. Henry Heimlich in a paper published in 1974 and are often referred to as "Heimlich maneuvers."

An alternative technique is the use of back blows to dislodge an airway obstruction caused by a foreign body. This technique is used in either the conscious or unconscious patient. The rescuer simply delivers four rapid and forceful blows to the upper portion of the patient's back. The heel of the hand is used to strike the patient between the shoulder blades over the spine. The rescuer's other hand can be used to help support the patient. Whenever possible, the patient's head should be lower than the chest to use gravity to facilitate removal of the foreign body (Fig. 9-9). This should be repeated as necessary or perform the abdominal thrust previously described.

Syncope (fainting)

Syncope is probably the most common medical emergency encountered in the dental office. It is usually brought on by fear, emotional upset, or pain. Essentially, fainting is a result of reduced flow of blood to the brain caused by dilation of blood vessels elsewhere in the body. If the patient is sitting upright, blood tends to pool in the lower portions of the body and the brain is left with a decreased blood supply. The supine position of the patient in the sit-down four-handed dentistry technique helps to prevent fainting, since the patient's head is kept on the same level as the lower part of the body.

The following are some common signs and symptoms of syncope:

Initial changes
1. The patient complains of feeling "funny"; warmth in neck and face is a common symptom. Dizziness and a feeling of nausea can occur.
2. The facial skin becomes pale (pallor) and clammy.

3. Pulse rate increases markedly (120 beats per minute).
4. Pupils of the eyes become enlarged (dilate).
5. Depth of respiration increases.

Advanced changes
1. Hands and feet become cold.
2. Pulse rate slows markedly (50 beats per minute) and is weak and harder to detect.
3. Pupils of the eyes enlarge markedly.
4. Loss of consciousness occurs; eyes may roll back under lids.
5. Respiration becomes shallow, irregular, and jerky.
6. Muscle convulsions occur in face, hands, and legs.

Since syncope is a condition that deprives the brain of an adequate blood supply, this should be attended to immediately. The steps in treatment are as follows:

1. Remove all articles from the patient's mouth.
2. Place the patient in a slightly lower than supine position with the head lower than the legs. Women in the third trimester of pregnancy should be placed on their side while in this position. Remove the head support if a contour chair is used.
3. Establish an open (patent) airway.
4. Loosen tight clothing around the neck.
5. Administer oxygen.
6. Stimulate patient's breathing by crushing an ammonia inhalant and holding it under the oxygen mask for a moment.
7. Provide other support measures such as placing a cold towel on the patient's forehead or using a blanket or drape to cover a shivering patient.

This treatment should be continued until the patient recovers completely, with normal respiration, skin color, and awareness of the surroundings.

Often syncope can be anticipated in apprehensive patients. The fear of a dental injection is probably the most common cause of fainting. Use of the hidden syringe transfer and careful injection techniques can help prevent syncope in these patients.

Hyperventilation

Hyperventilation is essentially an excessive breathing pattern that results in a marked decrease in carbon dioxide levels in the blood. Although unconsciousness rarely occurs, the patient may feel dizzy, faint, or have impaired consciousness. The major predisposing factor is anxiety. If a patient's anxiety is managed properly through psychosedative techniques, hyperventilation rarely occurs.

Typically, apprehensive patients will begin to breathe more rapidly and deeply in response to their own anxiety. The signs and symptoms that can occur are as follows:

1. Pounding of the heart (palpitation)
2. A feeling of a "lump" in the throat
3. A tight feeling in the chest
4. Deep rapid breathing
5. Tingling of the hands, feet, and lips

An apprehensive patient who starts to breathe excessively with a deep, rapid breathing pattern should be treated as follows:

1. Place the patient in an upright position.
2. Loosen tight clothing around the neck and remove all articles from the patient's mouth.
3. Reassure the patient and coach the individual to breathe slowly (4 to 6 breaths per minute). If the patient does not respond, proceed to step 4.
4. Have the patient breathe into a paper bag or headrest cover sealed over the mouth and nose until recovery occurs (Fig. 9-10). Rebreathing exhaled air, which has a higher level of carbon dioxide, helps to hasten the recovery process.

Treatment of the patient at future dental appointments should include consideration of treating the patient's anxiety before initiating dental procedures.

Cardiopulmonary arrest

The very serious emergency of cardiopulmonary arrest can occur anywhere at any time. If the patient does not receive treatment within 4 to 6 minutes, permanent brain damage can occur. If treatment is not rendered within 10 minutes, the patient can die.

The initial treatment for cardiopulmonary arrest is similar to that used for syncope. Namely, the patient is placed in Trendelenburg's position, all articles are removed from the mouth, and tight clothing around the patient's neck is loosened. The operating team need not know whether the patient is going into syncope or cardiopulmonary arrest before treatment is initiated. The goal is the same for both conditions, that is, *to provide an oxygen supply to the brain.*

Cardiac arrest rarely occurs in the absence of respiratory arrest. Therefore both conditions are treated simultaneously by the cardiopulmonary resuscitation (CPR) technique.

In a dental office, the patient is not usually monitored with an electrocardiogram during dental treatment. Consequently, a patient who shows signs of cardiopulmonary arrest is treated according to the rules that apply to unwitnessed cardiopulmonary arrest, even though the operating team may see the patient collapse.

If a patient should collapse during dental treatment, the following steps are recommended:

1. Quickly remove all articles from the patient's mouth.
2. Shake the patient's shoulders and shout, "Are you all right?" If patient does not respond, proceed to step 3.
3. Place the patient in Trendelenburg's position (described previously) and summon assistance from other staff members (or even from other patients in the office if you are alone). Have the helpers bring the emergency drug kit and oxygen supply unit as soon as practical.
4. Open the airway using the head tilt procedure previously described (p. 120). Pull the mandible forward if necessary to establish an airway.
5. Check for breathing by placing an ear close to the patient's nose and mouth. If no breathing is present, proceed.
6. Have helpers summon an ambulance while the rescue team begins artificial ventilation using the mouth-to-mouth technique:
   A. Maintain the head tilt.
   B. Pinch the patient's nose to seal it.
   C. Seal your mouth firmly over the patient's open mouth (Fig. 9-11).
   D. Blow into the patient's mouth rapidly four times to ventilate the lungs.
   E. Do not wait for full deflation of the lungs between ventilations.
   F. Watch for a chest rise during ventilation to be sure the airway is open.
7. Following the four ventilations, check for the presence of a carotid pulse (Fig. 9-12). If there is a definite pulse, continue to ventilate the patient with one ventilation every 5 seconds (12 per minute) until the patient can breathe without assistance. Continue to check for a pulse between ventilations. If there is no definite pulse, proceed as follows with external cardiac compression.
8. Quickly place the patient on the floor, if possible, for more effective compression of the chest.
9. If two people are available, one person should inflate the lungs once every five compressions of the heart performed by the other rescuer. Compressions are carried out as follows:
   A. Place the heel of one hand over the lower half of the breast bone (sternum) 2 inches above the notch formed by the lower border of the rib cage on the patient's midline.
   B. Place the other hand over the first hand and interlock the fingers (Fig. 9-13).
   C. Be sure that only the heel of the first hand is in contact with the patient's chest.
   D. While kneeling beside the patient, place your shoulders directly over the sternum and lock your arms straight (Fig. 9-14).

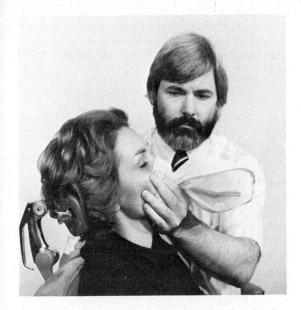

Fig. 9-10. Hyperventilating patient breathing into headrest cover.

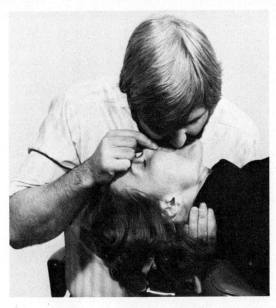

Fig. 9-11. Ventilation of patient by sealing nostrils, maintaining head tilt, and blowing air into the patient's mouth.

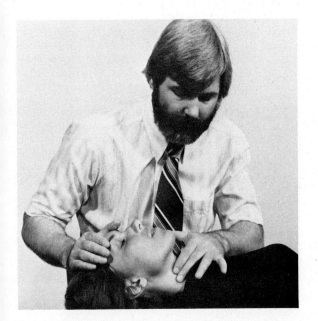

Fig. 9-12. Checking for a carotid pulse.

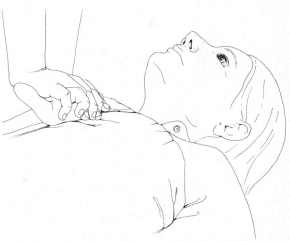

Fig. 9-13. Using heel of lower hand to compress patient's chest. Upper hand is used to lift fingers of lower hand to avoid injury to ribs during compression.

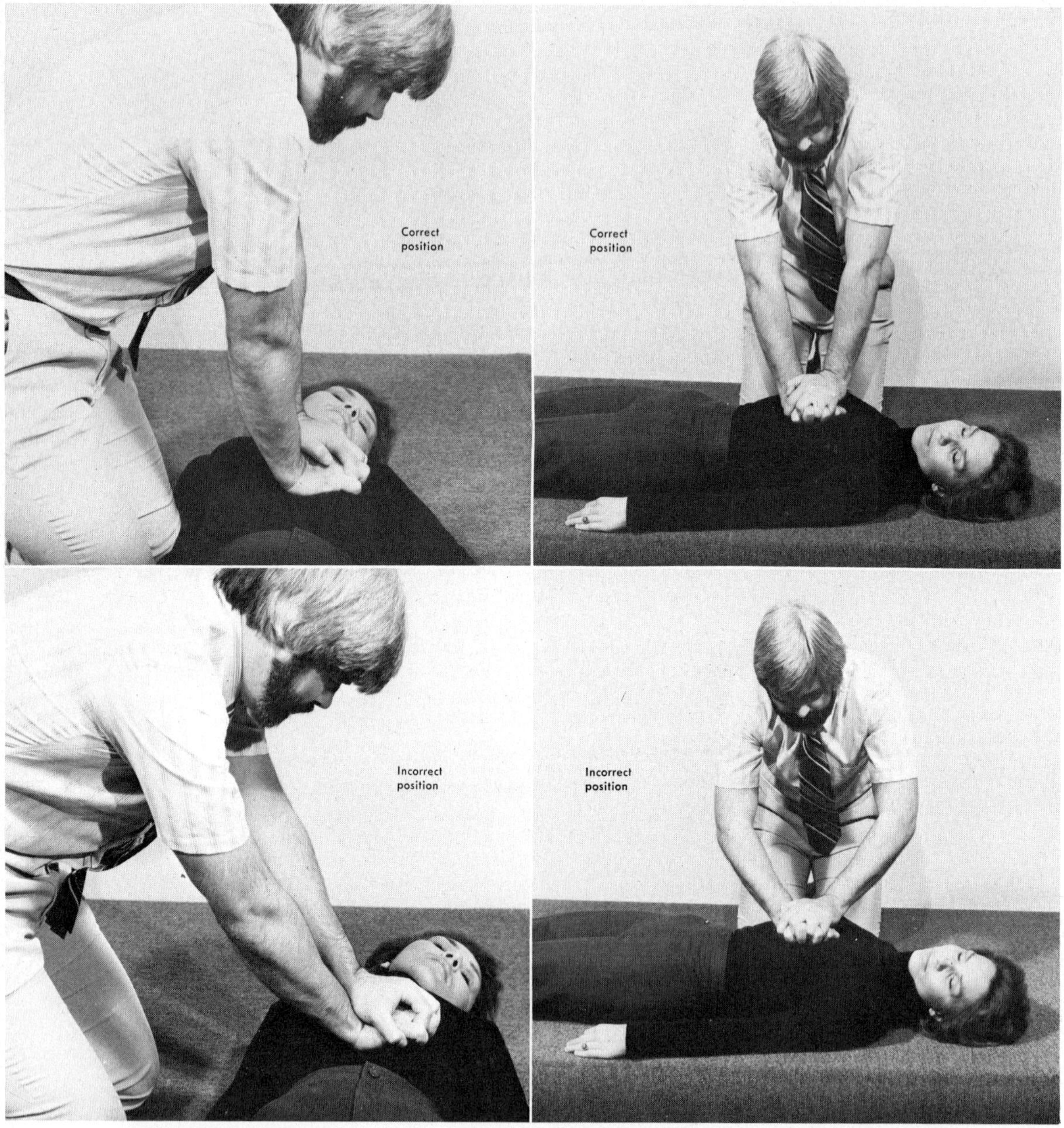

Fig. 9-14. Position of rescuer for compression of chest during cardiopulmonary resuscitation (CPR). **A** and **B,** Correct position. **C** and **D,** Incorrect position.

E. Apply pressure directly downward so that the sternum is depressed 1½ to 2 inches. Use your body weight to apply pressure, using a rocking motion from the hips.

F. Maintain contact with the patient's chest when pressure is relaxed between compressions.

G. Count five compressions, then have the other rescuer inflate the lungs once, as described previously.

This rescue effort is continued until the patient recovers or until medical personnel with more advanced training arrive. It is emphasized that all dental personnel should receive training in cardiopulmonary emergency treatment. This training should include practice sessions using resuscitation manikins. Time is of the essence in this type of emergency. The rescue team must be well prepared should such an emergency occur. Reading about this rescue technique is no substitute for actual rescue practice.

Epilepsy

Epilepsy is a disorder of the central nervous system that results in mild to severe episodes of convulsive seizure. The medical history should reveal this condition so that the operating team can anticipate the possibility of a seizure during dental treatment. Fear, pain, and even flashing lights can trigger a seizure. Convulsive seizures are transient but can be rather violent while they are occurring. Patients must be protected from harming themselves during the convulsion. A soft cloth folded several times can be inserted in the patient's mouth to help protect oral tissues from harm during the seizure (Fig. 9-15). Rescuers should never put their fingers between the patient's teeth during the convulsion stage.

Move all equipment and instruments out of the way to protect the patient. Limited, not forceful, restraint should be used to minimize excessive movements of the patient's arms and legs. Allow some minor movement of the patient's extremities to prevent injury to the joints.

After the seizure activity stops, the dental team should be prepared to provide basic life support for the patient. The patient can lapse into central nervous system depression, which can result in respiratory depression. Oxygen support or even the head tilt maneuvers described previously may be required. Once the patient recovers, it is advisable to have an adult accompany the person home.

Angina pectoris and coronary occlusion

Two other serious heart problems are angina pectoris and coronary occlusion. Often the patient is aware of this condition and carries medication to treat the attack. Essentially these conditions result from an inadequate blood supply to the heart muscle through the coronary artery. Severe chest pains occur, which often spread to the arms and up to the mandible. The treatment is to place the patient's dosage (usually 1 to

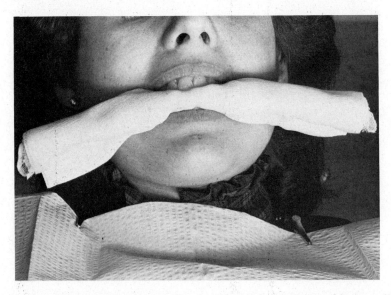

Fig. 9-15. Soft cloth placed between upper and lower teeth to protect soft tissues during epileptic seizure.

3 tablets) of nitroglycerin under the tongue. If this does not relieve the symptoms, the patient should inhale the vapors from a crushed amyl nitrite ampule. Both of these agents dilate the coronary artery, which increases the flow of blood to the muscle tissue of the heart. Once the nitroglycerin takes effect, oxygen can be administered to the patient to aid the recovery.

Hypoglycemia

Hypoglycemia is a condition frequently associated with patients with diabetes. Specifically, it is an abnormally low level of glucose (sugar) in the blood. In the patient with diabetes this usually occurs if the amount of insulin that is administered is excessive for the amount of food eaten. The result is that the patient's blood sugar is decreased so that the patient becomes weak and nervous, vision deteriorates, and the skin becomes pale and clammy. The patient can eventually lose consciousness. If the operating team is alert to the patient's diabetic condition, treatment is very simple. The patient should be offered some food with a high sugar content. Every emergency kit should contain a candy bar or lumps of sugar for this purpose. If the patient loses consciousness, basic life support measures should be carried out to ensure an adequate airway and adequate circulation. An intravenous injection of 50% dextrose solution should be administered. *Do not attempt to administer sugar by mouth to an unconscious patient.*

Anesthetic toxicity

An overdose of anesthetic solution in the patient's bloodstream causes anesthetic toxicity. This can occur because the anesthetic was inadvertently injected into a patient's blood vessel or because too much anesthetic solution was injected into the patient at one time. The result is that the patient will be stimulated immediately after the injection. Nervousness, talkativeness, and restlessness are early signs of stimulation of the central nervous system with anesthetic

solution. The patient may soon begin to convulse. The convulsive episode is often followed by a depression of the central nervous system, which results in respiratory depression and unconsciousness until the anesthetic is detoxified in the system.

Early recognition of the patient's condition is the key to treatment. This is why *a patient must never be left alone after an injection of an anesthetic solution.* Early signs of moderate stimulation should lead the dentist to administer an anticonvulsant intravenously until the patient is calmed. Oxygen should be administered. If severe respiratory depression and unconsciousness occur, emergency measures such as mouth-to-mouth resuscitation or forced oxygen treatment should be carried out until the anesthetic solution clears from the system and the patient recovers.

SUMMARY

The greatest emphasis in the discussion of emergency treatment has been placed on the techniques of providing the collapsed patient with an oxygen supply to the brain. In all medical emergencies the ABCs of first aid should be remembered and exercised:

A = Airway—open an airway

B = Breathing—establish respiration, if needed, with resuscitative measures

C = Circulation—support circulation with external cardiac compression and cardiovascular drugs

All other treatment measures are secondary to these ABCs that can save a life.

A periodic practice session and review of emergency procedures should be a regular part of the activities in a dental office.

BIBLIOGRAPHY

American Heart Association, Inc., Task Force on CPR Instructional Materials: CPR: cardiopulmonary resuscitation workbook, New York, 1975, The Association.

Malamed, S.F.: Handbook of medical emergencies in the dental office, ed. 2, St. Louis, 1982, The C.V. Mosby Co.

FOUR-HANDED DENTISTRY*

*Note: Text material and illustrations for this section were adapted from Chasteen, J.E.: Four-handed dentistry in clinical practice, St. Louis, 1978, The C.V. Mosby Co.

CHAPTER 10

THE CONCEPT OF FOUR-HANDED DENTISTRY

Since the early 1940s, considerable interest in the mode of dental practice has developed. The interest has centered on two basic issues that confront the practicing dentist every day: (1) minimizing stress and fatigue for the dentist during the process of delivering dental services to patients and (2) increasing the productivity of a dental practice while maintaining a high standard of quality in the services delivered.

The very nature of dentistry creates a high potential for the development of stress and fatigue for the practicing dentist. To provide quality dental services for patients, the dentist has to constantly maintain a high level of concentration throughout the working day. In addition, the achievement of clinical excellence is predicated on the dentist's ability to (1) meet the wide variety of dental needs of individual patients and (2) perform delicate manual skills within fine tolerances while working with limited access and visibility in the oral cavity. These clinical demands are superimposed on demands to meet a busy patient schedule and to manage the practice itself. Trying to meet the combination of clinical and management demands can result in severe stress and fatigue. The four-handed dentistry concept derives its name from the fact that the hands of both the dentist and the dental assistant are used to provide patient care. This method of practice is more efficient and reduces stress and fatigue for the dentist over an entire practice life span.

A second reason for practicing four-handed dentistry is to provide the dentist with a means of becoming more productive through increased efficiency in the dental practice. The issue of increased productivity in a dental practice is of great interest to dentists because of its economic implications and because of the ever-increasing demand by the public for dental services. In effect, four-handed dentistry is part of good practice management.

PRINCIPLES OF FOUR-HANDED DENTISTRY

The term *four-handed dentistry* has evolved over the past 25 years to the point at which it now represents an entire concept of delivering dental services. A sound concept on which a modern dental practice should be based, it consists of four basic principles:

1. Operating in a seated position
2. Employing the skills of trained dental auxiliaries
3. Organizing every component of the practice
4. Simplifying all tasks to the maximum

Sit-down dentistry

Several significant studies have been made on body mechanics in relation to the work environment. Spe-

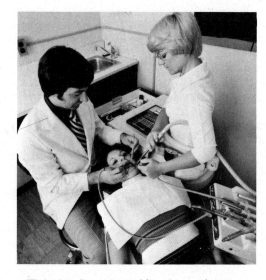

Fig. 10-1. Properly positioned operating team.

cifically, performance patterns of the dentist and assistant during a working day have been studied in detail. A seated position for the dental team has been found to be generally more favorable from the standpoint of body mechanics. In fact, statistics from life insurance companies reveal that the life expectancy for a dentist who operates in the seated position is 17% greater than that for a dentist who operates in a standing position. Industrial studies have further indicated that a seated worker uses 27% less energy than one who performs the same task in a standing position.

However, merely sitting down while practicing dentistry is not the whole answer to reducing stress and fatigue. *How* the dentist and assistant sit while operating is probably of greater significance than *whether* they sit or stand. The operating team working in a seated position of balanced posture is the real essence of sit-down dentistry (Fig. 10-1). Balanced posture for both the dentist and the assistant will be described in detail in Chapter 12.

Auxiliary utilization

To practice dentistry efficiently, the modern dentist has to make maximum use of the skills of dental auxiliaries. The days when a dentist could operate a busy practice alone have long since passed. Solo operating is an inefficient use of the practitioner's valuable time. Today dentists must engage in the delegation of duties to auxiliaries to increase the efficiency and productivity of a dental practice.

Duty delegation is exercised in two forms (1) total duty delegation and (2) partial duty delegation. Total-duty delegation is simply having an auxiliary perform an entire task such as taking radiographs, performing various business procedures, or taking impressions for study models. Partial-duty delegation is the process of having a dental auxiliary assist the dentist with a given task. Much of what a chairside assistant does through a typical work day falls in this category of duty delegation. Because partial-duty delegation is such a major part of chairside assisting, it will be emphasized throughout the text.

Clear evidence, dating back as far as the early 1940s, indicates that a dentist can increase productivity from 33% to approximately 78% by using the skills of a well-trained dental assistant at chairside on a full-time basis. The achievement of a significant increase in productivity while minimizing stress and fatigue requires that the dentist (1) employ a well-trained, skillful chairside assistant and (2) make a firm commitment to practice the principles of four-handed dentistry discussed in this text.

Half the efficiency of a dental assistant is the result of working with a well-organized, competent dentist who is willing to practice four-handed dentistry. Dentists should note this fact when they evaluate the performance of their assistants.

Practice organization

The process of organization is a never-ending one. As a practice grows and changes or when initial plans fall short of expectations, reorganization of certain aspects of the practice is warranted. Once the major elements are organized, the operating team can begin to refine the operation of the dental office in terms of the organization of the dental operatories and the method of delivering dental services to the patient. This level of organization is critical to the success of the four-handed dentistry concept. The following are some key areas requiring organization:

1. Dental operatory contents and arrangement
2. Complete preplanning of treatment to provide for efficient delivery of dental services
3. Planning work patterns to standardize as many procedures as possible; this enables the operating team to work in a predictable sequence
4. Placement of instruments and materials on preset trays in an arrangement that is convenient to use and consistent with the sequence of the standardized work pattern

All these areas will be discussed later in greater detail.

Work simplification

Just as the term implies, *work simplification* is the process of finding an easier way to do any task. "Work simplificaton is learning to work smarter, not harder!" In major industries, work simplification studies have been used for years in an effort to make workers more comfortable, more productive, and safer during the working day. The principles used in industry can be adapted in varying degrees to the practice of dentistry. Dentistry is hard, tension-producing work, and every effort should be expended to make it more comfortable for the operator, the auxiliaries, and the patient. As a result of work simplification studies, four basic processes that the dental team can follow to make dentistry easier have been established. These are traditionally identified as (1) rearrangement, (2) elimination, (3) combination, and (4) simplification.

Rearrangement. Equipment, instruments, and materials that are essential to operating procedures should be positioned in a favorable relationship to the operating team. This is an important step in work simplification. The environment in the operatory should be adapted to the operating team's needs, rather than having the team adapt to the environment (Fig. 10-2). Favorable positioning of these items helps minimize movements of the operating team. For example, an amalgamator that is located out of easy reach of the dental assistant causes unnecessary movement and delay in every amalgam procedure done in the operatory.

The rearrangement of treatment plans and patient scheduling can add to the convenience of many treatment regimens. Steps in various treatment procedures can often be rearranged to enhance the smooth flow of the procedure and minimize unnecessary movements of the operating team. Common procedures, such as those used in fabricating amalgam restorations, can be streamlined to minimize instrument exchanges,

bur changes, and delays while materials are prepared.

The dental assistant plays a key role in the arrangement of instruments and materials on preset trays and in the storage cabinetry. Maintenance of a favorable arrangement of these items is clearly the responsibility of the dental assistant.

Elimination. The practicing dentist begins the process of work simplification by engaging in task analysis. Every procedure, system, movement, and piece of equipment should be analyzed to assess its value and necessity in daily office activities. A great deal of time and effort can be saved by eliminating unnecessary movements, procedural steps, instruments, and equipment.

The dentist has a tendency to make many more movements than necessary to accomplish tasks. Excessive reaching for instruments, supplies, and to make operating-light adjustments can be eliminated by having a chairside assistant deliver instruments to the operator and adjust the light. As mentioned previously, the arrangement of equipment in favorable

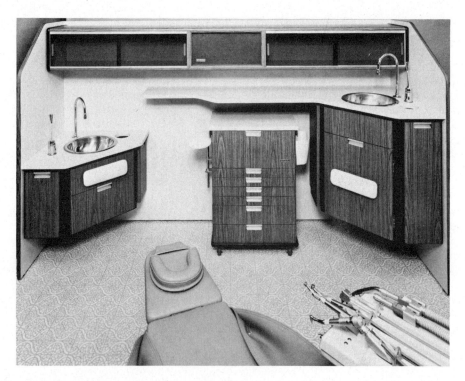

Fig. 10-2. Favorable operatory design, conducive to practice of four-handed dentistry. (Courtesy Health Science Products, Inc., Birmingham, Ala.)

locations around the operating area can reduce unnecessary movements for both members of the operating team.

Often steps in a procedure can be eliminated so that valuable chair time can be put to more productive use. The following are some examples of such eliminations:

1. Unnecessary bur changes in a procedure can be eliminated by using more than one handpiece with the burs already placed ahead ot time. An exchange of handpieces between the dentist and assistant is much quicker than waiting for a bur to be changed when only one handpiece is used.
2. Unnecessary instrument exchanges can be eliminated by using an instrument to the maximum before returning it to the dental assistant. Frequent switching of instruments is a rather common time-consuming habit among dentists.
3. Supplies and materials that may save steps in a procedure can be used whenever possible. For example, the use of preformed aluminum shell crowns can eliminate or at least minimize the contouring of crowns during a procedure. Using premeasured materials, such as alginate and amalgam capsules, and disposable items can eliminate unnecessary steps.

Often a dentist, when reviewing the contents of an instrument setup, discovers that some of the equipment is not used routinely and consequently could be eliminated. Thus the number of instruments to be purchased and processed can be reduced. Plan for the usual, not the unusual or occasional, need for certain instruments.

Common areas in which the process of elimination can save time and cost are the equipment, supplies, and devices stored in the operatory. Suffice it to say that many items that are seldom used or, in some instances, not used at all, can be eliminated from the operatory. These items simply add to the clutter and tend to bog down the entire operation.

Combination. Using one step or instrument to serve multiple functions has real value in work simplification. A major step in reducing the number of instruments to purchase, process, and transfer during a dental procedure was the advent of double-ended instruments. Even greater reductions in the number of instruments required for a given procedure will be made when the operator becomes proficient at using an instrument for more than one purpose. Amalgam condensers are handy for placing cement bases and driving interproximal wedges into place, as well as for condensing amalgam. To have all sizes of margin trimmers available on a tray setup is really not necessary, since one size usually suffices in most restorative situations.

Separate air and water syringes should be replaced with a combination air-water syringe, to serve all rinsing and drying needs while minimizing movements of the operating team. Stronger zinc oxide–eugenol cements, in selected situations, can serve as both a liner and cement base, thus eliminating the added step of placing a liner before the cement base.

Simplification. The simplification aspect of the entire work simplification process is the actual determination of how a job should be done. Simplification is listed last because it should take place after all the rearranging, eliminating, and combining activities have been completed. The basic idea of simplification is to minimize the number of variables in every aspect of the practice. It is a streamlining process geared to promote predictable routines in the work pattern.

Plan for the usual, not the unusual. The majority of procedures and activities in a dental office can be standardized. Standardization involves analyzing a procedure to determine the steps necessary to accomplish the task and then arranging them in a smooth sequence that will minimize movements, verbal communication, and delays. The next step is to determine what instruments and materials will be used in the procedure. The selected instruments are then as-

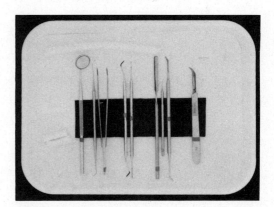

Fig. 10-3. Simple but well-organized preset tray. (From Chasteen J.E.: DAU manual of four-handed dentistry, Ann Arbor, Mich., 1977, University of Michigan School of Dentistry.)

sembled on a preset tray in the order in which they are to be used, from left to right. Instruments such as the mirror, explorer, and cotton pliers are used at various stages of a procedure and placed in the first three positions on the left side of the tray (Fig. 10-3). This standardization process simplifies a procedure by making the operator predictable. The dental assistant can easily follow a standardized sequence, thus minimizing delays, verbal communication, and misunderstanding. The standardized procedure will be smoother than a haphazard approach to accomplishing a task.

Ultimately this effort will create a more constant flow from the start to the completion of a procedure and usually result in a greater productivity. Furthermore a new chairside assistant can adapt more readily to any dentist's techniques if they are standardized.

It is highly recommended that in offices with multiple operatories each operatory be standardized by identical equipment and an identical arrangement. This permits the same predictable work pattern to be followed in each operatory without change. Special equipment that may not be used routinely can be moved from one operatory to another as needed (for example, electrosurgery units, nitrous oxide machines, and bead sterilizers). If these items are used routinely, each operatory should be outfitted with them. All operatories should be the operating team's "favorite." This not only makes the work pattern easier to maintain but also simplifies the scheduling of patients by permitting their placement in the various operatories regardless of the service to be rendered.

MOTION ECONOMY

The practice of dentistry cannot be discussed without repeated references to conservation of motion. Movements consume time and can produce fatigue. This does not imply that all movement is undesirable; that which is productive, purposeful, and not harmful to the health of the operating team is entirely acceptable. However, movements that place the dentist or assistant in a contorted posture for substantial periods of time are unnecessary and harmful over a long period of time. It is generally agreed that dentists and assistants who are physically able to exercise daily should be encouraged to do so.

As a result of research on the subject of time and motion in dentistry, a classification of common movements used during dental procedures was developed. For purposes of discussion throughout this text, reference will be made to this classification:

Class I: Movement of only the fingers
Class II: Movement of the fingers and wrist
Class III: Movement of the fingers, wrist, and elbow
Class IV: Movement of the entire arm from the shoulder
Class V: Movement of the entire arm and twisting of the trunk

This classification is helpful in the discussion of motion economy and analysis of work patterns. The basic idea of motion economy is to design an office facility and work patterns that will minimize the number of Class IV and V movements required for any procedure. These movements are the most fatiguing and time-consuming. They require the operator to look away from the brightly illuminated operative field and then to refocus; this can result in eye strain and subsequent headache. A dentist can substantially reduce the number of Class IV and V movements through the effective utilization of a chairside assistant.

In most instances, use of Class I, II, and III movements is preferable for both the operator and assistant because they involve less muscular activity, save time, and allow the eyes to remain fixed on the operative field.

Implementation of the work simplification and motion economy concepts should not be interpreted as an attempt to convert the operating team into statuelike figures at chairside. On the contrary, it is an attempt to guide the team into a comfortable, relaxed method of working that is free of wasted movements. As an example, studies have shown that as much as 15% of chair time is consumed by the patient's rinsing and expectorating into a cuspidor. The economic impact of this alone on the practice is significant. Elimination of the cuspidor from the operating routine and substitution of the high-velocity evacuator is a giant step in the direction of motion economy.

ELEMENTS OF FOUR-HANDED DENTISTRY

The performance of four-handed dentistry requires certain basic elements for it to be effective. These elements are a mixture of mechanical, technical and attitudinal factors that must be combined if the concept is to succeed. These elements are as follows:

1. Positive team attitude
2. Favorable work environment
3. Favorable positioning of the patient and operating team
4. Simplified instrumentation

5. Standardized operating procedures
6. Use of preset trays
7. Efficient instrument delivery
8. Effective oral evacuation and debridement
9. Proper time management

Positive team attitude

Both the dentist and the dental assistant must make a commitment to work together as a team. Working in a team configuration requires skills that must be acquired by both team members. Teamwork skills take time to develop. Each member of the team must be willing to openly communicate with one another and to help each other succeed on a daily basis. Dental personnel who do not make this committment often find themselves in frustrating circumstances that can lead to failure.

Favorable work environment

A wide variety of equipment and treatment room configurations work well in the four-handed dentistry concept. Regardless of which configuration is selected, the end result should be that both the dentist and the assistant can gain access and visibility during any procedure while maintaining comfort throughout the work day. Chapter 11 offers specific guidelines that have proven to be helpful in this regard.

Proper positioning of the patient and operating team

Studies have been done to identify the most favorable working positions to use while working in the different segments of the oral cavity. Guidelines are presented in Chapter 12.

Simplified instrumentation

Dentists develop their own methods of accomplishing a given task. They may select a battery of instruments that differs from other dentists, but the same result is achieved. One goal that should be strived for is to reduce the number of instruments to only those needed for the procedure at hand. Using instruments and materials to the maximum and using them for several functions usually results in fewer instruments being included on a preset tray. This is consistent with work simplification principles discussed earlier in this chapter.

Standardized operating procedures

Most procedures performed in general practice are rather straightforward and can be done with minimal variation. As mentioned previously, common procedures can be standardized to the extent that the dental team can perform them in a predictable and efficient manner. A little planning and arranging is required, but the effort is certainly worthwhile for both the dentist and the assistant.

Use of preset trays

The convenience of placing the most common items needed for a dental procedure on a preset tray during instrument processing is significant. Specific details of how preset trays are prepared and used during a procedure are presented in Chapter 6.

Efficient instrument delivery

The transport of instruments and other items to and from the patient's oral cavity constitutes a great deal of movement by the dentist who works alone. One of

Table 10-1. The concept of four-handed dentistry

Sit-down dentistry	Auxiliary utilization	Organization	Work simplification
Proper equipment	Delegation of as many duties as possible	Time management	Rearrangement
Proper positioning of patient and operating team	Instrument transfer	Treatment planning	Elimination
	Oral evacuation and debridement	Design of facilities	Combination
	Retraction	Business procedures	Simplification
	Preparation of dental materials	Staff recruitment and assignments	
	Preparation of operatory and patients	Recall	
		Inventory control	
		Establishment of work pattern	
		Preset tray system	

the most effective ways of reducing the amount of movement by the dentist during a procedure is to develop an efficient instrument transfer method in which the chairside assistant transports needed items to the hands of the dentist near the patient's oral cavity. Guidelines for effective instrument transfer are presented in Chapter 14.

Effective oral evacuation and debridement

Control of fluids and debris during a dental procedure is mandatory for favorable visibility and for patient comfort and safety. Details on rinsing and evacuating the patient's mouth are presented in Chapter 13.

Proper time management

Time is the most valuable commodity in a dental practice. Effective use of time allows the dentist to provide the best care for the most people. Any effort that is made to eliminate the waste of the operator's time is worthwhile. The disorganization of treatment areas, poor appointment scheduling, lack of standardized procedures, and interruptions of the dentist are common examples of poor time management that should be eliminated.

SUMMARY

Four-handed dentistry is a concept of performing dental procedures in a comfortable, stress-free, and effective manner for both the assistant and the dentist. The principles and elements outline in Table 10-1 are all part of this concept. Four-handed dentistry is not intended to mean "hurry up dentistry." Its purpose is to provide a method of treating patients at a steady pace without frustrating delays and unnecessary fatigue. The dental assistant is truly an integral part of this concept.

BIBLIOGRAPHY

Chasteen, J.E.: Four-handed dentistry in clinical practice, St. Louis, 1980, The C.V. Mosby Co.

Chasteen J.E.: DAU manual of four-handed dentistry, ed. 2, Ann Arbor, Mich., 1982, University of Michigan, School of Dentistry.

Green, E.J., and Brown, M.E.: Body mechanics applied to the practice of dentistry, J. Am. Dent. Assoc. **67:**679-697, 1963.

Green, E.S., and Lynam, L.A.: Work simplification: an application to dentistry, J. Am. Dent. Assoc. **57:**242-252, 1958.

Golden, S.S.: Engineering comfort into dentistry, Mechanical Engineering **86:**38-42, August 1964.

Hoffman, D.A.: Time and motion study in dentistry, Bull. Greater Milwaukee Dent. Assoc. **23:**101-102, July 1957.

Howard, W.W.: Dental practice planning, St. Louis, 1975, The C.V. Mosby Co.

Kilpatrick, H.C.: Work simplification in dental practice, ed. 3, Philadelphia, 1974, W.B. Saunders Co.

Klein, H.: Civilian dentistry in war-time, J. Am. Dent. Assoc. **31:**648-661, 1944.

Robinson, G.E., et al.: Four-handed dentistry manual, ed. 2, Birmingham, Ala., 1971, University of Alabama School of Dentistry.

Schmid, W., and Stevenson, S.B.: Dynamic instrument placement and operator's and assistant's stool placement, Dent. Clin. North Am. **15:**145-155, 1971.

Waterman, G.E.: Effective use of dental assistants, Public Health Rep. **67:**390-394, 1952.

CHAPTER 11

THE DENTAL
TREATMENT ROOM

The dental treatment room or operatory is the primary work environment for the dentist and the dental assistant. Its size, layout, and contents should be designed and organized to facilitate comfort and convenience for the operatory team. In other words, the work environment should be adapted to the workers instead of having the workers adapt to the environment.

Once the functional aspects of a treatment room have been included in the design, an attractive decor should be superimposed to create a pleasant ambience to the room. Factors such as lighting, color, textures, window treatments, sound systems, and floor coverings must be considered in decorating the treatment area. Room decor has a significant psychological effect on both the patient and the operating team.

ROOM DESIGN

New innovations in office design have expanded the thinking of dentists to create treatment areas instead of conventional rooms. Today dental offices may have an open design (Fig. 11-1). This design concept eliminates walls between the treatment stations. This creates a feeling of openness that many dentists prefer. However, some dentists object to the lack of privacy associated with this design.

A compromise between the open design and the conventional treatment room is the semiopen design. This concept utilizes some higher barriers between treatment stations. These barriers may be partial walls or dental cabinetry (Fig. 11-2).

If a conventional design is used, it functions quite well if the size of the room is 9 × 11 feet. Two doors at the rear of the room create a favorable traffic pattern for the operating team. Two sinks add to the

convenience by providing two washing stations and auxiliary counter space (Fig. 11-3).

Regardless of which design exists in a dental office, the treatment area should be kept as simple as possible in terms of its content. Only items that are used routinely should be kept in this prime work space. A cluttered environment should be avoided.

Treatment areas should be kept spotlessly clean. Constant assessment of the room is necessary to ensure its desirable appearance. It is a good idea to sit in the dental chair occasionally to see what the patient sees during treatment. That dusty operating light or the cobweb on the ceiling becomes quite obvious from this position. The maintenance of the treatment areas is a responsibility of the dental assistant throughout the workday.

BASIC OPERATING EQUIPMENT

To suggest that there is only one equipment setup suitable for four-handed dentistry is just as hazardous as suggesting that there is only one automobile design for all drivers. However, certain fundamental design features are essential to allow the operating team to work comfortably and have favorable access to the patient's oral cavity. A variety of brands of equipment meet these basic requirements. The following is a discussion of basic treatment room equipment required in a general practice.

A basic equipment setup that is used in a modern dental office generally includes the following items:

Dental chair	Operating light
Dental unit	X-ray machine
Operating stools	Sinks
Storage cabinets	Radiographic viewbox
Air-water syringe	Communications system
Oral evacuator	Preset trays

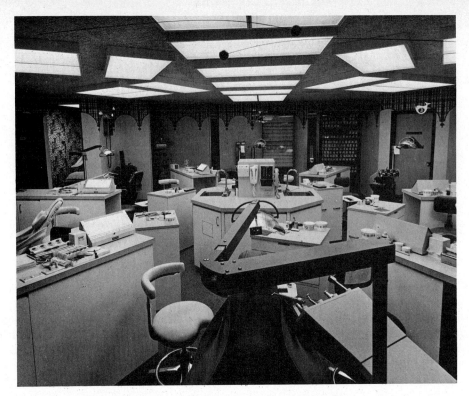

Fig. 11-1. Open clinic design. (From Wolff, R.M.: Dental Survey **49:**44-47, January 1973; courtesy Roy M. Wolff, Creve Coeur, Mo.)

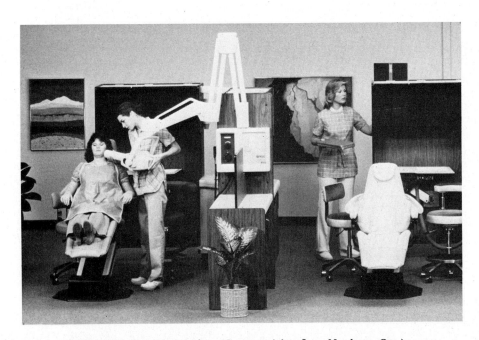

Fig. 11-2. Semiopen design. (Courtesy Adec, Inc., Newburg, Ore.)

Common optional items include the following:
Nitrous oxide machine
Ultrasonic scaler
Composite light (fiberoptic)
Vitalometer
Bead sterilizer

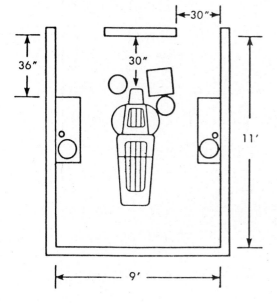

Fig. 11-3. Conventional design.

Dental chair

The dental chair is the center of activity for all treatment procedures. Its design is critical to successful four-handed dentistry. The most important features of the chair are those that allow access to the patient's oral cavity while the operating team is seated in a comfortable position. Of lesser significance are the features that provide patient comfort, since the patient is in the chair for only a short time. Fortunately, a chair like the one shown in Fig. 11-4 provides both excellent operator access and patient comfort.

An analysis of a desirable dental chair reveals the following features:

1. The back of the chair should be thin and narrow in the headrest area (Fig. 11-5). This allows the dentist and the assistant to position themselves as close to the patient as possible without leaning and reaching to gain access. The ability to see into the oral cavity is determined by how close the operating team can get to the patient. Therefore the thin, narrow back design is absolutely essential, since it permits the operating team to get closer to the patient.

2. Dental chairs should allow the patient to be placed in a supine position (Fig. 11-4, *B*).

3. Once the patient is in the supine position, the chair base must allow the patient to be lowered so that the person's head is actually located in the lap of the dentist. Therefore the base of the chair should allow

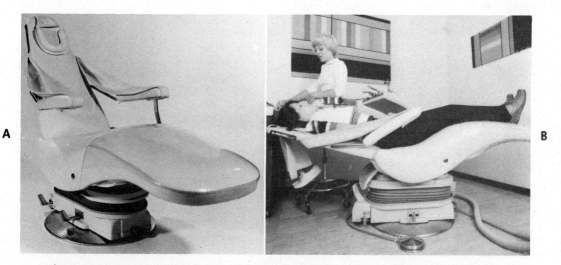

Fig. 11-4. A, Favorable dental chair. **B,** Chair that provides complete patient support and convenient access to adjustment controls. (**A** courtesy Den-Tal-Ez Manufacturing Co., Des Moines, Iowa; **B,** from Chasteen, J.E.: DAU manual of four-handed dentistry, Ann Arbor, Mich., 1977, University of Michigan School of Dentistry.)

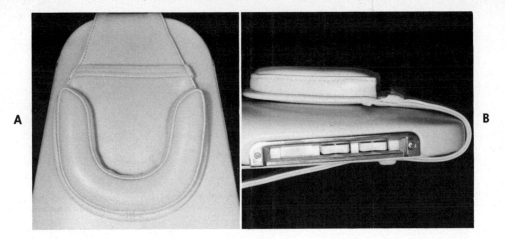

Fig. 11-5. Thin, narrow headrest area, permitting convenient access to patient. **A,** Top view. **B,** Lateral view.

the chair to be lowered to a position 14 to 16 inches above the floor.

4. The patient should be as comfortable as possible without sacrificing access and visibility. The chair shown in Fig. 11-4, *A* provides excellent support for the patient in the supine position. Note the support straps for the arms.

5. The controls should be located so that both the assistant and the dentist can reach them conveniently. A good arrangement is to have the control that raises and lowers the chair located on the chair base so that it can be activated with the foot. The back and seat tilt controls should be located along the side of the headrest area for easy access (Fig. 11-5, *B*).

An optional item available in newer dental chairs is a programmed-settings feature that allows the chair to be automatically placed in a preselected position with one touch of an activation switch. This adds to the convenience of seating and dismissing a patient. Another feature that is rather popular is a traverse function that moves the seat of the chair forward toward the foot board while the back of the chair is being reclined. This maintains the head of the chair at a uniform distance from any cabinetry or dental unit located behind the chair. Articulating headrests are also available on some chairs that allow the patient's head to be placed at various angles during treatment.

The dental chair can be kept clean with special upholstery cleaners or mild soap solutions. The crevices in the seat portion of the chair should be kept free of waste amalgam particles that may be dropped during an amalgam restorative procedure.

Dental unit

The dental unit is the control center for the dental handpieces. Its primary function is to control the flow of air and water to these instruments and to provide a holder to position them within reach of the operating team. Dental units vary in design and instrument configuration. Some units contain not only the dental handpieces but also items such as the oral evacuator, air-water syringe, saliva ejector, ultrasonic scaler, and the fiber optic composite light probe.

Since the dental assistant may encounter a variety of dental units in general practice, a review of the basic design concepts seems worthwhile. Three common concepts are in use today, grouped according to the location of the unit relative to the patient in the dental chair. Fig. 11-6, *A* is an example of a rear delivery system. Instruments are delivered to the dentist from the unit which is located behind the patient. Fig. 11-6, *B* is a side delivery unit, which is placed on the dentist's side of the chair. Side delivery units are mounted on either bracket arms or mobile carts. Fig. 11-6, *C* is an over the patient or transthorax delivery unit, which is located over the patient's chest between the dentist and the assistant.

Each concept has its own set of advantages and

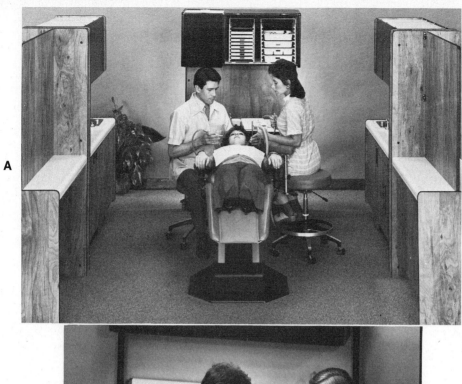

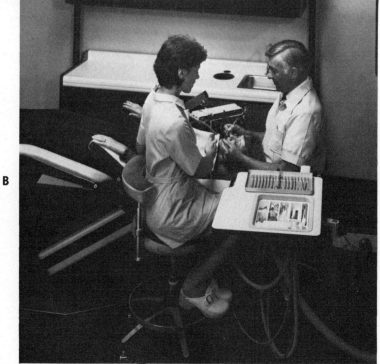

Fig. 11-6. Common dental unit designs. **A,** Rear delivery system. **B,** Side delivery system. (**A** and **B** courtesy Adec, Inc., Newburg, Ore.)   *Continued.*

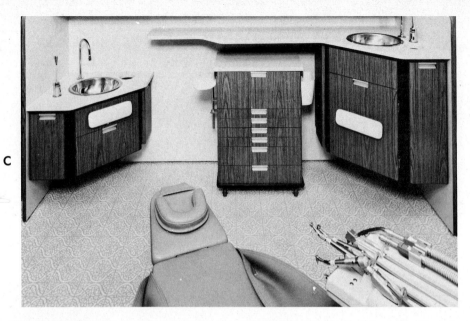

Fig. 11-6, cont'd. C, Transthorax delivery system. (**C** courtesy Health Science Products, Inc., Birmingham, Ala.)

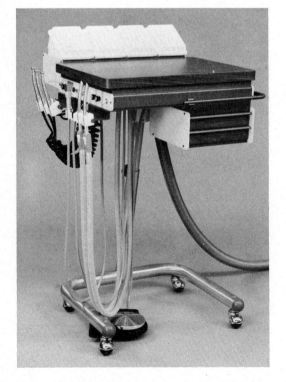

Fig. 11-7. Assistants' moble cart. Available with or without dental handpieces. (Courtesy Adec, Inc., Newburg, Ore.)

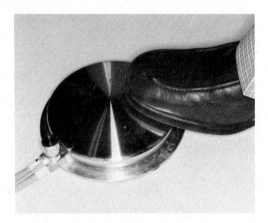

Fig. 11-8. Accelerator-style foot control. (From Chasteen, J.E.: DAU manual of four-handed dentistry, Ann Arbor, Mich., 1977, University of Michigan School of Dentistry.)

disadvantages, but all three function rather well in the four-handed dentistry concept if they are used properly in a favorable treatment room.

Dental units that do not house an air-water syringe, saliva ejector, or oral evacuator have to be used with a mobile cart that does contain these devices (Fig. 11-7). Generally the basic dental unit should contain at least two high speed handpieces, one conventional speed handpiece, and an air-water syringe. Some operating teams find it helpful to have two air-water syringes. One is located on the unit, and the other is mounted on the assistant's mobile cabinet.

Handpieces are controlled by two switches. One switch is located on the unit to program the handpiece to be used. The second switch is located in the foot control (Fig. 11-8), which the dentist uses to activate the handpiece and to make the bur spin at various speeds. If fiber optic handpieces are used, the light in the handpiece can be activated by the foot control. Some fiber optic handpieces light when they are touched by the dentist.

The maintenance of the dental unit involves routine cleaning and periodic inspection of pressure gauges to be sure that all instruments are working according to manufacturer's specifications.

Operating stools

The operating stools should be selected with as much care as would be taken to select lounge chairs for a cozy living room. Comfort is the key factor in stool selection. Remember that nearly a full working day is spent sitting on the operating stools.

The operator's stool should have the following features to ensure comfort and convenience (Fig. 11-9, *A*):

1. The seat should be padded adequately to support the operator. The seat can be flat-surfaced or contoured (saddle type).
2. A broad base with at least four casters on the stool is recommended to prevent tipping and allow mobility.
3. The seat should be adjustable from 14 to 21 inches. A lever located beneath the seat is used to activate a hydraulic system for raising or lowering the stool height.
4. The back support must be adjustable both vertically and horizontally to adapt to the individual operator.

The assistant's stool has to be designed a little differently from the operator's stool because of the position of the assistant at chairside. The following is a

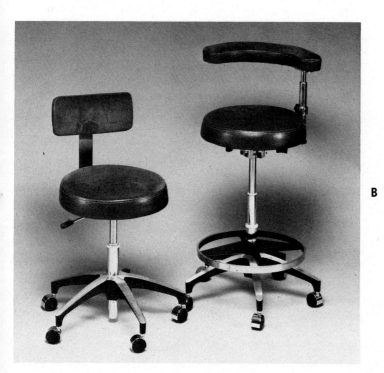

B

Fig. 11-9. A, Operator's stool. **B,** Assistant's stool. (Courtesy Adec, Inc., Newburg, Ore.)

list of features that are important to look for in selecting an assistant's stool (Fig. 11-9, *B*):

1. The base of the stool should be broad to prevent tipping. A stool with five casters is recommended. An adjustable foot ring is desirable to allow for the adaption of the stool to fit the lower leg length of the assistant.
2. The seat should be adjustable to a height of approximately 27 inches. This can be accomplished using the same hydraulic lever system found on operator stools.
3. The seat should be padded sufficiently for comfort.
4. A body support is recommended for the assistant's stool. This allows support for the upper portion of the trunk when the assistant leans forward. The body support must be adjustable horizontally and vertically.

The ability of the operating team to see into the oral cavity was mentioned during the discussion of dental chair design. Likewise, stool design and proper positioning contribute greatly to visibility. The design features listed permit the mobility, height adjustment, and body support necessary to achieve comfortable visual access to the oral cavity. Comfort and visibility are two critical goals that must be achieved if four-handed dentistry is to succeed. Obviously, equipment design is only part of gaining comfort and visual access to the oral cavity. Proper positioning of the patient and the operating team is discussed in detail in Chapter 12.

Storage cabinets

A great deal of chairside efficiency can be generated by organizing auxiliary instruments and materials in appropriate cabinetry in the operatory. Only commonly used items should be stored in the operatory. The main supply inventory should be kept in other storage areas in the office.

Dental cabinets can be divided into two categories. These are fixed cabinets that are attached to the wall (Fig. 11-10) and mobile cabinets that can be moved around the operatory on casters (Fig. 11-11). It is quite common to use a combination of both types to provide convenient storage.

Generally speaking, items that are kept in the fixed cabinetry are those used to prepare the operatory for treatment. Items such as preset trays and disposable

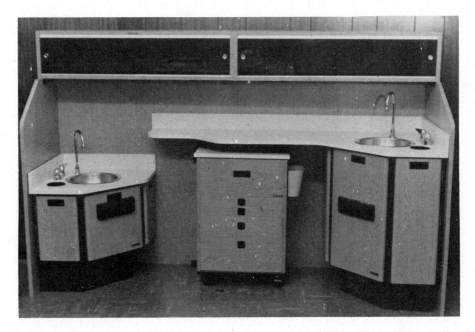

Fig. 11-10. Fixed cabinetry with space provided for storage of mobile cabinet. (Courtesy Health Science Products, Inc., Birmingham, Ala.)

paper goods are kept here. The mobile cabinet is reserved for auxiliary items needed during the treatment procedure.

Two of the most convenient mobile cabinet designs are the Alabama style and the North Carolina style cabinets (Fig. 11-11). These cabinets have a sliding top that can be pulled over the assistant's lap to create a convenient work surface. The preset tray is placed on this surface for maximum access during a procedure. There is a deep well under the top. The assistant has the easiest access to this storage space of any in the operatory. Therefore only the most frequently used auxiliary items should be kept here. These items include such articles as gauze sponges, cotton rolls, extra anesthetic cartridges, various bases and cavity liners, amalgamator, amalgam materials, and mixing pads. The operating team should analyze its procedures to determine what items should be kept in this prime storage space. Access can be gained to all areas of the well by simply sliding the top back and forth as needed.

The drawers should contain auxiliary instruments that can be used if an instrument from the preset tray is dropped during a procedure. Since these drawers are less convenient to reach, frequently used items should not be placed here. A good guide to cabinet organization is to place the more frequently needed items in the uppermost drawers and the less frequently needed items in the lower drawers. It should be emphasized that the reference to "frequently used items" is directed toward auxiliary items only. The primary instruments commonly used in any procedure will be placed on a preset instrument tray during sterilization procedures.

Air-water syringe (Fig. 11-12)

The combination air-water syringe is one of the greatest time- and motion-saving instruments developed in recent dental history. This instrument can deliver either a stream of air into the mouth to dry a preparation or a stream of water into the mouth for rinsing. A combination of air and water can be cre-

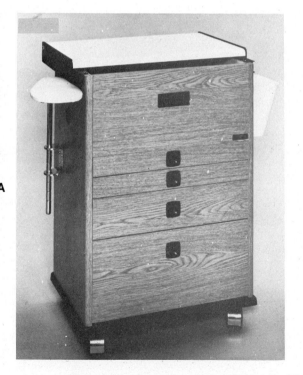
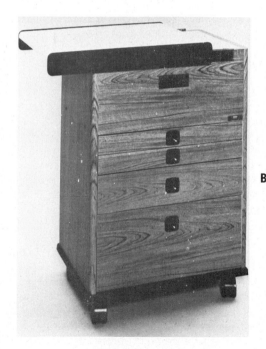

A

B

Fig. 11-11. Assistant's mobile cabinets. **A,** Alabama style. **B,** North Carolina style. (Courtesy Health Science Products, Inc., Birmingham, Ala.)

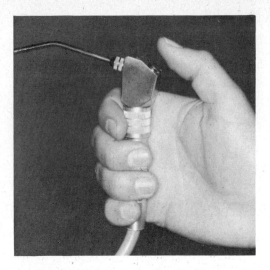

Fig. 11-12. Pistol-type air-water syringe.

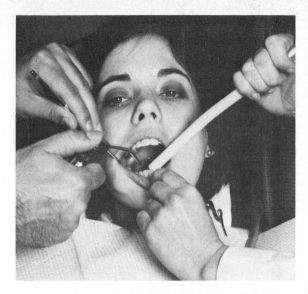

Fig. 11-13. Oral evacuator in use.

ated by activating both the air and water buttons at the same time. The water spray that is produced can be used to vigorously rinse the oral cavity.

In the past a separate syringe delivered only water and another delivered only air. The combining of these two syringes into one functional unit has made rinsing and drying a more convenient task.

The pistol-style syringe offers convenience in handling that cannot be matched by other designs. It is easy to transfer between operator and assistant, and it is comfortable to use. The activation buttons are located on the top of the syringe. The thumb is used to activate the syringe.

The syringe tip should be removable for sterilization. The tip should have a slight bend in it to assist in gaining access intraorally. In addition, the tip should be capable of swiveling 360 degrees to orient the tip to any area of the mouth. The proper use of the syringe and the method of transfer between the dentist and the assistant will be discussed in Chapter 14.

Oral evacuator (Fig. 11-13)

The oral evacuator is a suction instrument that is used to remove fluids and debris from the patient's mouth. Modern evacuation systems have virtually eliminated the need for the time-honored cuspidor. Oral evacuation is the responsibility of the chairside assistant. The technique of using the important instrument will be discussed in detail in Chapter 13.

Operating light (Fig. 11-14)

The operating light is an important factor in visibility. A ceiling-mounted type is preferred. The light should deliver at least 1200 footcandles of intensity to the oral cavity when it is 3 feet from the patient's face. Favorable light design will dissipate heat away from the patient. Since the positioning of the light is primarily the assistant's responsibility, the light should have handles on both sides for use by the dentist and the assistant.

Maintenance of the light is limited to cleaning the heat shield, disinfecting the handles between patients, and occasional bulb changes.

X-ray machine

X-ray machines are essential pieces of equipment in a dental office. The valuable diagnostic information provided through their use is critical to dental treatment. Dental offices may have an x-ray machine in all treatment areas or limit the x-ray service to one room.

The dental assistant should receive adequate training in the use of radiographic equipment. Many courses and excellent texts are available dealing with this important aspect of dental assisting.

X-ray machines require very little maintenance beyond disinfecting between patients.

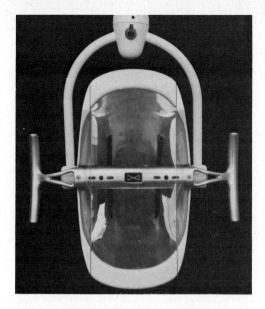

Fig. 11-14. Operating light.

Sinks

Two key points should be emphasized regarding sinks in the dental operatory. First, there should be two sinks in the operatory—one for the dentist and one for the assistant (Fig. 11-10). This eliminates wasted time spent in waiting for a turn to wash. Each sink should be located to provide convenient access to the operating team. Second, the water controls on the sink should be operated by a knee or a foot control (Fig. 11-15). This will prevent recontamination of the hands after washing by avoiding controls that require use of the hands to turn off the water. A good compromise is to use a hand control like the one shown in Fig. 11-16, which can be turned off using only the wrist. A few other considerations regarding sinks are as follows:

1. Small, stainless steel sinks are considered favorable because they require little space and are relatively easy to keep clean.
2. The dentist's sink can be either at stand-up or sit-down height, depending on personal preference. The assistant's sink is usually at stand-up height.
3. Each sink cabinet should contain a convenient disposal hole without a cover to permit easy discarding of towels.
4. Convenient soap and paper towel dispensers should be located at each sink.

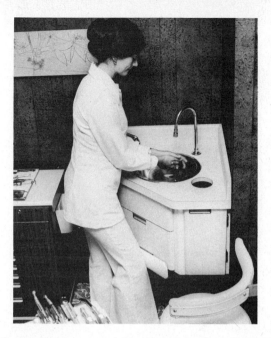

Fig. 11-15. Knee control for sink faucet. (Courtesy Health Science Products, Inc., Birmingham, Ala.)

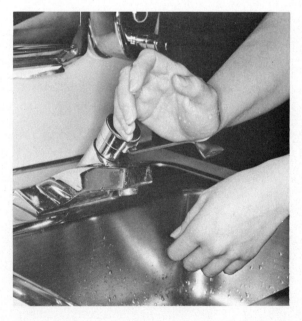

Fig. 11-16. Faucet control that can be turned off with the wrist.

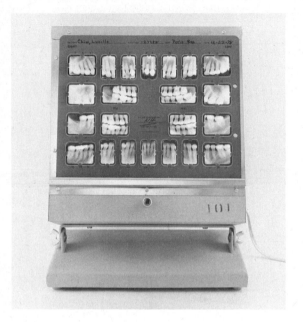

Fig. 11-17. Radiographic view box.

The team should wash in the presence of the patient just before starting an examination or treatment. This reassures the patient of the team's concern for cleanliness. If they wash in another room and then enter the operatory, the patient is not sure whether their hands have been washed or not. Hands should be rewashed whenever they touch an unclean object such as the telephone, hair or face, or the chair. Sinks should be cleaned, and disposal receptacles should be emptied several times a day to maintain a tidy appearance and prevent unpleasant room odors.

Radiographic view box (Fig. 11-17)

Dental radiographs can be more accurately interpreted by the dentist if they can be viewed with a diffused light source. The radiographic view box is such a light source.

View boxes are available in different shapes that fit the different sizes of radiographic mounts. The surface glass of the view box should be kept free of any spots or smudges that could be mistaken for dental disease when a radiograph is placed over it.

Communication system

Communication within the dental office is required for coordination of activities among the staff mem-

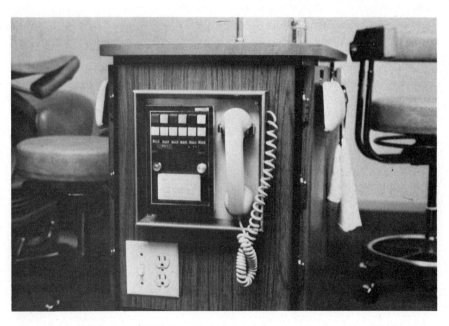

Fig. 11-18. Combination light signal and intercom system located in a treatment area.

bers. It is helpful to have some type of communication system located in each treatment room. This allows the dental team to communicate with other areas in the office. Color coded light signals and intercom systems are commonly used. The system shown in Fig. 11-18 is an example of a combination light signal and intercom system.

Each color coded light is used to designate a specific message such as "the next patient has arrived" or "the hygienist is ready for the dentist to examine a patient." The appropriate color is illuminated to convey the necessary message. The light is turned off when the message has been acknowledged.

Preset trays

A prime example of organization in the dental office is the establishment of a preset tray system. The basic idea of this system is to establish, item by item, what will be needed to perform a given procedure and then to make up several duplicates of the needed armamentarium to use as necessary throughout the day. For example, the dentist should decide what instrument setup is needed to do a composite restoration (Fig. 11-19). Several duplicates of this setup should be established to meet the requirements of a typical workday. The number of setups will vary with the needs of the individual dentist.

The instruments are kept on color-coded trays that identify the purpose of each setup. Each procedural setup is coded with a different color. Preset trays are usually established for every common procedure done in the dental office. This is not a limitation, but rather a trend. Certainly, preset trays should be established for as many procedures as the dental team thinks would be helpful. Since the preparation of preset trays is a part of processing dental instruments, further discussion is presented in Chapter 6.

Preset trays are kept in either a fixed cabinet located in each treatment room or in the sterilization room. The required tray is then retrieved and placed on the top of the mobile cabinet when it is needed.

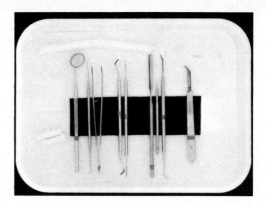

Fig. 11-19. Preset tray. (From Chasteen, J.E.: DAU manual of four-handed dentistry, Ann Arbor, Mich., 1977, University of Michigan School of Dentistry.)

SUMMARY

Dental offices vary considerably in design and in the equipment that is used. However, they are similar in the respect that all general practices require certain basic equipment items to function. This introductory discussion of the treatment room and its contents should serve to orient the new dental assistant to this important work area.

Dental assistants are encouraged to consult equipment manufacturer's manuals for details on the maintenance of each item in the treatment room.

BIBLIOGRAPHY

Chasteen, J.E.: Four-handed dentistry in clinical practice, St. Louis, 1980, The C.V. Mosby Co.
Cooper, T.M., and Dibiaggio, J.A.: Applied practice management: a strategy for stress control, St. Louis, 1979, The C.V. Mosby Co.
Kilpatrick, H.C.: Work simplification in dental practice, ed. 3, Philadelphia, 1974, W.B. Saunders Co.
Schmid, W., and Stevenson, S.B.: Dynamic instrument placement and operator's and assistant's stool placement, Dent. Clin. North Am. **15:**145-155, 1971.

CHAPTER 12

POSITIONING THE PATIENT AND OPERATING TEAM

A great deal of research has been done to determine the most favorable working position for the operating team and patient. The results of these studies have shown that the seated position is generally best for both the dentist and chairside assistant. Although there is no perfect operator-patient-assistant position, the sit-down approach fulfills the demands of most clinical problems.

However, comfortable, stress-free four-handed dentistry requires more than simply sitting down to operate. The manner in which the dentist and chairside assistant sit relative to the patient is the most significant factor in achieving comfort for the operating team. As with many other aspects of dentistry, it is not just a matter of doing, but rather how well it is done, for success to be achieved. Some dentists have abandoned efforts to practice dentistry in a seated position simply because they did not know how to sit properly. This chapter deals with several suggestions on how the operating team should be positioned relative to each other and the patient.

THE WORK CIRCLE

The focal point of activity in the treatment room is the patient's oral cavity. By placing the operating team and instrumentation close to the patient's head the following objectives can be achieved:

1. Favorable access to the operative field
2. Good visibility
3. Reduction of Class IV and V movements
4. Comfort for the operating team
5. Comfort and safety for the patient

Arranging the treatment room so that the operating team can work within an imaginary circle with a radius of approximately 20 inches around the patient's head is most helpful. This is referred to as the work circle (Fig. 12-1).

Zones of activity

The work circle can be divided into zones of activity, which are used to describe the working positions of both the equipment and operating team.

Four major zones of activity are visualized around a patient in a supine position. If one visualizes the patient's face as if it were located in the center of the

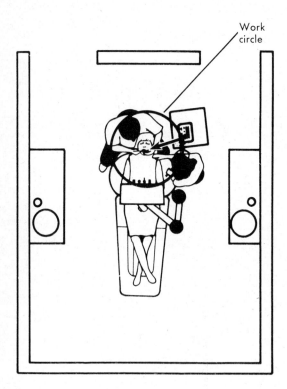

Work circle

Fig. 12-1. Work circle.

face of a clock, these zones may be designated as follows (Fig. 12-2):

Operator's zone (7 to 12 o'clock position)
Static zone (12 to 2 o'clock position)
Assistant's zone (2 to 4 o'clock position)
Transfer zone (4 to 7 o'clock position)

With this standard reference, the location of the operating team and equipment relative to the patient's face can be stated as positions on the clock. For example, the operator in Fig. 12-2, *A,* is in the 11 o'clock position, and the assistant is in the 3 o'clock position.

Operator's zone. The operator's zone is that part of the work circle where the dentist can be positioned to gain access to various segments of the patient's oral cavity. Patients enter and leave the dental chair through this zone.

Transfer zone. The transfer zone is the area where instruments and materials are transported to and from the oral cavity. It is also an excellent area for the location of the dental unit so that it is within easy reach of either the assistant or the dentist.

Assistant's zone. The assistant's zone is rather small because the dental assistant remains in the 3 o'clock position throughout a procedure regardless of the operator's position. It is critical to have a work surface extend into this zone over the assistant's

lap for convenience and reduction of excessive motion.

Static zone. The static zone is a nontraffic area where equipment such as a nitrous oxide machine or a mobile cabinet can be placed with the top extending into the assistant's zone. Rear delivery dental units are also placed in this zone.

POSITIONING THE OPERATOR

It is important to adapt the work environment to the operator, instead of having the operator adapt to a fixed environment. This concept requires the dentist to assume a favorable seated position and then arrange the patient, assistant, and equipment in relationship to that position.

The process of preparing for any chairside procedures should begin with the seating of the dentist in a position of "balanced posture," which is described according to the following characteristics:

1. The operator's stool height should be adjusted so that the top of the operator's thighs are parallel to the floor (Fig. 12-3).
2. The entire surface of the seat of the stool should be used to support the operator's weight.
3. A backrest to support the operator's back without interfering with movement of the arms is recommended.

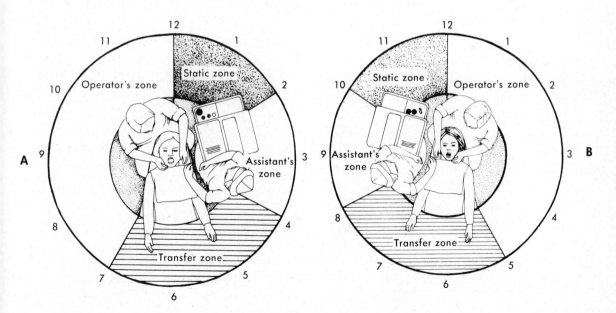

Fig. 12-2. A, Zones of activity for right-handed operator. **B,** Zones of activity for left-handed operator.

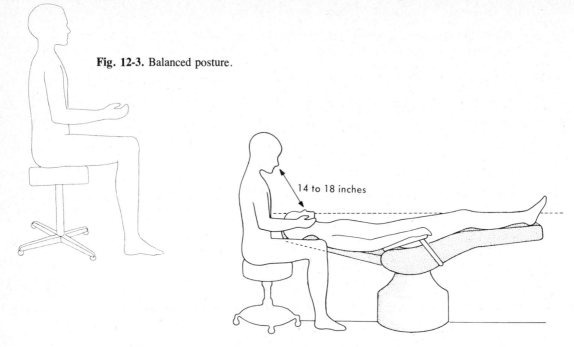

Fig. 12-3. Balanced posture.

14 to 18 inches

Fig. 12-4. Operator-patient relationship with operator in balanced posture and patient in supine position.

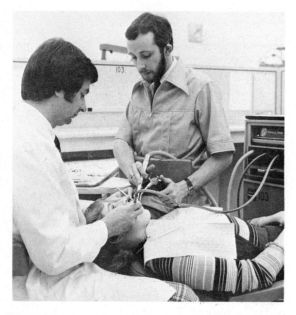

Fig. 12-5. Favorable working position for operating team.

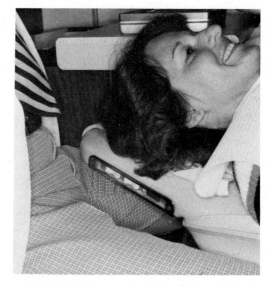

Fig. 12-6. Thin back of dental chair resting on top of operator's left thigh.

4. The patient should be positioned so that the operator's forearms are parallel to the floor when the hands are in operating position. The operative field should be located in the dentist's midline.
5. The elbows should be close to the body.
6. The operator's back and neck should be reasonably upright, with the top of the shoulders parallel to the floor.
7. A distance of approximately 14 to 18 inches between the operator's nose and the patient's oral cavity should be maintained (Fig. 12-4).

The essence of balanced posture is having the dentist positioned so that favorable body mechanics are at work, permitting comfort for the operator and minimizing fatigue.

This description of balanced posture is not intended to imply that the operator must sit in a statuelike manner but rather to establish a set of guidelines that is helpful in achieving comfort while the operator works at chairside.

POSITIONING THE PATIENT

One of the most important steps in adapting the work environment to the dentist is proper positioning of the patient relative to the balanced posture of the dentist. The patient is located so that the oral cavity is centered over the operator's lap at the height of the operator's elbow (Fig. 12-5). The dentist should not have to reach up to work in the oral cavity. Remember that the forearms of the dentist should be rather parallel to the floor when the hands are in working position in the patient's oral cavity. A thin back on

the dental chair permits most operators to fit their legs underneath the chair while working in the 10 to 12 o'clock positions (Fig. 12-6). However, a dentist with short, large thighs and a short upper body may have to place the chair back between the thighs to position the patient low enough to keep the forearms parallel (Fig. 12-7).

A lounge-style chair has proved to be a very favorable design for sit-down four-handed dentistry. Its low base and thin, narrow chair back allows the operator to be positioned close to the patient's oral cavity not only in the vertical relationship just discussed but also in the horizontal relationship of the dentist to the patient. A narrow chair back allows placement of the patient's head close to the edge of the chair back on the operator's side, thus improving access and visibility (Fig. 12-8). Access and visibility often involve fractions of inches. This fact should not be overlooked in purchasing the appropriate equipment for four-handed dentistry. The narrow chair back not only adds to the convenience of the dentist but also affords the chairside assistant similar access and visibility.

To benefit from the thin, narrow design of the chair back, the patient's head must be placed at the upper end of the chair and slightly to the operator's side. This is referred to as the working position for the patient (Fig. 12-9). Patients are placed in the working position regardless of their height. In other words, short

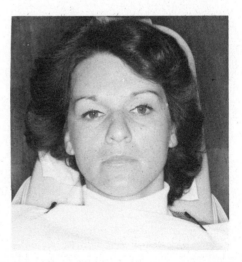

Fig. 12-8. Patient's head positioned on narrow portion of chair back to afford improved access and visibility for operator.

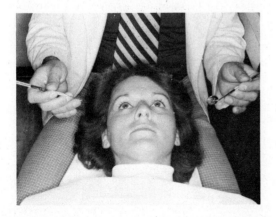

Fig. 12-7. Chair back positioned between operator's legs.

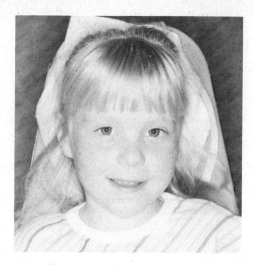

Fig. 12-9. Child patient's head placed in working position.

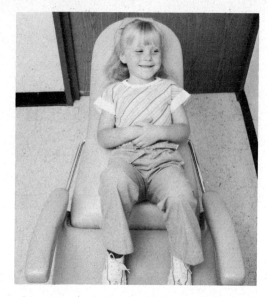

Fig. 12-10. Small child, with knees bent for comfort, positioned with head in working area of chair.

adults and children must be positioned in the chair from the head down. If they are always placed so that the buttocks are resting on the seat of the chair, the head of a short patient will be located in a wider portion of the chair back, tending to limit the access of the operating team to the oral cavity.

The force of gravity prevents the patient in a supine position from sliding down in the chair. Very small (3 to 4 years of age) children can simply bend their knees (Fig. 12-10).

Actually, a dental chair does not function as a chair per se in the practice of four-handed dentistry. For the most part, it becomes a kind of operating table when the dentist places the patient in supine position.

The following is a suggested technique for placing a patient in supine position:

1. Adjust the chair back so that it is at approximately 60 degrees to vertical.
2. Raise the chair to a height at which the patient can easily be seated.
3. Raise the arm of the chair.
4. Once the patient is seated, raise the chair approximately 10 inches. This allows room for the dentist to slide under the chair back.
5. Tilt the seat portion back so that the footrest area is raised approximately 6 to 8 inches.
6. Lower the back of the chair until the patient is about halfway toward a horizontal position. Pause a few moments to allow the patient to adjust.
7. Continue lowering the chair back until the following relationships exist:

A. An imaginary line drawn from the patient's chin to the top of the patient's ankles is parallel with the floor (Fig. 12-11).
B. The plane of the patient's forehead is also parallel with the floor (Fig. 12-12). The patient may have to tip his or her head as needed to achieve this relationship.
8. Lower the chair onto the operator's lap.

Placing a patient in the supine position is far more acceptable if the patient is not "thrown" into this position. With the chair back at 60 degrees before the patient enters the chair and a momentary pause halfway to supine position, the patient can adjust to the change. Some chairs with programmed positions tend to place the patient in a supine position too quickly, and the patient may object. Similar responses often occur when the patient is rapidly returned to the upright position at the conclusion of treatment.

In the supine position the patient's legs and head should be at the same level. The patient should lie flat in the chair with little bending at the waist. This duplicates the position that most people assume while sleeping for several hours without impairment of circulation. The patient whose legs are higher than the head is not considered to be in a supine position, and such placement for long periods of time is not recommended.

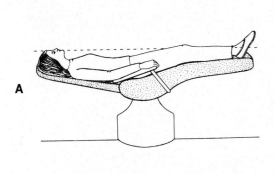

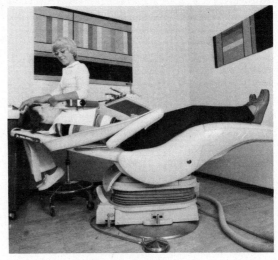

Fig. 12-11. A, Proper horizontal placement of patient in supine position. **B,** Patient in supine position.

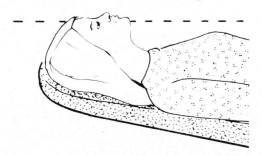

Fig. 12-12. Plane of patient's head approximately parallel with floor.

Once the patient is placed properly in the supine position, the chair base is lowered to place the head of the patient in the lap of the dentist. This height should be low enough so that the operator's forearms are reasonably parallel with the floor when the hands are in working position. Final adjustments for visibility and access to all quadrants of the mouth can be achieved by having the patient turn his or her head toward or away from the operator as needed. The patient's head can also be tilted backward or forward as needed to assist in improving visibility and access.

The supine position is considered a universal position for working in almost every area of the mouth. However, since every patient varies in oral anatomy and in the procedure to be done, some variations from supine position will be needed. The most notable case requiring this is that of gaining access to the most distal portion of the mandibular right quadrant. Sometimes better access to this area of the mouth is achieved by lowering the chair base to its lowest position. Then the chair back is raised until the operator's forearms are parallel with the floor when the hands are in working position. The chair seat is usually tilted somewhat backward, and the operator is placed in either the 7 or 9 o'clock position (Fig. 12-13). Access is further improved when the patient's head is turned slightly toward the operator and the chin is lowered.

At this point, it should be emphasized that once the patient is properly placed in either the supine position or some modification of it, assessment of proper patient positioning is accomplished by analyzing the operator and not the patient. The dentist should mentally go through the following positional checklist:

1. Thighs parallel to floor
2. Forearms parallel to floor
3. Elbows close to operator's side
4. Neck and back reasonably upright
5. Distance of 14 to 18 inches between the operator's nose and the patient's face
6. Operative field in dentist's midline

Adjustments in the position of the patient should be made until these relations are established. The chair-

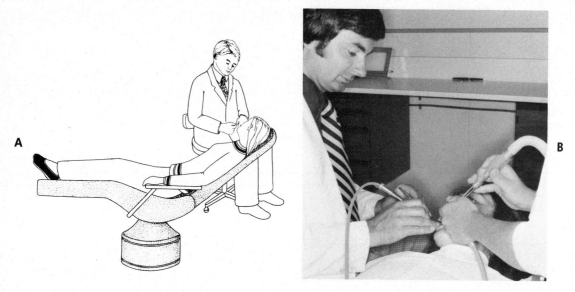

Fig. 12-13. A, Full view of operator-patient relationship while dentist is working in mandibular right posterior segment. **B,** Close-up of operator-patient relationship while dentist is working in mandibular right posterior segment.

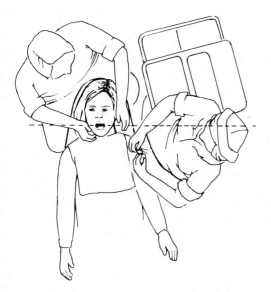

Fig. 12-14. Chairside assistant maintains 3 o'clock position while working in all areas of mouth.

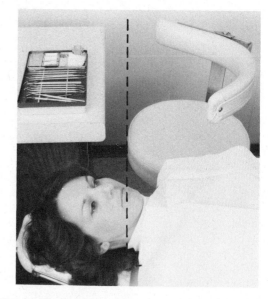

Fig. 12-15. Chairside assistant's stool properly positioned relative to patient's oral cavity.

side assistant can help the dentist by observing these relationships. The assistant who sees marked deviation from these guidelines can politely communicate this to the dentist by asking, "Are you comfortable?" This is a signal that perhaps a reassessment of position is in order.

POSITIONING THE DENTAL ASSISTANT

The dental assistant must be able to see and have favorable access to the oral cavity. The assistant has to retract tissues, evacuate fluids, keep the mirror free from water drops, debride the operative site, and view the progress of any procedure to anticipate the operator's needs. Although it is not absolutely necessary that the assistant see every detail that the operator can see, the assistant must at least be able to see the tooth or area being treated. The following are recommended considerations for positioning the dental assistant for all quadrants of the mouth:

1. The assistant should be in the 3 o'clock position for working in all quadrants (Fig. 12-14).
2. The assistant's stool should be placed so that the edge that is toward the top of the patient's head is in line with the patient's oral cavity (Fig. 12-15).
3. The stool should be as close to the dental chair as possible.
4. To enhance visibility, the height of the stool should be elevated so that the top of the assistant's head is 4 to 6 inches higher than that of the dentist while they are working in most areas of the mouth (Fig. 12-16). However, on occasion, improved vision can be achieved by lowering the stool so that the assistant's head height is the same as the operator's.
5. The assistant's back should be rather erect, with the body-support arm adjusted to support the upper body just under the rib cage (Fig. 12-17).

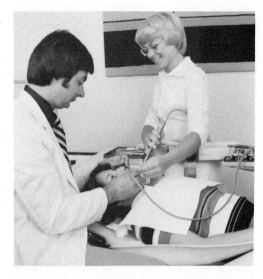

Fig. 12-17. Proper position for chairside assistant.

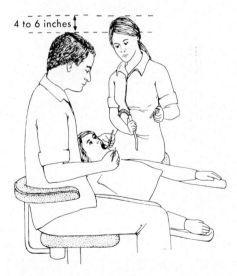

Fig. 12-16. Proper vertical relationship between the dentist and the assistant to enhance the assistant's visibility.

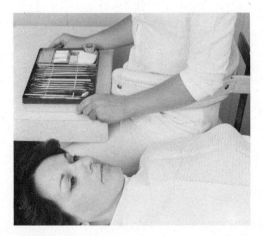

Fig. 12-18. Properly positioned assistant's stool allows tray to be within comfortable reach.

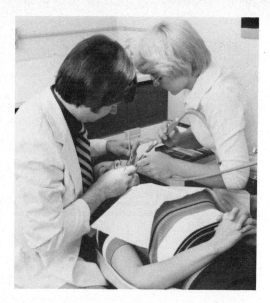

Fig. 12-19. Operating team leaning forward and blocking light.

6. The assistant's legs should be directed toward the head end of the chair with the sides of the thighs parallel with the chairback. The feet should rest on the foot support at the base of the stool.
7. When the assistant's stool is properly positioned, the mobile cabinet top can be placed over the lap of the assistant, thus putting instruments and materials within comfortable reach (Fig. 12-18).

LIGHTING THE OPERATIVE FIELD

Operating lights should deliver at least 1200 footcandles to the operative field at a distance of 3 feet from the patient's face. Most modern operating lights have this capacity.

In general, high light positions are used for working in mandibular areas and lower positions for maxillary areas. When both the dentist and assistant are properly positioned, they should not block the path of the operating light into the oral cavity. Leaning forward over the patient by either the operator or assistant is not only uncomfortable but also tends to obstruct the light and impair visibility (Fig. 12-19).

DISMISSING THE DENTAL PATIENT

After the dental procedure has been completed, all isolation materials should be removed, and a complete mouth rinse should be done to remove debris and freshen the patient's mouth. The patient's face should be wiped clean of any debris.

All operating equipment should be moved out of the way of the patient. The dental chair should slowly be returned to a rather upright position. The right arm of the chair should be raised. The patient should be encouraged to remain seated for a moment until the patient's circulatory system has had sufficient time to readjust to the upright position of his body. During that time the patient napkin can be removed. Individuals often appreciate the use of a hand mirror to inspect their appearance before departing the operatory.

SUMMARY

Access and visibility during a treatment procedure is essential. The guidelines presented in this chapter used in conjunction with favorable dental equipment are designed to enhance access and visibility. This can be accomplished while the operating team sits in comfort throughout most of the work day.

BIBLIOGRAPHY

Chasteen, J.E.: Four-handed dentistry in clinical practice, St. Louis, 1980, The C.V. Mosby Co.

Cooper, T.M., and DiBiaggio, J.A.: Applied practice management: a strategy for stress control, St. Louis, 1979, The C.V. Mosby Co.

Green, E.J., and Brown, M.E.: Body mechanics applied to the practice of dentistry, J. Am. Dent. Assoc. **67:**679-697, 1963.

Golden, S.S.: Engineering comfort into dentistry, Mechanical Engineering **86:**38-42, August 1964.

Kilpatrick, H.C.: Work simplification in dental practice, ed. 3, Philadelphia, 1974, W.B. Saunders Co.

CHAPTER 13

ORAL EVACUATION

It is interesting to note how the various elements that make up the concept of four-handed dentistry relate to each other. Comfort and access to the patient's oral cavity are essentially achieved by placing the patient in a supine position while the operating team sits as close to the patient's head as possible. However, it would be nearly impossible to treat a patient in the supine position successfully without some way to control the accumulation of saliva, blood, water, and debris in the posterior region of the mouth. Patients in the supine position would be extremely uncomfortable if such accumulations could not be removed.

The oral evacuation system removes fluids and debris from the oral cavity while the patient remains in the supine position throughout a dental procedure. Heretofore, the patient sat upright, and the dentist bent over to see and gain access to the mouth. Fluids and debris were removed by the patient's rinsing with a cup of water and expectorating into a cuspidor attached to the dental unit. The oral evacuator has eliminated the need for the cuspidor in four-handed dentistry.

The oral evacuator is a high-velocity vacuum system that creates enough suction to remove fluids and debris from the mouth. It works on a principle similar to that of the household vacuum cleaner. High volumes of air are moved into the vacuum hose at rather low negative pressure. A vacuum cleaner is capable of picking up debris when the opening of the hose is placed near, but not actually touching, the debris. Likewise, the oral evacuator can pull fluids into the evacuation hose without making contact with the pool of fluid. This phenomenon is possible because of the movement of massive volumes of the room air at normal pressure into the vacuum system, which has a low negative pressure.

Mobile evacuation systems are available. These are self-contained units that can be moved from one oper-

atory to another. Studies have demonstrated that these are less desirable than a central evacuation system, since they create an aerosol of bacteria from the evacuated oral debris. In addition, if more than one operatory is to be equipped with an evacuator, it is more economical and more practical to install a central system. Central systems are more hygienic, are easier to maintain, and require less space in the operatory.

Central evacuation systems consist of a main vacuum pump, vacuum lines to each operatory, and an evacuation hose that the assistant manipulates to remove oral debris. The vacuum pump is usually placed in the basement of the office near a sewer line. The vacuum lines draw debris from each operatory to the pump, where it is exhausted into the sewer (Fig. 13-1). Evacuation hoses are connected to the vacuum lines via a solids trap connector that catches most solids in the operatory (Fig. 13-2, A).

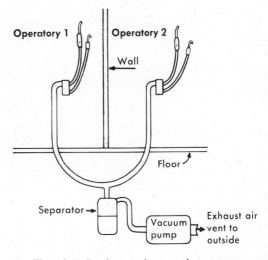

Fig. 13-1. Semiwet oral evacuation system.

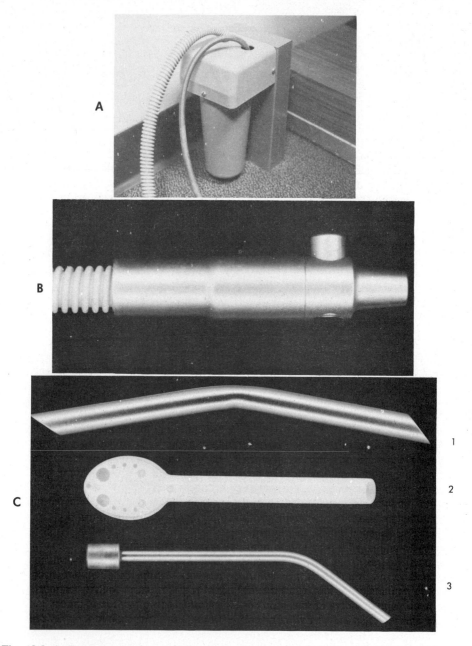

Fig. 13-2. A, Evacuator trap for solids. **B,** Oral-evacuator control. **C,** Evacuator tips. *1,* Universal style (stainless steel); *2,* spoon-shaped retractor; *3,* surgical style.

Most modern dental units have a trap attached to the unit assembly itself. This makes it convenient to retrieve a solid object such as an inlay that may be inadvertently picked up by the oral evacuator. The solids trap should be cleaned daily.

The evacuator hose in the operatory is a flexible hose that will not collapse when it is manipulated. It has a control on the operating end of the hose, which has an on-off switch to control air flow into the hose while the pump is running. An oral evacuator tip is inserted into this control for use in the oral cavity (Fig. 13-2, *B*). The evacuator tip is changed for each patient. An electrical control switch should be conveniently located on or near the dental unit so that the vacuum pump can be turned on or off with ease.

Maintenance of evacuation systems generally includes daily cleaning of the solids trap and flushing the vacuum hose and lines with a special cleaner. This routine procedure maintains cleanliness, prevents odors, and keeps the system from clogging with debris.

The oral evacuator control should be disinfected after each use along with handpieces and other parts of the dental units.

ORAL EVACUATOR TIPS (Fig. 13-2, *C*)

Several styles of oral evacuator tips are available. Some are made of plastic, and others are stainless steel. Some tips are disposable, and others are sterilizable. Every dental assistant soon establishes a preference for a style of evacuator tip. Regardless of personal preferences, the following are a few key features that must be considered in the initial purchase of evacuator tips.

Diameter of the opening

For the tip to draw fluids from the mouth properly, approximately 10 cubic feet of air must be drawn into the evacuator tip per minute at a negative pressure of about 5 inches of mercury created by the vacuum pump. The tip should have an opening approximately 10 mm in diameter to effectively draw this volume of air at this rather low negative pressure. The low negative pressure will help prevent the soft tissues of the mouth from being sucked into the tube and stopping its function. Yet the high volume of air rushing into the evacuator tip will effectively carry fluids out of the operative field. Drastic changes in the diameter of the opening will alter the effectiveness of the evacuation system.

Surgical tips are often used when suction is required in a small area. Such is the case during surgical procedures. The effectiveness is reduced considerably for generalized evacuation purposes but excellent for concentrated evacuation in and around surgical sites.

Metal versus plastic

Metal evacuator tips are durable and can be sterilized in the autoclave. However, patients sometimes complain about the coldness of the metal on their faces when air is constantly rushing through the tip, cooling the metal. Some of the plastic tips eliminate this minor problem; however, some of them cannot be put into the autoclave.

An important consideration in the selection of a plastic tip is its stiffness. One auxiliary function of the suction tip is to act as a retractor for the soft tissues while it is used to evacuate fluids from the mouth. Some of the thin-walled plastic tips are too flexible to serve as adequate retractors.

Plastic evacuation tips are recommended during electrosurgery. This is a safety precaution to prevent burning the patient should the electrosurgery probe come in contact with the evacuator tip.

Straight versus bent styles

Depending on the dexterity of the individual assistant, the suction tips that have a bend in the center are usually more convenient to use. The bend is an aid to the assistant in reaching around the cheek and tongue to properly place the tip and helps to avoid blocking the operating light (Fig. 13-3).

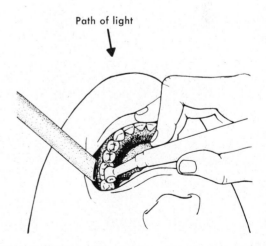

Fig. 13-3. Proper placement of an evacuator tip that will not block the path of light.

Design of the tip opening

Many unique and even bizarre designs for suction tip openings have been created to assist in retraction and prevent "tissue grabbing" while the evacuator is in use. Again, personal preference plays an important role here. If it works well in your hands—use it! However, a standard tip design with opposite bevels on each end (Fig. 13-4) will work very well in the hands of most people. Proper tip placement is the greatest factor in oral evacuation, and not the paraphernalia on the end of the tip.

Length of the tip

The length of the tip should be adequate to keep the assistant's hand out of the operating field but still able to reach all areas. A length of approximately 6 to 7 inches is recommended.

ORAL EVACUATION TECHNIQUE

The natural salivation of a patient during dental procedures plus the use of a constant water coolant sprayed into the patient's mouth from the ultraspeed handpiece have created a profound need for effective oral evacuation. In addition, rinsing techniques using the air-water syringe with the patient remaining in the supine position require the use of the oral evacuator. Both patient and dentist truly appreciate the assistant who masters an effective oral evacuation technique. Efficient evacuation prevents the patient from "drowning" in oral fluids and maintains a clear, visible operating field for the dentist.

The principal responsibility for oral evacuation falls on the chairside assistant. The following discussion of technique will serve as a guide to effective evacuation during most dental procedures. Slight modifications are needed from time to time in individual cases.

Holding the oral evacuator

Two popular methods are commonly used to hold the oral evacuator: (1) the thumb-to-nose grasp (Fig. 13-5, *A*) and (2) the modified pen grasp (Fig. 13-5, *B*).

Both methods give the assistant positive control of the evacuator tip. This is essential for the safety of the patient. Remember that a secondary function of the

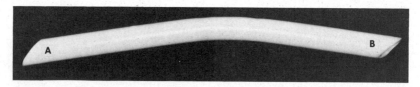

Fig. 13-4. Universal-style evacuator tip. End *A* is generally used in posterior areas and end *B* in anterior areas.

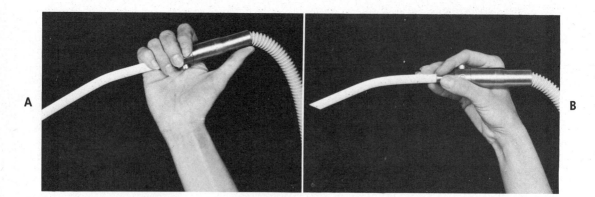

Fig. 13-5. Common methods of holding oral evacuator. **A,** Thumb-to-nose grasp. **B,** Modified pen grasp.

evacuator tip is to retract the soft tissues. This retraction requires a firm grip on the evacuator. Most assistants switch back and forth between the two grasps depending on the resistance of the tissues to retraction and the area being treated. The thumb-to-nose method is a more positive grasp that is used when more leverage is needed for retraction.

The assistant holds the evacuator in the right hand when assisting a right-handed dentist and in the left hand when assisting a left-handed dentist. The discussion here applies to the right-handed dentist.

Use of the universal evacuator tip

The universal, or standard, evacuator tip is the one commonly used for most dental procedures. It has two functional ends (Fig. 13-4). An important relationship to remember is which end of the beveled evacuator tip should be used in a given area of the oral cavity. Fig. 13-4 demonstrates that the bevels are in opposite directions on the ends of the tip. Generally, one end *(A)* is used in all posterior segments, and the other end *(B)* is used in all anterior regions (Fig. 13-6).

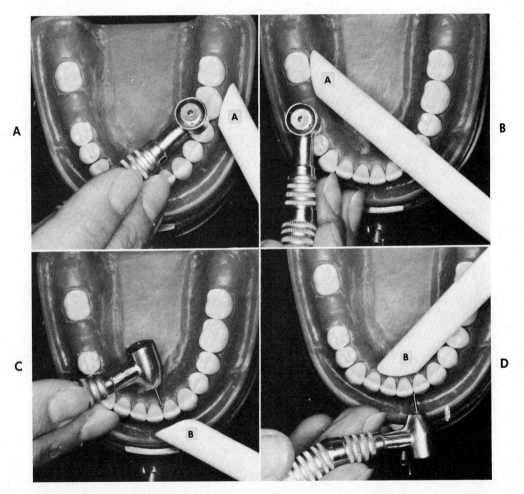

Fig. 13-6. Proper placement of universal-style evacuator tip. **A,** For posterior areas on assistant's side of patient's mouth. **B,** For posterior areas on dentist's side of patient's mouth. **C,** For anterior areas when dentist is using lingual approach. **D,** For anterior areas when dentist is using either labial or incisal approach. (End *A* is used in posterior areas; end *B* is used in anterior areas.)

When a dental handpiece is used with water coolant, the assistant must remove the water continuously to maintain a clear field of operation for the dentist. The following are six basic steps to follow in positioning the evacuator tip:

1. Select the appropriate end (*A* or *B*) for use in the segment being treated.
2. Hold the evacuator in either the thumb-to-nose or modified pen grasp.
3. If the operator is using indirect vision in a mirror, the suction tip is usually placed first to retract soft tissue and avoid trapping the mirror behind the tip. The mirror-evacuator relationship varies somewhat with the area being treated.
4. Place the tip as close as possible to the tooth being treated (usually sightly distal when an occlusal approach is used). In this position the evacuator draws the water coolant into the opening immediately after it cools the tooth being prepared.
5. Position the bevel on the suction tip so that it is parallel to the buccal or lingual surface of the tooth being prepared. This increases the efficiency of the evacuator. The tip is placed on the buccal aspect of posterior teeth being prepared on the assistant's side of the patient's mouth, and on the lingual aspect of posterior teeth that are prepared on the dentist's side of the patient's mouth (Fig. 13-6, *A* and *B*).
6. Place the upper edge of the tip slightly beyond the occlusal surface (Fig. 13-7). The evacuator tip should be thought of as a scoop to catch the water spray from the handpiece after it strikes the tooth being prepared. In

anterior preparations the same basic rules are applied, with the following exceptions:

A. If the dentist is preparing a tooth from a lingual approach, hold the beveled suction tip (end *B*) parallel with the labial surface of the tooth being prepared. The tip is held slightly beyond the incisal edge (Fig. 13-6, *C*).
B. If the dentist is preparing a tooth from either the labial or incisal approach, hold the tip parallel with the lingual surface. Again, place the tip slightly beyond the incisal edge (Fig. 13-6, *D*).

Evacuator tip placement

Fig. 13-8 demonstrates placement of the universal evacuator tip in various areas of the oral cavity for various approaches with the dental handpiece. Note the relationships between the handpiece, the tooth being prepared, the mouth mirror when used, and the evacuator tip.

One problem that is encountered by the dentist when using a mouth mirror for indirect vision is the collection of water drops on the surface of the mirror. The water drops obscure vision. This problem can be eliminated by holding the mirror as far from the tooth being prepared as possible. The assistant should maintain a constant stream of air blowing on the mirror to prevent water drops from collecting on the surface. The assistant can do this by using the left hand to operate the air-water syringe while the right hand operates the oral evacuator.

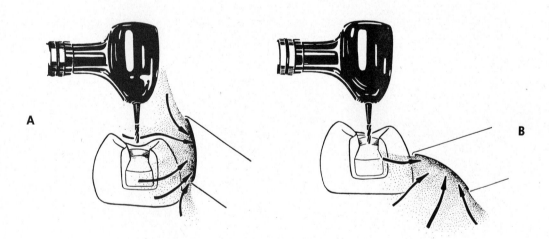

Fig. 13-7. Vertical orientation of evacuator tip relative to buccal (or lingual) surfaces for maximum efficiency. **A,** Opening of evacuator tip is placed slightly beyond occlusal surface for maximum efficiency. **B,** Placing opening too far cervically reduces efficiency.

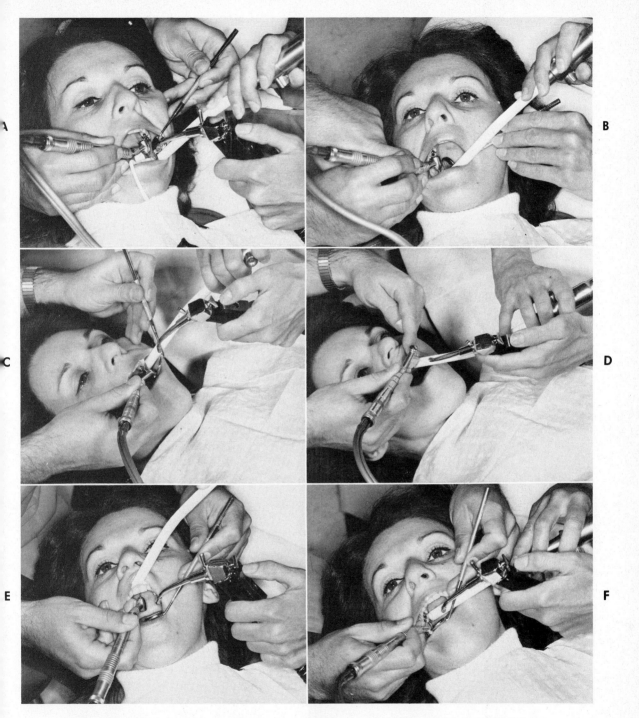

Fig. 13-8. Guide to proper evacuator tip placement. **A,** Lower left posterior segment. **B,** Lower right posterior segment. **C,** Upper left posterior segment. **D,** Upper anterior segment (labial approach). **E,** Upper anterior segment (lingual approach). **F,** Upper right posterior segment.

The mandibular lingual surfaces are difficult to treat. It is often helpful to have the assistant simply retract the tongue and evacuate intermittently as fluid accumulates in this area. Furthermore, use of a conventional-speed handpiece without water coolant is recommended for cavity refinement. Evacuator tip placement for the mandibular anterior area is similar to that shown in Fig. 13-8, *E* for the maxillary anterior area.

This technique has proved effective. In summary, it should provide the following results:

1. Removal of both fluids and debris from the oral cavity
2. Retraction of soft tissues for better access and visibility
3. Placement of the evacuator tip in such a way as not to interfere with access and visibility for the operator
4. Control of the suction tip by the assistant's right hand with the left hand free to retract, operate the air-water syringe, or transfer instruments to the operator
5. Comfort for the patient during dental procedures

ORAL RINSING TECHNIQUE

Oral rinsing maintains a clear operating field for the dentist and frees the patient's mouth of debris before dismissal. The two basic types of rinsing procedures are limited-area and complete-mouth rinsing.

Limited-area rinsing

As the name implies, limited-area rinsing is limited to a small area of the mouth being treated. It is used to maintain a clear operating field for the dentist as treatment progresses. The debris that accumulates in a tooth as a preparation proceeds can be removed quickly and conveniently, without significant delay in the procedure. This rinsing should be done automatically when the operator pauses during cavity preparation to inspect the detail of the cavity.

The limited-area rinse is accomplished by having the assistant operate the air-water syringe with the left hand and the oral evacuator with the right hand while the dentist retracts the cheeks or lips as needed to give the assistant access (Fig. 13-9). If the assistant can keep the syringe in the left hand during the preparation phase, limited-area rinsing and drying can be done rapidly every time the dentist pauses for cavity inspection. Note that four hands are at work. The dentist retracts while the assistant rinses, evacuates,

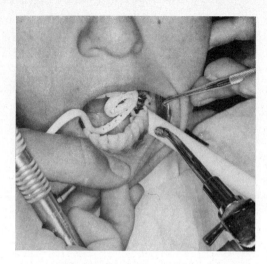

Fig. 13-9. Limited-area rinse.

and dries the preparation. Fluids that accumulate in the posterior region of the patient's mouth should be removed after each rinse.

Complete-mouth rinsing

The complete-mouth rinsing technique is designed to eliminate the need for patients to rinse and expectorate into a cuspidor. It is used whenever it is desirable to freshen the patient's entire mouth. Prolonged restorative procedures, periodontal treatment, and routine dental prophylaxis often require the use of this rinsing technique. Before the patient is dismissed after any dental procedure, it is a good idea to rinse the mouth completely, allowing the patient to leave the office with a comfortable, fresh feeling in the mouth. The method by which this can be accomplished is a matter of choice, but one of the most convenient is as follows:

1. The dentist operates the air-water syringe with the right hand and retracts the lips and cheeks with the mouth mirror held in the left hand.
2. The assistant retracts the lips and cheeks with the left hand and operates the oral evacuator with the right hand.
3. The combination of air and water produces a vigorous spray to dislodge debris.
4. Starting at the maxillary midline, the operator rinses the mouth by quadrants, finishing one side completely before proceeding to the other side (Fig. 13-10).
5. The pattern of rinsing should be to force the water to loosen and push debris posteriorly. The water collects in the posterior region, since this is the lowest part of the

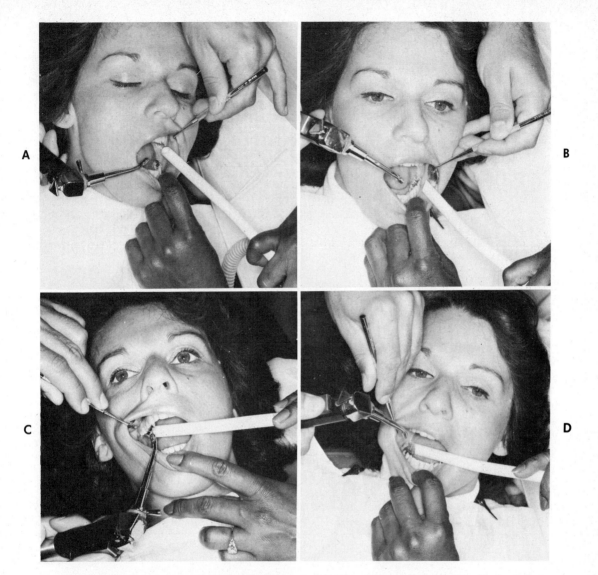

Fig. 13-10. Complete-mouth rinsing sequence. **A,** Maxillary left quadrant. **B,** Mandibular left quadrant. **C,** Maxillary right quadrant. **D,** Mandibular right quadrant.

mouth. The assistant can easily evacuate the accumulation, and the dentist can assist in the evacuation by gently blowing the accumulation of water into the evacuator tip with air from the air-water syringe.

6. The last action of the assistant with the evacuator tip should be to remove all the accumulated water in the posterior region until the evacuator just picks up the mucosa. This must be done quickly and gently. It ensures removal of all the water and leaves the patient dry and comfortable.

7. Immediately after removal of the water, it is helpful for the assistant to suggest that the patient swallow by stating, for example, "Now that your mouth is clean, you can swallow if you like." This reassures the patient that the mouth is clean and it is safe to swallow. Hence, the patient is less likely to look for a place to expectorate.

8. Patients who still feel the need to rinse at the end of treatment can simply use a cup of water and one of the sinks in the operatory before they leave.

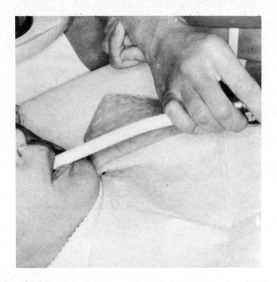

Fig. 13-11. Use of the evacuator tip in lieu of a cuspidor to flush the oral cavity.

An alternative follow-up rinsing method is placing water in the patient's mouth with the air-water syringe and instructing the patient to swish the water around vigorously. Then, the oral evacuator tip is placed in the patient's mouth and turned on. The patient expectorates by simply pushing the water forward into the tube. It is advisable to instruct the patient in this technique before placing water in the mouth (Fig. 13-11).

SUMMARY

Oral evacuation is one of the most important standard duties of the chairside assistant. Maintaining a clear operating field for the dentist and eliminating the need for a cuspidor to rinse the mouth can reduce the time required for a given procedure by as much as 15%.

The patient relies heavily on the dental assistant to remove the fluid from the mouth during a procedure to make treatment a more comfortable experience. Likewise, the dentist depends on the assistant to monitor fluid accumulation and remove it as needed. Most of the time assistants have a better line of sight into the most posterior areas of the oral cavity because of their working position. Therefore they are in a more favorable position to perform this task than is the dentist.

BIBLIOGRAPHY

Chasteen, J.E.: Four-handed dentistry in clinical practice, St. Louis, 1980, The C.V. Mosby Co.
Davies, M.H., and others: Criteria of air flow and negative pressure for high volume dental suction, Br. Dent. J. **130:**483-487, 1971.
Kilpatrick, H.C.: Work simplification in dental practice, ed. 3, Philadelphia, 1974, W.B. Saunders Co.
Robinson, G.E., and others: Four-handed dentistry manual, ed. 3, Birmingham, 1971, University of Alabama School of Dentistry.
Snedaker, R.F.: High volume evacuation, Philadelphia, 1971, W.B. Saunders Co.
Thompson, E.O.: Clinical application of the washed field technique in dentistry, J. Am. Dent. Assoc. **51:**703-713, 1955.
Thompson, W.R.: Principles of evacuative systems, Dent. Clin. North Am. 367-381, July 1967.

CHAPTER 14

INSTRUMENT TRANSFER

The elimination of unnecessary movement by the dentist while dental services are performed is one of the principles of work simplification. Techniques have been developed that are designed to transport instruments and materials to and from the patient's oral cavity with minimum movement by the dentist. Since hundreds of movements are required to perform dental services throughout each day, it makes sense to try to eliminate unnecessary movements and reduce the extent of movement by the operating team.

One of the principal chairside functions of a dental assistant is delivering instruments and material to the dentist as they are needed without delay. This requires a standardization of the operating sequence so that the assistant can anticipate the operator's needs as the procedure progresses. A smooth, efficient instrument transfer technique requires coordination and communication between the dentist and the assistant. The rewards for these team efforts result in less fatigue, a more continuous "flow" of the procedure, and a reduction in eyestrain for the dentist.

The instrument transfer techniques described in this chapter are designed to eliminate Class IV and V movements and allow the dentist's eyes to remain rather fixed on the brightly illuminated operative field. The discussion will center around the techniques used while assisting a right-handed dentist.

EFFECTIVE USE OF ASSISTANT'S LEFT HAND

Since the evacuator is handled with the right hand in most instances, the assistant's left hand is free for the following tasks during a dental procedure:

1. Retraction of soft tissue, to improve visibility and access for the dentist (Fig. 14-1, *A*)
2. Retrieval and exchange of instruments as they are needed (Fig. 14-1, *B*)
3. Operation of the air-water syringe to clear the operating field (Fig. 14-1, *C*)

4. Wiping the working end of instruments, such as scalers, spoon excavators, and cavity-liner applicators, as they are withdrawn from the patient's mouth (Fig. 14-1, *D*)

The phase of the treatment sequence and other circumstances determine how the assistant uses the left hand. A thorough knowledge of both the procedure and the dentist's established working pattern helps the assistant to be most effective with the left hand. A little common sense added to this knowledge is of value as well. For example, in difficult cases in which soft tissues are blocking visibility and access for the dentist, retraction would be the function of choice for the assistant's left hand. It would be senseless for the assistant to hold the next instrument ready for exchange in the left hand when the dentist cannot even see to manipulate the instrument already in use.

An alert assistant is mentally involved in the entire procedure along with the dentist so as to be readily aware of the operator's needs as the treatment progresses. There is no room for daydreaming or an idle mind in effective chairside assisting.

A general rule with regard to effective use of the assistant's hands is simply to remember the name of this entire assisting technique—*four-handed dentistry!* Not three-handed or two-handed dentistry, but four-handed dentistry. The assistant who is using only one hand during a procedure is probably not assisting the dentist enough.

COMMON INSTRUMENT TRANSFER METHODS

Following are criteria that can be used in selecting an instrument-transfer method:

1. The movement required by the operator for an instrument transfer should be limited to Class III movements at the most.
2. Transfer methods used should be suitable for most common dental instruments. These in-

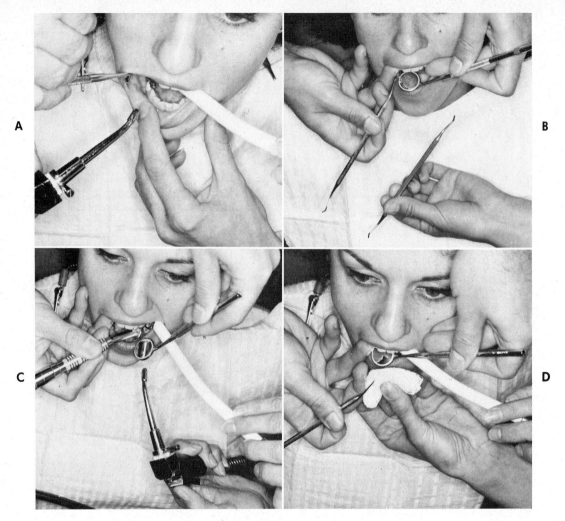

Fig. 14-1. Assistant's left hand can be used for **A,** retraction of soft tissue, **B,** instrument transfer, **C,** operating air-water syringe, and **D,** debridement of instruments with 2 × 2 inch gauze sponge.

clude hand instruments and instruments with attached hoses.

3. Transfer methods should not require the operator's vision to shift from the operative field to execute a smooth, stable transfer.

4. Whenever possible, transfers should require the use of only the assistant's left hand (for a right-handed operator). This leaves the assistant's right hand free to do other tasks, such as maintaining retraction, operating the evacuator tip, delivering materials to the oral cavity, or drying the operative field with the air-water syringe.

5. Any instrument transfer method that is selected should be easy to learn with a little practice. Stable transfers are mandatory for safety, since they are executed near the patient's face.

The three most common methods of transferring instruments between the dentist and assistant are (1) the hidden syringe transfer, (2) the two-handed transfer, and (3) the pickup-and-delivery method.

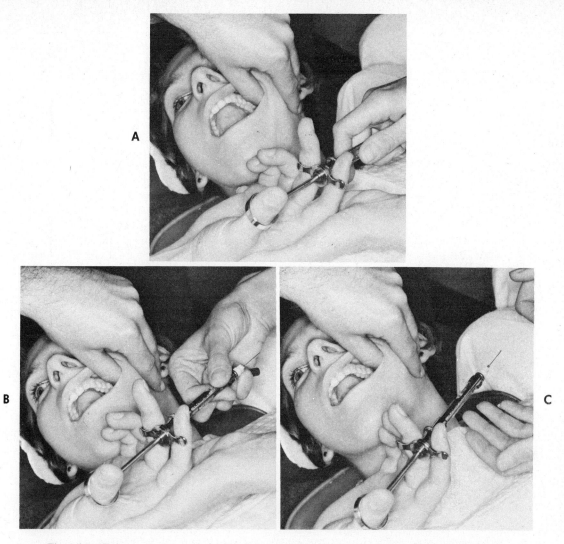

Fig. 14-2. Hidden syringe transfer. **A,** Delivery of syringe by assistant while stabilizing operator's hand. **B,** Cap removal and needle bevel orientation while assistant stabilizes operator's hand. **C,** Release of operator's right hand.

Hidden syringe transfer

Many dental patients fear the dental injection more than any other phase of dental treatment. It should be a challenge to the dental team to make the injection as pleasant as possible. One important part of this task is to keep the syringe out of the patient's line of sight during its preparation and delivery to the dentist. The syringe can be prepared before the patient arrives and then covered so that the patient cannot see it when entering the operatory.

After the injection site is prepared, the syringe should be delivered to the dentist in such a way that the patient cannot see it. Following is a method that is helpful in accomplishing the hidden syringe transfer:

1. Ask the patient to tip the head backward slightly.
2. Raise the operating light so that it is almost in the patient's eyes.
3. Apply the disinfectant.
4. The dentist should continue to look at the injection site while the assistant places the syringe securely in the dentist's hand. This is done below the level of the patient's line of sight.
5. The left hand of the dentist is used to retract the lips and cheeks, palpate anatomical landmarks, and hold the patient's head in the desired position.
6. These preliminary steps make it difficult for the patient to ''peek'' during the transfer. The patient who tries will probably see only the bright operating light.
7. The assistant loosens the protective cap on the needle.
8. The syringe is delivered to the operator's open hand. The assistant guides the operator's thumb into the thumb ring by holding the operator's right hand with her left hand. Stabilizing the operator's right hand during the transfer eliminates the need for the operator to watch the transfer take place (Fig. 14-2, *A*).
9. Once the syringe is positioned properly in the operator's hand, the cap is removed, and the needle bevel can be oriented properly for the area being anesthetized (Fig. 14-2, *B*).
10. Once the needle is properly oriented, the assistant releases the operator's right hand, to signal that the syringe is ready for the injection (Fig. 14-2, *C*).
11. The process is reversed for the return of the syringe to the assistant after the injection. The cap should be replaced after the syringe is removed from the transfer zone. The operating team should establish some landmarks on the dentist's right hand that can be used as a guide to proper placement of the syringe. Once this is accomplished, the same landmarks can be used every time the syringe is transferred.

This procedure is effective with both adults and children. The dentist's constant eye contact with the injection site eliminates the patient's desire to see what the dentist is looking at, which may result if the dentist watches the assistant transfer the syringe.

Two-handed transfer

Use of the two-handed instrument transfer technique requires the use of both the assistant's hands. This may or may not be a disadvantage, depending on the type of treatment being rendered or the phase of the procedure in which the transfer is needed. Sometimes the assistant's right hand is not needed for other tasks when an instrument is exchanged; in this case, two-handed transfer is useful and convenient. Heavy instruments, such as surgical forceps and elevators, are easier to transfer by the two-handed method.

Essentially, the technique requires the use of the right hand to pick up the unwanted instrument from the operator and then the left hand to deliver the new instrument (Fig. 14-3). The instrument that is delivered should be oriented so that it is in the appropriate working position when placed in the operator's

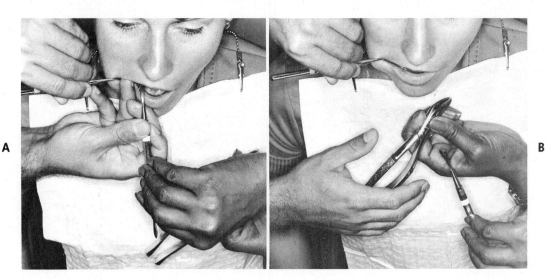

Fig. 14-3. A, Retrieval of unwanted instrument with assistant's right hand. **B,** Delivery of desired instrument with assistant's left hand.

hand. The unwanted instrument is returned to its proper position on the preset tray so that it can be located quickly if needed again later in the procedure.

Pickup-and-delivery method (one handed)

The pickup-and-delivery method of transferring instruments has gained great popularity because it meets all the criteria stated previously. Once the dental team masters this one-handed technique, they will recognize its superior convenience.

The basic description of the one-handed instrument exchange applies to the transfer of hand instruments, handpieces, and the air-water syringe. Forceps and scissors exchanges are made by the same fundamental method with a slight modification that will be described later.

The assistant's left hand is divided into two parts, according to the function of the fingers of the hand. The thumb and first two fingers working together form the "delivery" part of the hand, and the last two fingers form the "pickup" part of the hand (Fig. 14-4). When the dentist has finished using an instrument and wants to exchange it for another, the assistant picks up the unwanted instrument with the pickup fingers and delivers the new instrument with the delivery thumb and fingers (Fig. 14-5). The assistant accomplishes the entire exchange using the left hand. The right hand is free to operate other instruments or

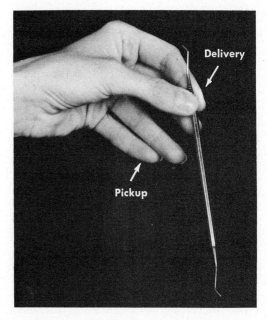

Fig. 14-4. Pickup and delivery portions of assistant's left hand.

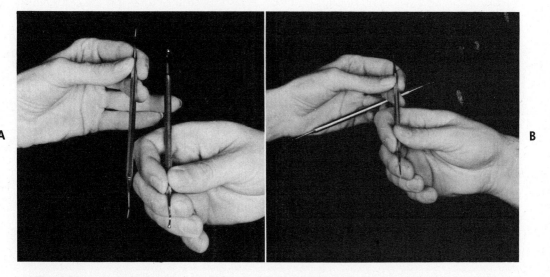

Fig. 14-5. A, Assistant's pickup fingers in position to retrieve unwanted instrument from operator. **B,** Delivery of new instrument with delivery portion of hand.

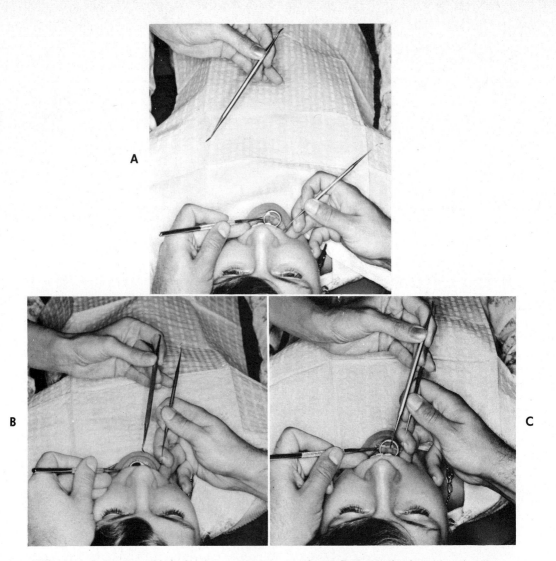

Fig. 14-6. A, Ready position of an instrument to be transferred. **B,** Paralleling instrument handles. **C,** Pickup fingers grasping unwanted instrument. **D,** Tucking retrieved instrument into palm and delivery of new instrument to operator. **E,** Rolling instrument between thumb and last two fingers to reposition it in delivery portion of hand. **F,** Instrument repositioned in delivery portion of assistant's hand, in readiness for another exchange if needed.

to retract. The sequence of the instrument exchange is as follows:

1. Hold the instrument to be delivered between the tip of the thumb and the first two fingers. The instrument must be held close to the end opposite from the one the operator will use after the instrument is delivered. Hold it 8 to 10 inches away in the ready position until a signal is given for the exchange to begin (Fig. 14-6, *A*).

2. Position the working end of the instrument so that it will be in the proper operating position for the area being treated. Cutting edges of hand instruments and the burs of handpieces should be directed downward for mandibular and upward for maxillary areas.

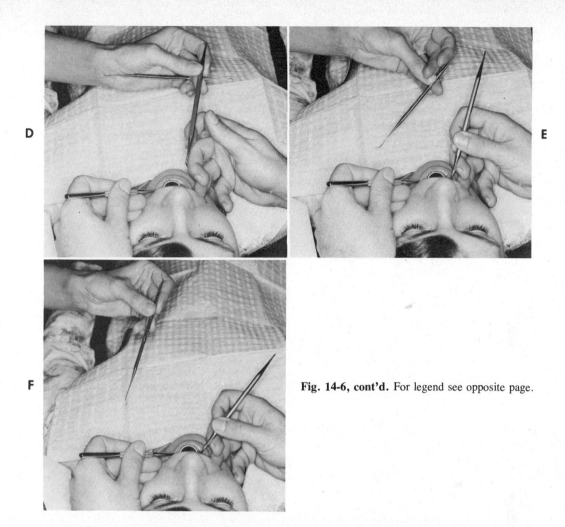

Fig. 14-6, cont'd. For legend see opposite page.

3. When the operator signals a readiness to exchange instruments, position the instrument close to the dentist's right hand and hold it so that the handle is parallel to the handle of the instrument in the dentist's hand (Fig. 14-6, *B*). This is important. The dentist should not have to reach for an instrument; it should be delivered close to the hand. Paralleling the instruments prevents tangling during the exchange.
4. Next, extend the pickup fingers and grasp the instrument in the operator's hand at the end opposite the working end (Fig. 14-6, *C*).
5. Fold the pickup fingers into the palm, and lift the hand slightly above the operator's hand. These movements lift the unwanted instrument from the dentist's hand and tuck it into the assistant's palm (Fig. 14-6, *D*).

6. Once the unwanted instrument is tucked into the palm, deliver the new instrument by simply lowering it into the operator's hand.
7. If the same two instruments are to be exchanged again immediately, reposition the retrieved instrument from the pickup fingers into the delivery fingers. Roll the instrument between the thumb and pickup fingers and shift it to the delivery fingers in readiness for the next exchange (Fig. 14-6, *E* and *F*).

The handpiece can be exchanged for another instrument in the same manner (Fig. 14-7). Caution should be exercised in orienting the hoses when two handpieces are exchanged to avoid tangling them during the exchange.

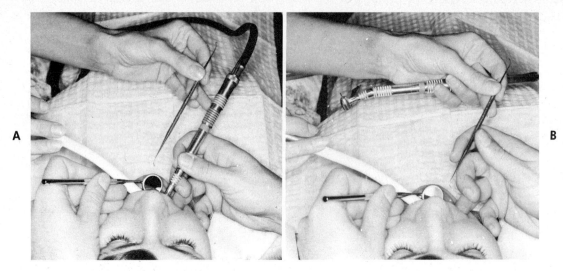

Fig. 14-7. A, Retrieval of handpiece from operator. **B,** Delivery of explorer.

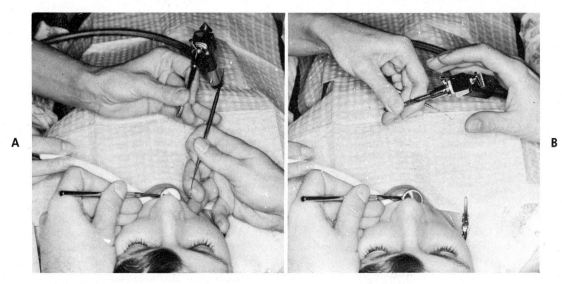

Fig. 14-8. A, Retrieval of unwanted instrument. **B,** Delivery of air-water syringe.

The assistant conveniently transfers the air-water syringe to the dentist by holding the nozzle of the syringe in the delivery fingers. If the dentist is already holding a hand instrument, it can be removed with the pickup fingers as just described. Deliver the handle of the syringe by bending the wrist slightly as the dentist positions the hand to receive it (Fig. 14-8). Scissors and forceps are delivered in a similar fashion, except that the operator's hand must be positioned as shown in Fig. 14-9 to receive these instruments.

When nonlocking cotton pliers are used to pick up or deliver various items to and from the oral cavity, a modification in the transfer must be made. For example, if articulating paper is delivered to the dentist

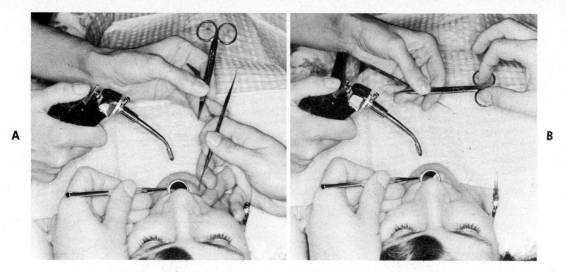

Fig. 14-9. A, Retrieval of unwanted instrument. **B,** Delivery of scissors.

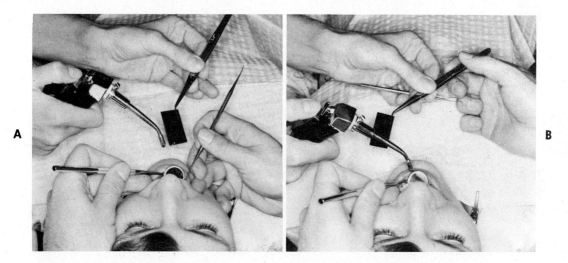

Fig. 14-10. A, Retrieval of unwanted instrument. **B,** Delivery of cotton pliers and contents.

in nonlocking cotton pliers, the assistant must deliver the pliers to the dentist while pinching the beaks together with the delivery fingers and thumb to avoid dropping the paper. The pliers are delivered so that the dentist can grasp and hold the beaks together before the assistant releases them (Fig. 14-10). Pickup of the same pliers is made by the pickup fingers at the working end of the pliers, again to avoid dropping the articulating paper. Many dentists prefer to use non-

locking cotton pliers, so this transfer method is often needed.

At the beginning of each procedure the dentist often wishes to inspect the area to be treated with a mirror and explorer. The assistant can deliver both of these at the same time with a two-handed exchange, since no other instruments must be handled during this beginning phase. The dentist can signal readiness to receive the instruments by placing the open hands

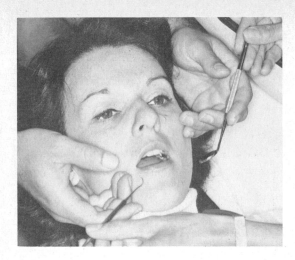

Fig. 14-11. Simultaneous delivery of mirror and explorer.

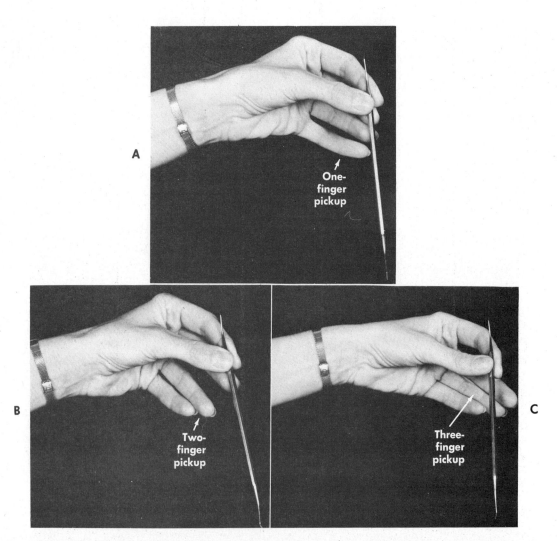

Fig. 14-12. Alternative hand positions for retrieving instruments from operator. **B** is recommended.

on each side of the patient's mouth. This not only tells the assistant, ''I am ready,'' but also fixes the hands in a standard position to receive the instruments (Fig. 14-11).

A definite relationship exists between a well-organized preset tray and effective instrument transfer. The preset tray should be kept in order throughout a procedure, and each instrument should be returned to its proper position on the tray after it is used. This orderliness will permit the assistant to select needed instruments quickly without unnecessary delays. The experienced assistant can mentally visualize the position of every instrument on the preset tray after working with the setup several times. Once this is mastered, instrument transfers can become smooth and efficient.

HELPFUL HINTS
Pickup-and-delivery modifications

Alternate methods of doing the pickup-and-delivery instrument transfer are available for chairside assistants who experience difficulty in using the last two fingers of the left hand for picking up the unwanted instrument. In these cases either the last finger or the

last three fingers can be used to form the pickup portion of the hand (Fig. 14-12). The use of the last two fingers for this purpose is encouraged because of greater stability in both the pickup and delivery positions of the hand.

Pickup-and-delivery practice

The chairside assistant bears most of the responsibility for executing a smooth instrument transfer. Use of the technique requires practice to develop the necessary skill. Since the operator is not always available for practice sessions, the following practice method is recommended:

1. Hold an instrument in the delivery position of the left hand.
2. At the same time, hold another instrument in the right hand with a pen grasp, simulating the operator's right hand.
3. Then make repeated exchanges of instruments from the left hand to the right hand after repositioning the retrieved instrument in the left hand (Fig. 14-13).

This exercise is designed to develop both the pickup-and-delivery skills of the left hand. In addition,

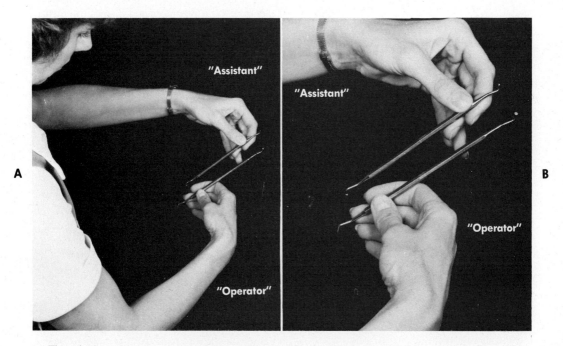

Fig. 14-13. A, Dental assistant's hand position for practicing pickup-and-delivery method of instrument transfer. **B,** Assistant's right hand represents operator's right hand during practice session.

the repositioning maneuver with which an instrument is shifted from the pickup fingers to the delivery portion of the left hand is developed.

Finger signal

Repeated verbal communication can become tiring for both the dentist and assistant. A dentist can soon tire of calling for instruments as they are needed throughout a workday. Also, the assistant can tire of unnecessary requests for instruments. Use of a standardized operating sequence helps reduce the need for this type of communication and enhances the flow of the procedure. The operator who standardizes the sequence becomes predictable, and the chairside assistant can anticipate needs.

Once the assistant has an instrument ready to transfer, the operator can signal readiness to receive the instrument by simply withdrawing the instrument from the operative field by bending the index finger and shifting the instrument away from the oral cavity (Fig. 14-14). This eliminates the need to use such verbal indicators as "ready," "now," or "OK" every time an instrument exchange is needed.

Depending on the area being treated, the dentist can help the assistant with the exchange by maintaining a finger rest and "presenting" the instrument to the assistant. Maintenance of the finger rest fixes the

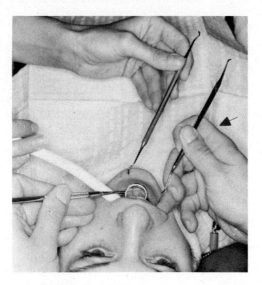

Fig. 14-14. Finger signal to begin exchange.

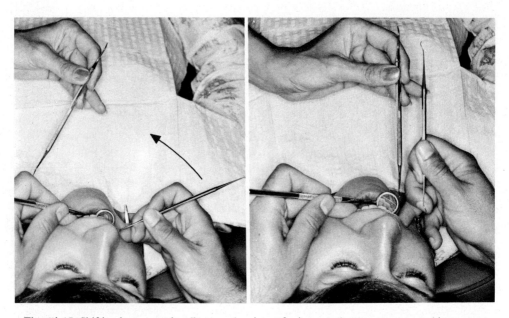

Fig. 14-15. Shifting instrument handle toward assistant for improved access to unwanted instrument during exchange.

hand in a predictable position, so that an instrument can be delivered at a fixed point without the assistant having to guess where the hand will be located as the exchange begins. This also eliminates the need for the operator to look at the instruments as the exchange is made and thus helps to reduce the eye fatigue discussed previously.

If the operator's hand is located far to the patient's right side, it is helpful to present the handle portion of the instrument to the assistant during the finger-signal phase. This is accomplished by simply shifting the handle slightly toward the assistant when the signal is given (Fig. 14-15). This helps the assistant parallel the instrument handles as the exchange begins.

The operator should never present an instrument to the assistant past the patient's midline. Placing the instrument handle too close to the assistant only complicates the exchange. Placing the handle at a 45° angle to the midline seems to be the most favorable.

Common problems and solutions

Crowding. Sometimes a chairside assistant can be overzealous in having an instrument ready for transfer to the dentist by holding it too close to the operator's hand while another instrument is still being used by the operator. This "crowding" can be distracting. In addition, it often leads to false starts of an exchange if the operator withdraws the instrument from the oral cavity, since the assistant may misinterpret this movement as a finger signal to begin the exchange. It is suggested that the chairside assistant hold an instrument ready at a distance of 8 to 10 inches from the operator's hand, in anticipation of an instrument transfer. Once a positive finger signal is given, the instrument is brought close to the operator's hand and the handles of the instruments are then paralleled to begin the exchange.

Shorting. Shorting is the delivery of an instrument to the operator in such a way that the hand receives it too close to the working end (Fig. 14-16, *A*). This usually occurs if the assistant does not hold the instrument in the delivery portion of the hand far enough from the working end (Fig. 14-16, *B*). With practice the assistant should be able to judge where to grasp the instrument before delivery.

Tangling. Tangling of instruments during an exchange is usually caused by failure to parallel the handles before an exchange (Fig. 14-17).

Disorientation. Before delivery to the operator, instruments should be oriented in the working position that is correct for the area being treated. The

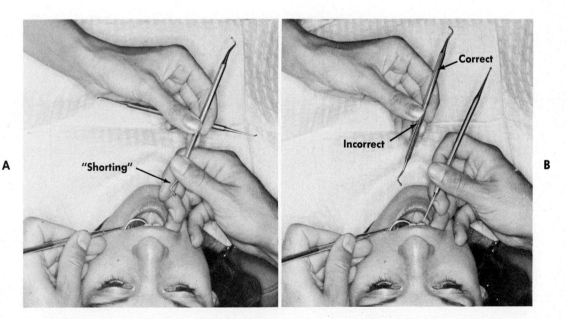

Fig. 14-16. A, Delivery of an instrument to operator too close to working end, or shorting. **B,** Cause of shorting. Assistant does not hold instrument far enough from working end.

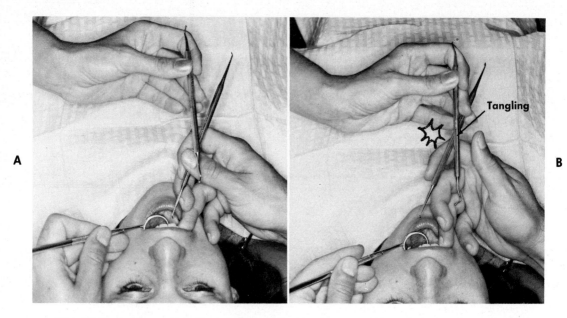

Fig. 14-17. A, Nonparalleled instrument handles may lead to tangling of instruments during exchange. **B,** Instruments tangled during transfer attempt.

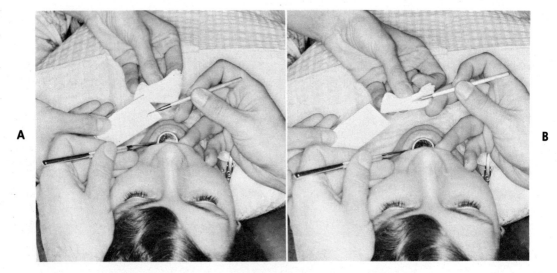

Fig. 14-18. A, Delivery of cavity liner on mixing pad in assistant's right hand. **B,** Wiping insertion instrument with 2 × 2 inch gauze sponge between applications of liner.

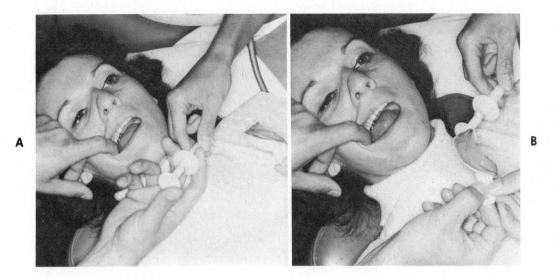

Fig. 14-19. A, Delivery of syringe filled with impression material. **B,** Delivery of impression tray.

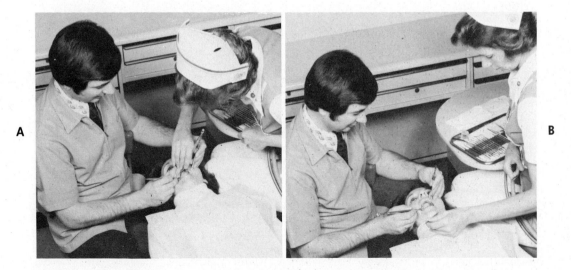

Fig. 14-20. A, Dental assistant leaning excessively to insert amalgam in an area of the mouth that is more accessible to operator. **B,** Operator inserting amalgam in same preparation while both members of operating team remain in balanced posture.

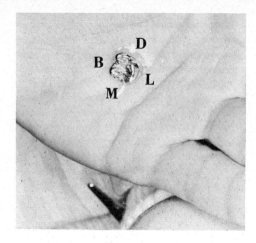

Fig. 14-21. Restoration placed cement side down and oriented properly.

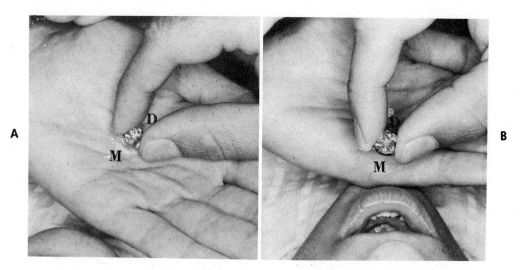

Fig. 14-22. A, Mandibular restoration picked up with operator's palm down and **(B)** carried to oral cavity.

operator should not have to shift an instrument in the hand after it has been delivered. The working end should be pointing upward for maxillary areas and downward for mandibular areas.

PREPARATION OF DENTAL MATERIALS

One of the challenges to an operating team is to establish favorable timing for the various phases of a procedure to promote flow. One of the most common interruptions in flow is during the preparation of den-

tal materials. Once a procedure has been standardized, the operating team should plan the preparation of materials so that they are ready for use when the operator needs them. This requires planning, coordination, and communication.

The dental assistant's having materials set up in advance, knowledge of the procedure in progress, and use of a standardized sequence all contribute to minimizing delays associated with the preparation of dental materials.

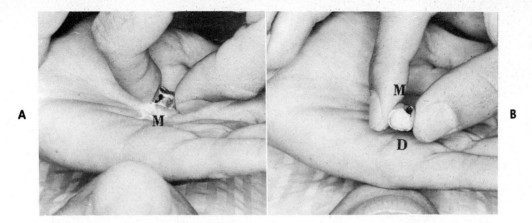

Fig. 14-23. A, Maxillary restoration picked up with operator's hand rotated so that palm is turned away from patient's face. **B,** After restoration is picked up, operator's hand is rotated so that palm is down, with restoration in proper orientation for upper arch.

DELIVERY OF DENTAL MATERIALS

Generally, materials should be delivered to the operator over the chest area of the patient.

Cements and liners. Cements and liners can be delivered on a mixing slab or pad, along with an insertion instrument. It is helpful for the assistant to hold the mixing pad in the right hand and a 2 × 2 gauze in the left hand. The dentist has convenient access to the material, and the assistant can then wipe the tip of the insertion instrument as needed (Fig. 14-18).

Impression materials. Impression materials can be delivered directly to the operator in syringes and impression trays (Fig. 14-19).

Amalgam. The question of whether the assistant should deliver dental amalgam to the operator for insertion or place it in the prepared cavity often arises. It is really a matter of convenience. The assistant who can see and reach the prepared cavity conveniently should place the material directly in the cavity, thus eliminating unnecessary instrument exchanges. However, rather than go through uncomfortable contortions to insert the material, the assistant should deliver it to the operator for insertion (Fig. 14-20).

Restorations to be cemented. Once cement has been applied to a gold restoration or orthodontic band, it should be delivered to the operator in the open palm of the assistant's left hand. The restoration should be oriented cement side down and with proper mesiodistal orientation (Fig. 14-21). The operator can then pick up the restoration between the thumb and index finger without touching the cemented surface. This is most significant during the transfer of inlay restorations. Mandibular restorations should be picked up with the operator's palm down (Fig. 14-22). Maxillary restorations can be picked up with the palm rotated away from the patient's face (Fig. 14-23). Use of this maneuver keeps the operator from having to reorient the restoration after picking it up from the assistant's hand.

SUMMARY

The development of a smooth instrument-transfer technique is based on the concept of work simplification. The operating team can use either of the techniques discussed in this chapter; however, maximum use of the pickup-and-delivery method whenever possible is recommended to promote predictability and efficiency.

BIBLIOGRAPHY

Robinson, G.E., and others: Four-handed dentistry manual, ed. 3, Birmingham, 1971. University of Alabama School of Dentistry.

OPERATIVE DENTISTRY

CHAPTER 15

CLASSIFICATION AND MEDICATION OF CAVITY PREPARATIONS

Operative dentistry has traditionally been considered that area of dental practice primarily concerned with the preservation and restoration of tooth tissue. In the area of operative dentistry the majority of carious lesions and tooth fractures are treated. Most restorations that are fabricated by operative dentistry techniques are primarily contained within the confines of the tooth itself. The public simply identifies operative restorations by referring to them collectively as "fillings." Restorations that serve to contain the majority of the crown area of the tooth, such as gold crowns, porcelain jackets, and fixed bridges, are often considered a part of crown and bridge prosthodontics. Crown and bridge procedures are discussed in Chapter 20.

There are several different categories of operative restorations. The methods used to fabricate these restorations vary from one dentist to another. However, each dentist must use basically the same fundamentals to produce a successful result. These fundamentals are discussed with regard to the amalgam restoration, esthetic restoration, cast gold inlay restoration, and gold foil restoration in subsequent chapters in this section.

CAVITY CLASSIFICATION

Several years ago the dentist G.V. Black developed a system of classifying dental caries according to its location on the tooth surface. Clinical experience has demonstrated that caries occurring in tooth surfaces with developmental pits and fissures differs in its progression from caries occurring on the smooth surfaces of the teeth. As a result, the two different types of caries are treated differently and are classified by

where they most commonly occur on the teeth. A summary of Black's cavity classification is shown in Table 15-1.

Cavity classification is only useful when teeth have a limited extension of decay on the various tooth surfaces. Teeth that are extremely mutilated by decay do not fit into Black's classification scheme. Each dentist generally establishes a personal method of referring to extensively destroyed teeth.

Cavity classification is one method the dentist uses to assess fees for services. For example, different fees are assessed for Class I amalgam restorations than for Class II amalgam restorations. A basic understanding of this classification scheme will be helpful for the dental assistant in business office procedures.

CAVITY PREPARATIONS

A cavity preparation is a systematic cutting of tooth structure in which any unwanted portion of the hard layers of the tooth is removed. These unwanted portions of the tooth are usually one or more of the following:

1. Carious tooth structure
2. Fractured tooth fragments
3. Enamel not supported by dentin
4. Enamel pits and fissures that are considered vulnerable to carious activity

The design of the prepared cavity must provide suitable containment of the restorative material. The preparation must hold the restorative material firmly in place. Proper preparation design will also help prevent fracture of the restorative material or of the tooth when the tooth is subjected to biting forces.

All cavity preparation designs include three basic

Table 15-1. G.V. Black's classification of cavities

Class	Description	Appearance
I	Cavities beginning in the pit and fissure areas of teeth A. Occlusal surfaces of posterior teeth	
	B. Buccal or lingual surfaces of posterior teeth	
	C. Occasional defects in either the incisal or occlusal two thirds of all teeth	
	D. Lingual surfaces of incisors	
II	Cavities on proximal surfaces of *posterior teeth*	
III	Cavities on proximal surfaces of *anterior teeth* that do not involve the inangle	

Continued.

Table 15-1. G.V. Black's classification of cavities—cont'd

Class	Description	Appearance
IV	Cavities on proximal surfaces of *anterior teeth* that require restoration of the incisal angle	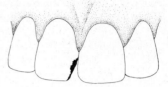
V	Cavities on the cervical one third of all teeth that originate on a smooth surface	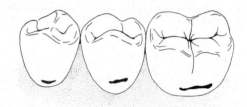

Modifications (used in various regions of the United States)

Class	Description	Appearance
II	Cavities on one proximal surface of a posterior tooth	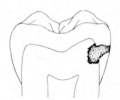
VI	Cavities on incisal edges or cusp tips that are not included in Black's original classification	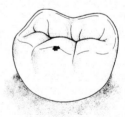
VI	Cavities on *both* proximal surfaces of *posterior teeth*, which when restored will be joined across occlusal surface by restoration	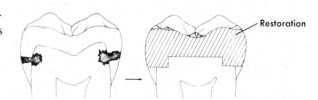

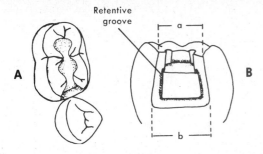

Fig. 15-1. A, Outline form of Class II amalgam preparation. B, Class II amalgam preparation viewed into proximal box, demonstrating that preparation is wider at base (*b*) than at occlusal surface (*a*).

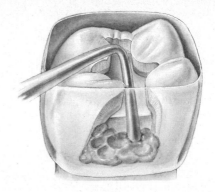

Fig. 15-2. Insertion of amalgam in its moldable state into a slightly "undercut" preparation. (From Howard, W.W., and Moller, R.C.: Atlas of operative dentistry, ed. 3, St. Louis, 1981, The C.V. Mosby Co.)

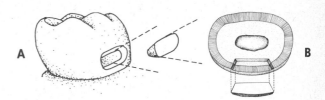

Fig. 15-3. A, Class V inlay preparation demonstrating "draw." B, Cross section of A.

considerations: (1) outline form, (2) resistance form, and (3) retention form.

Outline form. Outline form is the overall shape of the preparation along the external surface of the enamel, or the cavosurface margin. The outline form is determined by the size and shape of the carious lesion and by the need for a suitable design that will hold a restoration firmly in place. The concept *extension for prevention* also determines outline form. This is the extension of the preparation so as to eliminate deep occlusal fissures and to place the margins of the restoration in areas that are easy for the patient to keep clean (Fig. 15-1).

Resistance form. Resistance form is the internal shape of the cavity preparation. This shape is designed to protect both the restoration and the tooth from fracture when biting forces are applied to the restored tooth.

Retention form. Retention form is the relationship that exists between the different walls of the preparation, which creates a mechanical retention of the restorative material. The walls of an amalgam restoration are generally parallel to slightly undercut in their relationship to each other. Retention is also enhanced by the addition of retentive grooves in the walls of cavity preparations (Fig. 15-1). All cavity preparations that have proper outline, resistance, and retention form provide the foundation for a successful restoration.

• • •

The basic internal design of a cavity preparation is dictated by the restorative material to be used in it. All restorative materials that are placed in a prepared cavity while they are in a soft, moldable state require a different internal design from restorative materials that are placed in the prepared cavity in a completely hard state.

Moldable materials such as amalgam, acrylics, composites, and gold foil require a cavity design that will hold them in place by mechanical lock. Mechanical lock is provided when such a soft, moldable material is packed into a cavity that has its cavity walls parallel or slightly undercut in relation to each other. The soft material hardens while in the preparation after it has been properly shaped during its soft stage (Fig. 15-2).

Hard substances such as cast gold and porcelain restorations (inlays) are held in place by the "grasping action" of the dentin and enamel walls of the cavity preparation. These restorations are hard substances at the time of insertion into the prepared cavity. The preparation design must not only provide a grasping action by the tooth but also allow the restoration to be conveniently slid into place. Once the restoration is in place, it must adapt tightly to the cavity walls. Thus the internal design of a cavity preparation for a gold or porcelain inlay must have its walls tapered from the base of the preparation to the cavosurface margin. This is called "draw" (Fig. 15-3). The taper should be enough to allow the insertion of the inlay into the preparation but not so much that the inlay readily falls out of the preparation. Inlays are sealed in the cavity preparation by the use of a variety of cementing agents.

Specific cavity designs for each type of restoration will be shown during the discussion of each individual operative procedure.

MEDICATION OF THE CAVITY PREPARATION

Cavity medication is the cleaning of the cavity preparation and the placement of appropriate agents in the prepared cavity that will assist in the maintenance of a healthy pulp.

One of the great variables in cavity preparation design is the depth of the cavity after the caries is removed. This is determined by the size of the carious lesion. Regardless of what type of restorative material is to be used, every cavity preparation design must include a strong consideration of the health of the dental pulp. Shallow cavity preparations are treated differently from those that involve removal of extensive amounts of carious dentin. Generally, most cavity preparations can be placed in four categories according to the depth of the prepared cavity. Each category is medicated differently before the restorative material is placed over the medication.

Four categories of cavity depth

1. A cavity preparation that has ideal minimal depth to retain the restorative material (Fig. 15-4, *A*).
2. A cavity preparation that had to be extended beyond the ideal minimal depth to remove caries (Fig. 15-4, *B*). However, there is still no serious invasion of the pulp.
3. A cavity preparation that nearly exposes the dental pulp after caries is removed (Fig. 15-4, *C*). A thin layer of healthy dentin still covers the pulp. This is commonly referred to as a near-exposure cavity preparation.
4. A cavity preparation that extends so deeply into the dentin that an actual exposure of the pulp can be observed (Fig. 15-4, *D*). These pulp exposures must be minimal in size if there is to be any hope for the pulp to survive.

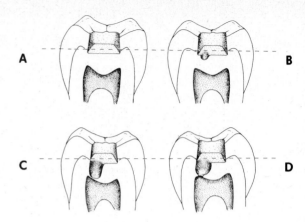

Fig. 15-4. Four categories of cavity depth. **A,** Ideal depth just beyond dentinoenamel junction. **B,** Extension of cavity depth slightly deeper than ideal. **C,** Near-exposure of pulp. **D,** Pulp exposure.

Treatment of the minimal-depth cavity preparation

The cavity preparation of minimal depth can be medicated adequately by cleaning the prepared cavity with a vigorous spray of an air-water mixture from the air-water syringe found on most standard dental units. The cavity is isolated and dried with the air-water syringe. The dentin is then coated with a thin layer of cavity varnish (Fig. 15-5, *A*). Varnish is easily applied with tiny cotton pellets held in cotton pliers. Two thin coats of varnish are more effective than one thick coat. Cavity varnish seals the open ends of the dentin tubules with a glazelike covering.

Remember that the dentin tubules represent microscopic "tunnels" that extend from the pulp out to the now prepared cavity. The varnish closes the end of each tubule within the cavity preparation to prevent further irritation of the tooth by oral fluids that may seep under the restoration in the future.

Treatment of the more extensive–depth cavity preparation

A cavity preparation with a depth greater than the ideal minimum for retention is rinsed thoroughly with the air-water syringe and dried. A coat of varnish is applied as described previously. The excessive lost dentin is replaced up to the ideal cavity preparation depth by a cement base (Fig. 15-5, *B*).

Cement base can be made from several new cement materials currently available (Fig. 15-6). By far the

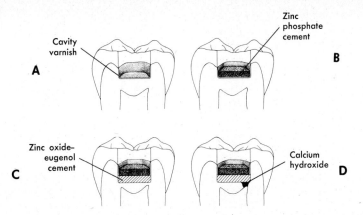

Fig. 15-5. Method of cavity medication. **A,** Dentin is sealed with cavity varnish in minimal-depth cavity preparations. (NOTE: Varnish is much thinner than shown.) **B,** Slightly deeper than normal cavity depth requires the use of both varnish and a cement base. **C,** Near-exposure preparations are treated with a thin layer of soothing zinc oxide–eugenol cement before varnish, and a cement base is placed. **D,** Small exposures of the pulp are first covered with a layer of calcium hydroxide to stimulate reparative dentin formation; then the tooth is medicated as in the near-exposure cavity preparation.

most popular cement base material has been zinc phosphate cement (p. 235).

Two physical properties of a cement base are of major importance: it should be a poor thermal conductor and have adequate compressive strength. The cement base must not transfer changes in temperatures from outside the tooth to the inner dentin layer. Such changes in temperature inside the tooth, if allowed to occur, would be painful. The primary reason for using a cement base at all is to place a poor thermal conductor (the cement base) between the deeper layer of dentin and the metal restoration (an excellent thermal conductor). Thermal changes in the minimal-depth cavity are usually not significant; however, thermal changes deeper in the dentin can be painful and damaging to the delicate pulp. The cement base should also be strong enough to resist being crushed under compression. Compressive strength that will resist biting forces is essential for the support of the restoration that is placed over it. If the cement base collapses under biting pressure, the restoration over it will surely fracture.

Zinc phosphate cement has been the cement base of choice for years because it has low thermal conductivity and high compressive strength and it is inexpensive. However, many of the newer cements currently available may eventually replace zinc phosphate because they are more convenient to prepare.

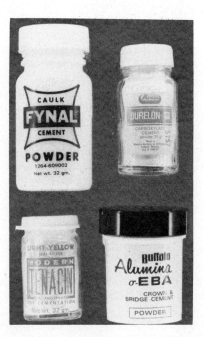

Fig. 15-6. Common cement-base materials currently available.

Cement bases are also used under nonmetal restorative materials such as silicate, composites, and acrylic. These materials do not present a thermal conduction problem because they are not metals. However, each of these materials is somewhat chemically irritating to the pulp when placed in deep cavity preparations. The cement base provides a barrier between the irritating restorative material and the pulp. (Zinc phosphate cement base can be prepared by simply adding more powder to the consistency used for cementation [p. 235].)

The use of cavity varnish on the exposed dentin before placement of a zinc phosphate cement base helps to protect the pulp from the cement itself. Zinc phosphate cement is slightly acidic for a period of time after it is inserted into the cavity preparation. Thus the varnish layer prevents the phosphoric acid from penetrating into the dentin tubules and causing pulpal irritation.

Treatment of the near-exposure cavity preparation

Whenever dentin is lost to the extent that the pulp is nearly exposed, additional precautions must be taken to protect this delicate tissue. Near-exposure cavity preparations are cleaned and dried with cotton pellets. Drying with cotton pellets avoids overdrying, or desiccating, the dentin, which is injurious to the pulp.

The cavity is medicated with a thin layer of zinc oxide–eugenol cement over the deepest portion of the cavity preparation. Zinc oxide–eugenol cement has a soothing effect on the dental pulp. In addition, it affords further protection of the pulp from the temporarily acidic zinc phosphate cement that is placed over it. Most zinc oxide–eugenol cements do not have the compressive strength that zinc phosphate cement does, and therefore they are not used widely for the entire cement base. Recent improvements in the strength of zinc oxide–eugenol cements will probably permit their use as a cement base and eliminate the need for the zinc phosphate cement in the future.

For the present, however, most near-exposure cavity preparations are treated by placing (1) a thin layer of zinc oxide–eugenol cement, (2) then a coat of cavity varnish over both the cement and the remaining dentin, and (3) zinc phosphate cement over the varnish to replace the lost dentin up to the level of the ideal cavity preparation depth (Fig. 15-5, *C*).

Treatment of the cavity with the pulp exposed

Unfortunately, some patients do not seek dental treatment until caries has advanced to the depth of the pulp. When the decayed dentin has been removed, the pulp is uncovered. The dentist must then decide whether to attempt to save the vitality of the pulp or proceed with endodontic treatment. The decision is based on the size of the exposure, the preoperative symptoms, the status of the pulp itself, and the age of the patient.

If the factors appear favorable, a procedure called *pulp capping* is done. Pulp capping is an attempt to stimulate healing of the injured pulp tissue. The cavity preparation is cleaned thoroughly with moist cotton pellets. Mild pressure applied to a moist cotton

Table 15-2. Summary of cavity medications

Cavity depth	Order of cavity medication (from pulp to restorative material)
Ideal	Rinse and air dry, then: 1. Cavity varnish 2. Restorative material
Slightly deeper than ideal	Rinse and air dry, then: 1. Cavity varnish 2. Cement base (zinc phosphate 3. Restorative material
Near-exposure of pulp	Rinse and dry with cotton pellets, then: 1. Thin coat of zinc oxide–eugenol cement 2. Cavity varnish 3. Cement base (zinc phosphate 4. Restorative material
Small pulp exposure	Rinse and dry with cotton pellets, then: 1. Calcium hydroxide (over exposed area) 2. Thin layer of zinc oxide–eugenol cement 3. Cavity varnish 4. Cement base 5. Restorative material
Extensive pulp exposure in young permanent teeth and primary teeth*	Pulpotomy procedure, then: 1. Zinc oxide–eugenol cement base (IRM) 2. Restorative material

*See Chapter 23 for explanation of the pulpotomy procedure.

pellet for a few minutes will stop any bleeding from the pulp. Dry cotton pellets are used to dry the preparation. Again it is important not to desiccate the tooth by air-drying. After the tooth is dry, a layer of calcium hydroxide is applied to the exposed area and the adjacent dentin. The tooth is then treated as a near-exposure cavity preparation; a layer of zinc oxide–eugenol cement is placed over the calcium hydroxide, the cavity preparation is varnished, and the zinc phosphate cement base is placed (Fig. 15-5, *D*).

Calcium hydroxide stimulates the dentinoblasts that are present in the pulp to produce new dentin over the area of exposure. This reparative process requires several months to a year to be complete. The pulp of a tooth that has been pulp capped should be tested periodically to determine its status.

Once cavity medication procedures have been completed, the final restorative material can be prepared and placed in the cavity preparation.

PULPOTOMY

Pulpotomy is a procedure that involves partial removal of the dental pulp after it has been extensively exposed. This is in contrast to the pulpectomy, which involves the complete removal of the pulp.

Pulpotomy procedures are usually done on primary and young permanent teeth (Chapter 23). Success rates drop markedly when attempts are made to treat permanent teeth of individuals past their teens. Extensive pulp exposures in older adult teeth are usually treated with a pulpectomy procedure (Chapter 22).

• • •

Table 15-2 provides a summary of the traditional scheme of cavity medication. Much of this scheme will probably be simplified as some of the newer cements are studied as to their effectiveness as cement bases. For example, the polycarboxylate cements (Durelon, Poly-C) are being tried as bases in all cases requiring a cement base. Since this cement is relatively nonirritating, its use would eliminate the need for the many medication layers discussed previously. The dentist could simply place a polycarboxylate base in a near-exposure–type cavity preparation and then insert the final restoration.

BIBLIOGRAPHY

Charbeneau, G.T., and others: Principles and practice of operative dentistry, ed. 2, Philadelphia, 1981, Lea & Febiger.

Howard, W.W., and Moller, R.C.: Atlas of operative dentistry, ed. 3, St. Louis, 1981, The C.V. Mosby Co.

CHAPTER 16

AMALGAM RESTORATIONS

The silver amalgam restoration is the most common restoration used by dentists today. Amalgam is defined as any metal alloy that has mercury as one of its components. Since most dental amalgam contains approximately 65% silver, it is referred to as silver amalgam. The public refers to these restorations as "silver fillings."

The amalgam restoration has been in use since 1833. Its widespread use is primarily the result of the fact that it is a highly successful restoration. In addition, it is a rather easy material to manipulate and is a relatively inexpensive restoration for the patient.

Silver amalgam has its limitations. It must not be subjected to excessive biting forces, and it must be well supported by tooth structure. Teeth that have been subjected to massive destruction through fracture or dental caries cannot be adequately restored for long periods of time with amalgam. These teeth are candidates for gold restorations if maximum success is to be achieved.

COMMON AMALGAM INSTRUMENTS AND SUPPLIES

There are certain instruments and accessories that are specifically required for the fabrication of an amalgam restoration (silver filling). These, along with some of the general operative instruments already discussed, are assembled on a preset tray or placed in the assistant's mobile cabinet for use during the procedure.

Amalgamators (Fig. 16-1)

The amalgamator is a machine that mixes mercury with silver alloy to produce amalgam. Most of the amalgamators available utilize a capsule-and-pestle system to achieve proper mixing. Mercury and silver alloy are placed in a small capsule in premeasured amounts with the use of a proportioner. A small pestle, or mixing rod, is placed in the capsule, and the capsule is closed. The loaded capsule is inserted into the amalgamator, which shakes the capsule back and forth, causing the pestle inside to mix the mercury and alloy together. Amalgamators are equipped with a timer to control the mixing time. This mixing process is called trituration. The trituration time has to be increased when the volume of amalgam to be mixed is increased. A word of caution is in order with regard to the amount of amalgam to be mixed at one time. Most capsules are only large enough to accommodate a maximum of two alloy tablets to be triturated at a time. Attempts at triturating more than two tablets at a time often result in an inadequately triturated amalgam. There is not enough room for pestle movement in most capsules when more than two alloy tablets are mixed. Manufacturers' charts should be consulted for recommended trituration times.

Premeasured disposable mixing capsules are available through various alloy manufacturers (Fig. 16-1). The capsules contain a premeasured alloy powder and the proper amount of mercury. The two components are kept separate by a foil membrane inside the capsule. The assistant ruptures the membrane by squeezing the capsule before inserting it into the amalgamator. These are very convenient for the assistant but expensive for the dentist.

Amalgam carriers (Fig. 16-2)

After the amalgam material is mixed (triturated) in the amalgamator and mulled, it has to be transferred to the cavity preparation in small increments to ensure proper filling of the preparation. Amalgam carriers are very convenient for this purpose.

Carriers are filled with amalgam by pressing the opening of the instrument into the mix. This forces the material into the barrel of the carrier. After transfer to the prepared tooth, the material can be expelled from the barrel by pressing a lever or a plunger that activates a small piston in the barrel. The piston pushes the material out of the barrel into the preparation. The carrier is refilled repeatedly until the preparation is completely filled with amalgam.

Both syringe and lever-action carriers are available. The lever style is available in both single- and double-ended models. Some manufacturers offer carrier models with different barrel sizes.

Amalgam condensers (Fig. 16-2)

The amalgam condenser is an instrument with a flat surface on the working end that is used to press amalgam against the cavity walls and floors.

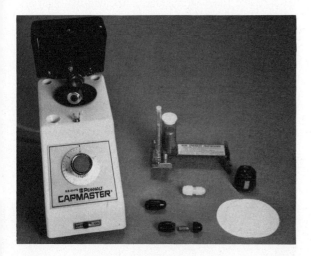

Fig. 16-1. Amalgam mixing accessories: amalgamator, mixing capsule (closed), mixing capsule (open), a premeasured mixing capsule (white), squeeze cloths, dappen dish, and mercury-alloy proportioner.

There are both automatic and hand-operated condensers. The hand instruments are more popular by far. They are usually double-ended, with one end being smaller than the other. Hand condensers are available in different styles and sizes.

Dentists usually prefer to begin condensation with a smaller condenser until the preparation is one-half to two-thirds full. The remaining additions of amalgam material are condensed with a larger condenser. This ensures excellent adaptation of the restorative material to cavity walls and in retentive areas.

Squeeze cloth (Fig. 16-1)

This small piece of cotton cloth is used to squeeze the freshly prepared mix of silver amalgam. Such a squeezing procedure was needed in older types of silver alloys that were mixed with an excess of mercury to improve the mixing process. After mixing, the preparer twisted the amalgam in a squeeze cloth, which allowed the excess mercury to escape through the weave of the cloth.

Advances in the manufacture of newer silver amalgam alloys have reduced the need for excess mercury in the mixing process. Hence the need for a squeeze cloth has diminished. However, assistants will find the squeeze cloth helpful in keeping the prepared amalgam together in one mass for ease in loading the amalgam carrier. The dappen dish can also be used for this function.

Matrix bands (Fig. 16-3)

Matrix bands are thin strips of stainless steel sheet metal that are used to create a form around a prepared tooth (Fig. 16-4, *B*). These matrix bands are needed

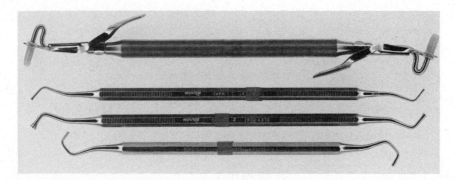

Fig. 16-2. Amalgam instruments. Top to bottom: amalgam carrier, No. 1 Ward condenser, No. 2 Ward condenser, No. 6B Clev-Dent back-action condenser.

only for cavity preparations that are not completely surrounded by tooth structure. Examples of such preparations are Classes II, III, and VI and those for teeth that are even more extensively destroyed. Class I and V cavity preparations are completely sur-

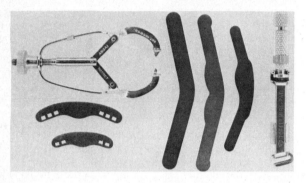

Fig. 16-3. Matrix retainers and bands. *Left to right:* Tofflemire retainer with assorted bands, Ivory retainer with bands.

rounded by tooth structure and do not require the use of matrix bands.

A matrix band serves the dentist in the same manner that a form for concrete serves the construction worker. It contains the restorative material in a desired place to give it shape. After the restorative material acquires its desired shape, the matrix, or form, can be removed. Circumferential matrix bands are those that completely surround the circumference of the tooth. The universal circumferential band is one of the most popular.

Amalgam is inserted into the cavity preparation with an amalgam carrier. Then it is pressed into place to adapt the material tightly against the cavity walls and the matrix band. This process is called condensation. Condensation provides a good seal to prevent excessive leakage of the restoration in the future. Condensation also improves the strength of the amalgam to resist fracture. To achieve adequate condensation in cavity preparations that have open aspects, the dentist uses the matrix band as a metal wall to pack

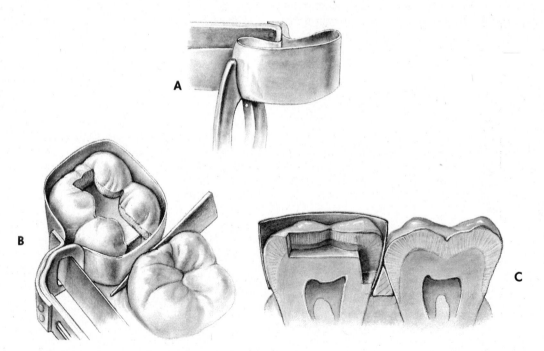

Fig. 16-4. Placement of the matrix band and wedge. **A,** Contouring the band with contouring pliers. **B,** Matrix and wooden wedge in place. **C,** Longitudinal section of the prepared cavity, matrix, and wedge. (From Howard, W.W., and Moller, R.C.: Atlas of operative dentistry, ed. 3, St. Louis, 1981, The C.V. Mosby Co.)

the amalgam against. Without the matrix band, the amalgam material would simply flow out of the open aspect of the preparation when condensation pressure is applied to the material (Fig. 16-14).

Matrix retainers

Matrix bands are held in place around a prepared tooth either by spot-welding the band before its placement or by an adjustable clamp called the matrix retainer. Fig. 16-3 shows two styles of retainers. The Tofflemire retainer is by far the most popular retainer in use today.

The Tofflemire retainer is used with the various styles of circumferential matrix bands.

Contouring pliers (Fig. 16-4, *A*)

Matrix bands can be shaped to better assume the contour of the prepared tooth by the use of contouring pliers. The matrix band is squeezed in the beaks of the pliers, which press it into the desired shape.

Interproximal wedge (Fig. 16-4, *B*)

Although the matrix band is held tightly against the tooth by the retainer, a small amount of amalgam can still escape, under condensation pressure, out of the preparation between the tooth and the band. This is not of major significance except in the cervical areas

Table 16-1. Indications for use of the interproximal wedge

Amalgam preparation cavity classification	Matrix band needed?	Number of wedges
Class I	No	None
Class II	Yes	1
Class III	Yes	1
Class V	No	None
Class VI	Yes	2
Larger than Class VI	Yes	2 if both mesial and distal aspects are involved
Exceptions: Preparations with cervical margins on distal aspect of last molars or on teeth with adjacent teeth missing	Yes	Wedge only cervical margin adjacent to another tooth

of preparations on proximal surfaces. These areas are rather inaccessible to carving, and the potential for excess amalgam to become lodged interproximally is great. Excess amalgam along the cervical margin is commonly referred to as an overhang. Overhangs are damaging to the surrounding tissues if they are allowed to remain (Fig. 21-10). All other areas of the restoration can easily be trimmed with carving instruments, because the operator has access to these areas.

The best way to treat an overhang is to prevent it in the first place. This can be done with an interproximal wedge. The wedge is usually a triangular-shaped wooden or plastic stick that is inserted between the teeth after the matrix band is placed. The wedge is forced tightly into place between the teeth (Fig. 16-4, *C*). The wedge then acts as a brace to hold the matrix band tightly against the tooth to ensure that amalgam cannot escape into the interproximal area during condensation.

Another benefit of the wedge is that when it is in place, it separates the teeth slightly to compensate for the thickness of the matrix band. The amalgam is then inserted and condensed. When the matrix band is removed, there is a space the thickness of the matrix band between the new restoration and the adjacent tooth, which is closed as the separated teeth move back together. Dentists use their own judgment in determining the amount of separation that is desirable.

A wedge is needed in an interproximal space only where there is a prepared cervical margin. Hence a Class II amalgam preparation would require one wedge, and a Class VI would require two wedges. Wedges cannot be used when there is no adjacent tooth to wedge against, as on the distal aspect of the last molars and in areas of missing teeth. Overhangs that might occur in these regions are readily accessible to carvers for removal.

Table 16-1 provides a review of the need for matrix bands and interproximal wedges in amalgam preparations.

Preparation of the Tofflemire matrix assembly

Since the Tofflemire, or circumferential, matrix assembly is the most common amalgam matrix used, an explanation of how to assemble it for use in various quadrants of the oral cavity is warranted.

Fig. 16-5 demonstrates the parts of the Tofflemire retainer. These parts function as follows:

frame The main body of the retainer to which the vise, spindle, and adjustment knobs are attached.

vise A clamplike device that holds the ends of the matrix band in the retainer.

spindle A screwlike rod used to lock the ends of the matrix band in the vise.

outer knob An adjustment knob used to tighten the spindle against the band in the vise.

inner knob An adjustment knob used to slide the vise along the frame to either increase or decrease the size of the matrix band loop.

guide slots Slots that enable the matrix band loop to be positioned in the direction of choice.

For purposes of orientation, there are two important aspects of the retainer that must be recognized, as shown in Fig. 16-6. These views are identified as follows:

occlusal aspect The opening of the guide slots on the end of the retainer, as well as the diagonal slot in the vise, are not visible.

gingival aspect The opening of the guide slots on the end of the retainer, as well as the diagonal slot in the vise, are visible.

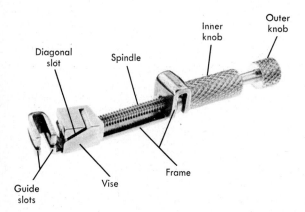

Fig. 16-5. Parts of Tofflemire matrix retainer.

Once the dental assistant can identify the parts of the retainer and their functions, as well as recognize the occlusal and gingival aspects of the retainer, the preparation of the matrix assembly is simplified.

The procedures for preparing the Tofflemire retainer and the matrix band are as follows:

Phase I: Preparing the retainer

1. Hold the retainer by the vise in the left hand so that the gingival aspect is visible.
2. Turn the outer knob clockwise until the end of the spindle is visible in the diagonal slot in the vise (Fig. 16-7, *A*).
3. Turn the inner knob until the vise moves to within approximately $3/16$ inch of the guide slots at the end of the retainer.
4. Now turn the outer knob counterclockwise until the tip of the spindle just disappears from view in the diagonal slot in the vise. The retainer is now ready to receive the matrix band (Fig. 16-7, *B*).

Phase II: Preparing and inserting the matrix band

1. Identify the occlusal and gingival edges of the universal matrix band (Fig. 16-7, *C*).
2. Bring the ends of the band together so that a loop is formed.
3. With the gingival aspect of the retainer toward you, slide the joined ends of the band, occlusal edge first, into the diagonal slot of the vise.
4. At the same time, thread the joined band through the guide slot next to the vise.
5. Continue threading the joined band so that it emerges from between the prongs of the guide slots.

NOTE: If the loop is positioned above the retainer, it is prepared for use in either the patient's lower left or upper right quadrants (Fig. 16-7, *D*). On the other hand, if the loop is positioned below the retainer, it is prepared for use in either the patient's lower right or upper left quadrants (Fig. 16-7, *E*).

Another and perhaps more convenient way of identifying the correct orientation of the band is to hold

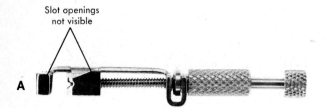

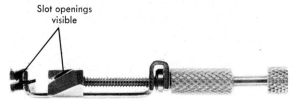

Fig. 16-6. Tofflemire matrix retainer. **A,** Occlusal aspect. **B,** Gingival aspect.

the retainer so that the guide-slot end is away from you. If the retainer and band assembly are to be used for lower teeth, the guide-slot openings are positioned downward toward the gingiva. The band loop is positioned to the right of the retainer if it is to be used on the patient's right side (Fig. 16-8, *A*). If the retainer is to be used on the patient's left side, the band loop would be positioned to the left of the retainer (Fig. 16-8, *B*).

If the retainer is to be used on upper teeth, the guide-slot openings are positioned upward toward the gingiva. Again, the band loop is positioned to the

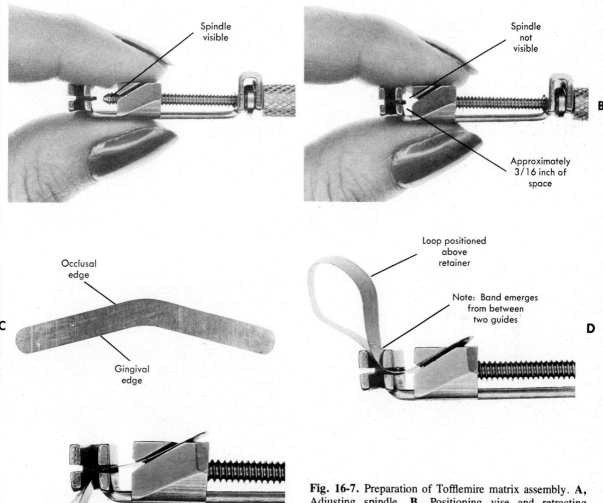

Fig. 16-7. Preparation of Tofflemire matrix assembly. **A,** Adjusting spindle. **B,** Positioning vise and retracting spindle. **C,** Universal matrix band. **D,** Inserting matrix band for lower left or upper right quadrants. **E,** Inserting matrix band for lower right or upper left quadrant.

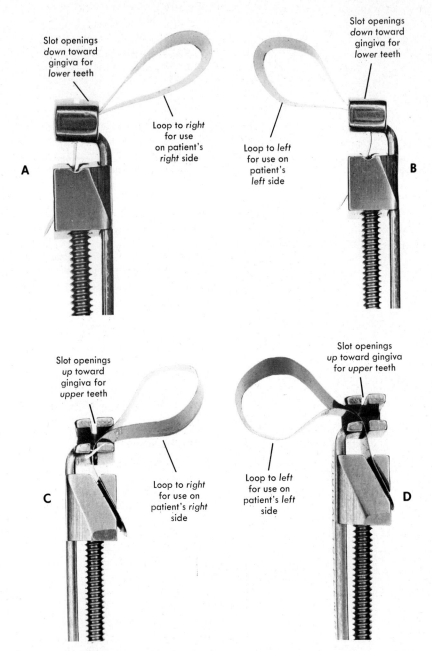

Fig. 16-8. Common configurations of Tofflemire matrix assembly. **A,** Used in lower right quadrant. **B,** Used in lower left quadrant. **C,** Used in upper right quadrant. **D,** Used in upper left quadrant.

right of the retainer for use on the patient's right side (Fig. 16-8, *C*) and to the left of the retainer for use on the patient's left side (Fig. 16-8, *D*).

6. Once the loop is positioned, seat the band completely in the slots.
7. Turn the outer knob clockwise to clamp the band in the vise.
8. If the loop has been flattened somewhat by placement in the retainer, the handle end of a mouth mirror can be used to make the loop round again, as shown in Fig. 16-9.
9. Once the loop is rounded, the size of the loop can be made larger or smaller by turning the inner knob as needed. The diameter of the tooth being restored dictates the approximately size of the loop.

It is helpful to the dental assistant to know that most dentists place the Tofflemire matrix assembly on the tooth being restored in a conventional way. When the assembly is placed, the retainer is located on the buccal aspect of the tooth being restored. Furthermore, the gingival aspect of the retainer is always placed toward the gingiva to facilitate easy removal once the amalgam has been inserted in the tooth.

The preparation of the matrix assembly should be accomplished as a part of the operatory preparation sequence so that delays can be avoided when the matrix is needed during the procedure.

Amalgam carvers

Every dentist has favorite amalgam carvers. Some of the more popular designs are shown in Fig. 16-10.

Generally carvers can be divided into two categories: occlusal and smooth-surface carvers. The Ward carver is an example of a smooth-surface carver. The long, narrow blade allows dentists to contour the smooth-surface aspects of an amalgam restoration readily (Fig. 16-10).

The 26 spoon and the cleoid-discoid carvers facilitate the carving of the occlusal aspect of a restoration. Their design permits easier establishment of cusp inclines and occlusal grooves and fossae in the restoration (Fig. 16-10).

Anatomical burnishers (Fig. 5-14)

Anatomical burnishers are smooth-tipped hand instruments that are used to smooth and enhance the occlusal anatomy of the amalgam restoration. They are used immediately after the carving phase if the dentist chooses to employ them. It is not a mandatory procedure.

Finishing burs

These special steel burs are used to polish amalgam, gold, and composite materials. The difference between a regular bur and a finishing bur is found in the number of cutting edges (flutes) on the bur. The

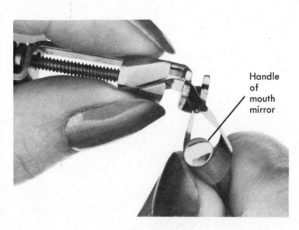

Handle of mouth mirror

Fig. 16-9. Rounding loop using handle end of mirror.

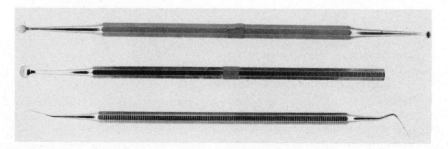

Fig. 16-10. Amalgam carvers. *Top to bottom:* cleoid-discoid (No. 7C), No. 26 spoon, Ward's carver.

finishing bur has two to three times as many flutes as does the regular bur. The additional flutes leave a glossy surface on restorations when moderate pressure is applied.

The burs are used in the conventional-speed handpiece. They are available in HP and RA styles (Fig. 5-5, *C*).

THE AMALGAM RESTORATIVE PROCEDURE
Amalgam cavity preparations

Amalgam cavity preparation designs incorporate the principles discussed previously with regard to outline, retention, and resistance forms. Fig. 16-11 shows some conventional cavity preparation designs.

Armamentarium

The instrument selection and arrangement will vary considerably between one operator and another. The armamentarium in Fig. 16-12 is an example of a typical setup for any amalgam procedure. Any materials that cannot be processed on the preset tray should be kept in an immediate-access area to be used as auxiliary items.

If rubber dam isolation is to be used, a separate preset tray is required in addition to the armamentarium shown in Fig. 16-12.

Fabrication of an amalgam restoration: Class II example

Although the specific technique used in the fabrication of an amalgam restoration may vary from one dentist to another, virtually all techniques follow the same fundamental steps. When a dentist restores a tooth with a Class II amalgam restoration, the following fundamental steps are employed:

1. Anesthesia administration
2. Isolation
3. Cavity preparation
4. Cavity medication
5. Matrix placement
6. Insertion
7. Initial carving
8. Matrix removal
9. Final carving
10. Postoperative instructions

Anesthesia administration. The appropriate area is anesthetized with the standard anesthetic setup and technique described in Chapter 7.

Isolation. The area to be treated is isolated with one of the isolation techniques described in Chapter

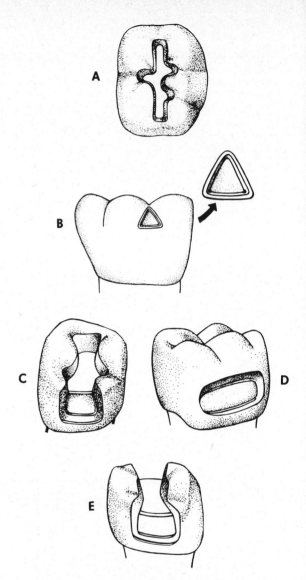

Fig. 16-11. Common classes of cavity preparations used for amalgam restorations. **A** and **B**, Class I. **C**, Class II. **D**, Class V. **E**, Class VI (Table 15-1).

8. Good isolation technique is extremely important because it provides maximum visibility and access to the operating area. In addition, the quality of the finished restoration is enhanced because proper isolation prevents contamination of the restorative material.

Cavity preparation. Most dentists follow a pattern in cavity preparation. The first phase is cutting

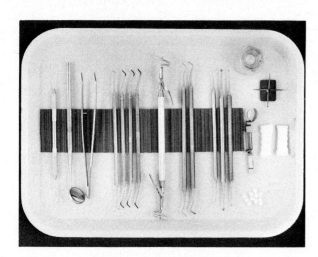

Preset tray

Cowhorn explorer, No. 3
Mouth mirror, No. 4
Cotton pliers
Spoon excavator
Enamel hatchet 8E
Gingival margin trimmers, No. 12 and No. 13
Amalgam carrier
Condensers, No. 1 and No. 2
Ward's "C" carver
Cleoid-discoid carver, No. 7C and No. 5C
Tofflemire matrix assembly
Dappen dish
Burs: F.G. No. 35 and No. 56, R.A. No. ½ and No. 4
Cotton rolls
Wedges
Cotton pellets

Add-on items

Cavity medicaments
Premeasured amalgam capsules
Amalgamator
Articulating paper (often a
    preset tray item)

Fig. 16-12. Amalgam restoration armamentarium.

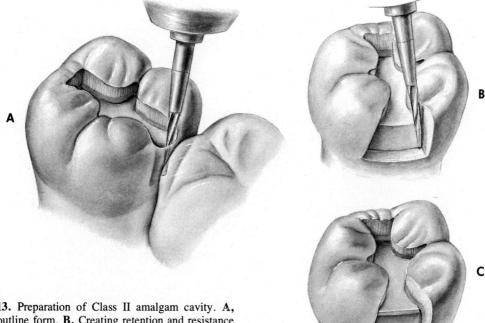

Fig. 16-13. Preparation of Class II amalgam cavity. **A,** Gaining outline form. **B,** Creating retention and resistance form. **C,** Finished preparation. (From Howard, W.W., and Moller, R.C.: Atlas of operative dentistry, ed. 3, St. Louis, 1981, The C.V. Mosby Co.)

through the hard enamel layer—called *opening the cavity*. This is often done with a No. 35 inverted cone bur. These burs are efficient instruments for cutting through the very hard enamel layer. After being opened, the cavity is enlarged to gain the necessary outline, retention, and resistance forms. This is accomplished very well with any of the side cutting burs, such as a No. 56 plain fissure bur or a No. 171 plain tapered fissure bur (Fig. 16-13, *A* and *B*).

The refinement of the cavity preparation is accomplished by scraping the walls and floors with enamel hatchets and/or gingival margin trimmers.

If the carious lesion extends beyond the desired form of the cavity preparation, the caries is removed with slow-speed round burs and spoon excavators. This is a precautionary measure to avoid removing more tooth structure than absolutely necessary.

After the cutting and refining procedures have been completed (Fig. 16-13, *C*), the cavity medication phase begins.

Cavity medication. Cavity medication is discussed in detail in Chapter 15. If the caries has extended beyond the normal cavity preparation depth, cement bases are used to replace the destroyed dentin.

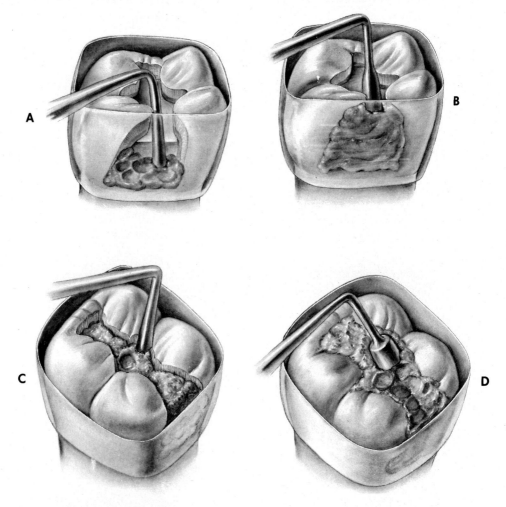

Fig. 16-14. Insertion and condensation of amalgam in prepared cavity. Small increments of amalgam are inserted and condensed in cavity until cavity is overfilled. (From Howard, W.W., and Moller, R.C.: Atlas of operative dentistry, ed. 3, St. Louis, 1981, The C.V. Mosby Co.)

Matrix placement. Matrix bands are placed around the prepared tooth to create a form, or mold, into which the soft amalgam is placed.

Once the band is in place around the tooth, it must be forced against the cervical margin of the proximal box with an interproximal wedge (Fig. 16-4).

Every dentist has his own preference as to how the matrix should be placed. A conventional relationship is to place the retainer so that it will be along the buccal surfaces of the teeth when it is in position. The wedge is usually inserted from the lingual aspect (Fig. 16-4, *B*). (It should be noted that if a cavity prepara-tion has both mesial and distal proximal boxes to be restored, two wedges are needed.)

Insertion. Once the matrix band and wedge are in place, the amalgam is triturated (mixed) and brought into the cavity preparation with an amalgam carrier.

The dental assistant can place the amalgam directly into the preparation while the dentist condenses it into place, or the assistant can alternately exchange the carrier and condenser with the dentist as the amalgam is placed and condensed in the preparation.

Condensation of the amalgam has two basic pur-poses: (1) to adapt the material to the cavity walls and

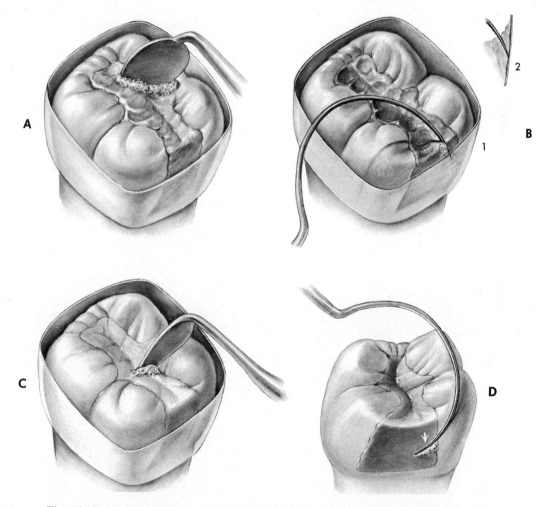

Fig. 16-15. Carving amalgam. **A,** Carving away excess amalgam. **B,** Relieving marginal ridge. *1,* Relationship of explorer tip to matrix band *(2).* **C,** Carving occlusal anatomy. **D,** Carving smooth surface margins. (From Howard, W.W., and Moller, R.C.: Atlas of operative dentistry, ed. 3, St. Louis, 1981, The C.V. Mosby Co.)

(2) to eliminate excess mercury from the mix to strengthen the restoration. Condensation is most commonly done by hand, with a condenser or plugger. Amalgam is added in small increments and condensed until the cavity is slightly overfilled. Fig. 16-14 demonstrates this process.

Initial carving. Before the matrix band is removed, the excess amalgam on the occlusal surface can be carved away with a cleoid-discoid carver (Fig. 16-15, *A* and *C*). In addition, a small portion of amalgam must be removed between the matrix band and the marginal ridge of the restoration (Fig. 16-15, *B*). This minimizes the possibility of fracturing the new restoration during band removal.

During all carving procedures the assistant should keep the evacuator tip close to the restoration so that the amalgam shavings are removed as soon as they are carved away. This is especially important when rubber dam isolation is not used.

Matrix removal. The matrix band retainer and wedge assembly are usually removed in the following order: (1) retainer, (2) wedge, and (3) band. The wedge and the band can be removed with cotton pliers or a small hemostat. The band must be removed in a bucco-occlusal direction to avoid fracturing the still soft amalgam restoration.

Some dentists prefer to cut the ends of the matrix band after the retainer is removed. Then the remaining band fragment is pulled in a lingual direction to remove it.

Final carving. While the amalgam is still soft, it is advisable to carve the less accessible areas first to remove any amalgam that may have squeezed out of the cavity preparation during condensation. These areas are the buccal and lingual proximal margins as well as the cervical margins. A smooth surface carver such as Ward's "C" carver or the explorer are used for this purpose (Fig. 16-15, *D*).

The occlusal portion of the restoration is then carved so that it contacts the opposing tooth properly when the jaws are closed together. If a rubber dam has been used for isolation, it must be removed before the occlusion (bite) is established. The cleoid carver is an excellent choice for this procedure. The various anatomical grooves and cusp inclines can be formed very nicely with this instrument.

The dentist checks proper occlusion by having the patient close the teeth together while holding a piece of articulating (carbon) paper on the biting surface. A heavy blue mark on the restoration will indicate that the restoration is "high" and that it must be reduced to blend into the normal biting pattern of the patient.

Some dentists prefer to wipe the completed restoration with a moist cotton pellet after carving. This helps to leave a smooth surface on the restoration until it is polished at a future appointment.

Postoperative instructions. Amalgam requires 24 hours to reach its maximum hardness. During this time the patient should be cautioned to protect the new restoration during meals. Hard-textured foods should be avoided. Most amalgam alloys reach sufficient hardness within 6 to 8 hours to withstand forces generated by chewing on soft-textured foods.

This precaution is not as critical in small occlusal restorations or in Class V restorations.

Classes I, V, and VI restorations

The Class VI restoration (Table 15-1) is fabricated in the same manner as the Class II except that two wedges are required to adapt the cervical aspect of the band on both the mesial and distal surfaces of the preparation.

Classes I and V restorations do not require the use of a matrix band, since the entire cavity preparation is surrounded by walls of tooth structure. The preparation can be filled with amalgam and condensed into place by simply forcing it against these cavity walls.

Any restorations placed entirely on smooth surfaces will require only the use of a smooth surface carver to properly shape the restoration (Ward's, Wall's, Hollenbeck).

Polishing the amalgam restoration

The amalgam restoration can be polished any time after the 24-hour hardening period. Polishing smooths the surface of the metal so that plaque will not adhere to it readily and makes the restoration more attractive.

A standard method of polishing is to lightly grind the occlusal portion with various sizes of round finishing burs. Smooth surfaces are polished with sandpaper disks.

The grinding procedure is followed by polishing the metal with a rubber cup and a thin silex paste. After a thorough rinsing, a high luster can be imparted to the restoration by polishing the metal with a thin paste of water or tin oxide and water. The rubber cup is filled with one of these pastes and run at a fairly high speed. The assistant should direct a constant stream of air toward the tooth during this procedure. This dries the paste to a fine powder that will provide a beautiful finish to the metal restoration.

Pin-retained amalgam restorations

On occasion, the dentist is confronted with a restorative problem that requires the use of amalgam in substantially destroyed teeth. For amalgam to be successful, it must be retained within the confines of the remaining tooth. When retention is reduced by loss of tooth structure, the amalgam can be retained by the use of retention pins along with the remaining tooth tissue.

All the pin techniques that are utilized today involve drilling holes into the dentin using a special twist drill provided by the manufacturers of pin kits that are available. Starter holes must be drilled between the pulp and the external portion of the root (Fig. 16-16). After the starter holes have been drilled, the appropriate type of twist drill is used to complete the holes.

Three common types of pins are in use today: cemented pins, friction pins, and threaded pins.

Cemented pins (Markley) (Fig. 16-17). Holes that are slightly larger than the pin are drilled into the dentin. A special twist drill is used for this purpose. Standard dental cement is spun into the hole with a Lentulo spiral mounted in a conventional-speed contra-angle. The pin is dipped in cement and inserted into the pinhole. The cement is allowed to harden, and the restorative material is placed around the pin or pins if more than one are used.

Friction pins (Unitek) (Fig. 16-18). These pins require no cement. They are held in place by friction only. A hole smaller than the pin is drilled into the dentin with a special twist drill. Pins are driven into the small hole with a pin driver tapped gently with a gold foil mallet.

Threaded pins (Whaledent) (Fig. 16-19). These pins are held in place by twisting the threaded pin into a slightly smaller hole made by a twist drill. The threaded pin acts like a wood screw. The threaded pin is twisted into the pinhole with either a small hand wrench or a special pin driver that attaches to the

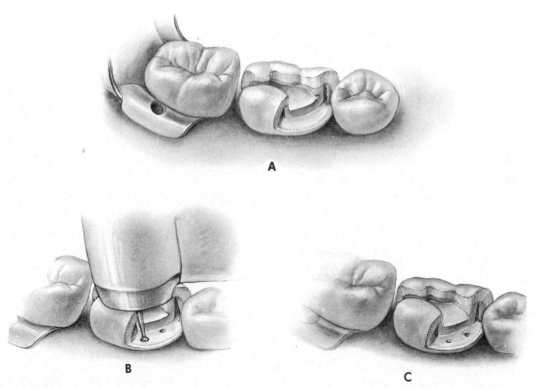

Fig. 16-16. Retention pin placement. **A,** Prepared cavity. **B** and **C,** Placing starter holes. (From Howard, W.W., and Moller, R.C.: Atlas of operative dentistry, ed. 3, St. Louis, 1981, The C.V. Mosby Co.)

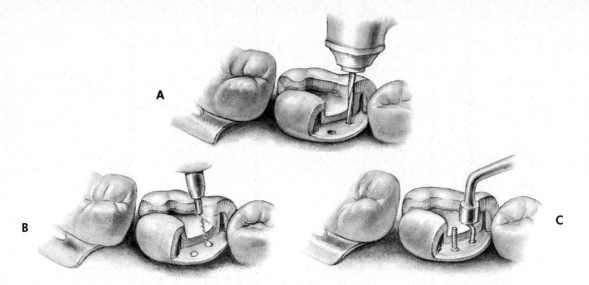

Fig. 16-17. Cemented pins. **A,** Placing pinholes. **B,** Inserting cement in pinholes with lentula spiral. **C,** Placing pins with amalgam condenser. (From Howard, W.W., and Moller, R.C.: Atlas of operative dentistry, ed. 3, St. Louis, 1981, The C.V. Mosby Co.)

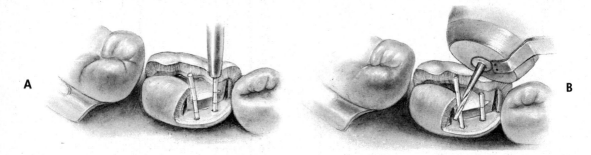

Fig. 16-18. Friction pins (Unitek). **A,** Placing pins in previously drilled holes with pin driver. **B,** Cutting pins to proper length using ultraspeed handpiece. (From Howard, W.W., and Moller, R.C.: Atlas of operative dentistry, ed. 3, St. Louis, 1981, The C.V. Mosby Co.)

conventional handpiece. Added retention can be gained with these pins by dipping them in cyanoacrylate adhesive (Permabond) before twisting them into the pinholes.

• • •

After the pins are inserted, the matrix band and retainer are placed, and amalgam is condensed around the retention pins to restore the tooth.

After the matrix band is removed, the amalgam is carved with conventional instrumentation.

It should be noted that the use of retention pins is not limited to amalgam restorative procedures. Pin retention is commonly used with extensive esthetic restorations which will be discussed in Chapter 17.

SAFETY PRECAUTIONS

Research has shown that there is a potential hazard to the health of dental personnel who come in contact with mercury or mercury-containing substances such as amalgam. Dental assistants are vulnerable since

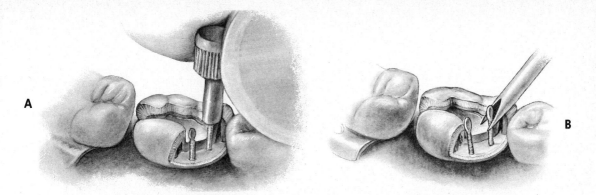

Fig. 16-19. Threaded pins (Whaledent). **A,** Placing threaded pins using special wrench. **B,** Bending pins with special instrument provided with kit. (From Howard, W.W., and Moller, R.C.: Atlas of operative dentistry, ed. 3, St. Louis, 1981, The C.V. Mosby Co.)

they mix mercury with the silver alloy and dispose of the excess amalgam material.

Although mercury can be absorbed through the skin, poisoning commonly results from aspiration of mercury vapors in the lungs. Mercury poisoning results in a wide variety of signs and symptoms depending on the total accumulation of mercury in the body.

The vulnerability of dental personnel in general practice is significant because the amalgam restorative procedure is the predominant service provided by the general practitioner. As a result, the following measures are recommended to minimize the risk of mercury poisoning:

1. Use premeasured amalgam capsules to reduce the contact with mercury and to minimize the risk of mercury spillage.
2. Use an amalgamator with a protective cover to confine any capsule leakage to a limited area. Placement of the amalgamator in a covered area of a cabinet also helps to confine contamination to a small area.
3. Scrap amalgam left over from a procedure should be stored in a tightly sealed plastic container which has 1 inch layer of glycerin, water or x-ray fixer covering the scrap.
4. Scrap amalgam and spilled mercury should not be allowed to accumulate in cabinetry, in the crevices of the dental chair or on the floor of the operatory.
5. Use of squeeze cloths to express free mercury from an amalgam mix should be avoided. (Newer amalgam materials do not require this step in the mixing procedure)

6. Use of a water spray and central evacuation during the removal of an existing amalgam restoration is encouraged to avoid the creation of mercury dust into the breathing zone of the operating team.
7. Exclude all food, drink, and smoking materials from the work area.
8. Use of monitoring devices to assess the contamination level of the work area should be considered.
9. Periodic analysis of urine samples of dental personnel is also recommended.

SUMMARY

Approximately 70% of the procedures done in a general dental practice are amalgam restorations. The dental assistant who works in a general practice must be thoroughly familiar with the instruments, supplies, and procedures as well as safety precautions related to the amalgam restorative process.

BIBLIOGRAPHY

Carter, L., and Yaman, P.: Dental instruments, St. Louis, 1981, The C.V. Mosby Co.

Charbeneau, G.T., and others: Principle and practice of operative dentistry, ed. 2, Philadelphia, 1981, Lea & Febiger.

Howard, W.W., and Moller, R.C.: Atlas of operative dentistry, ed. 3, St. Louis, 1981, The C.V. Mosby Co.

Johnson, K.F.: Mercury hygiene, Dent. Clin. North Am. **22:**3, July 1978.

Rao, G.S., and Hefferen, J.J.: Toxicity of mercury. In Smith, D.C., and Williams, D.F., editors: Biocompatibility of dental materials, vol. 3, Biocompatibility of dental restorative materials, Boca Raton, Fla., 1982, CRC Press, Inc.

CHAPTER 17

ESTHETIC RESTORATIONS

The restoration of tooth surfaces that are readily visible during normal oral functions presents an interesting challenge to the dental team. There is an increasing demand for esthetics in dental restorations that are placed in these visible surfaces. Few patients will tolerate an unsightly metal restoration being placed in a visible surface of an anterior tooth or in the facial aspect of the maxillary premolars. Although metal restorations would function very well in these teeth, their poor esthetic quality discourages their use.

Dentistry has had continuous research projects devoted to the development of a restorative material that would have a favorable appearance and would last a reasonable length of time under the influence of the oral environment. In addition, the material must not be harmful to the tooth. Although the perfect material to meet these requirements has yet to be developed, three types of materials have been used for esthetic restorations with varying degrees of success: silicate cement, acrylic resin, and composite resin. All these materials are favorable from an esthetic standpoint.

Because of the unique environment in which these materials are placed, they all ultimately fail for one reason or another. Dental restorations are subjected to chemicals produced by oral bacteria, chemical substances found in saliva, and various foods and beverages. The alternate heating and cooling of these restorations, along with the chemical substances just listed, have a damaging effect on esthetic restorative materials. The restoration will slowly disintegrate, begin to leak oral fluids into the cavity preparation, or discolor. All the materials mentioned will ultimately discolor after a period of time.

Regardless of which restorative material is selected for an esthetic restoration, the same basic cavity preparation designs are used for each of them. The same armamentarium is used for all three of these materials with the exception of the specific equipment required to mix the material selected.

In the past materials such as silicate cements and unfilled resins (acrylic) reigned as the principle esthetic restorative materials. Today composite resins (filled resins and microfilled resins) and glass ionomer cements are predominantly used. These materials seem to resist the undesirable effects of the oral environment better than either silicate cement or acrylic.

The following represents the basic instrument and supply items needed to fabricate these restorations.

COMPOSITE RESTORATIVE MATERIALS

Two major categories of composite resin materials are used in esthetic restorations: filled resins and microfilled resins. The primary difference between them is the type and size of the filler particles in them. Both are referred to as composites because they are a combination of acrylic and filler particles. Some products rely on a chemical reaction between a base material and a catalyst material for the material to set. Other products are placed in a prepared cavity and hardened by the use of either ultraviolet or visible light.

The paste-paste system

Composite materials are marketed in different forms. One of the most widely used forms is a paste-paste system (Fig. 17-1). The manufacturer provides two different pastes in small jars. One paste is usually called the universal or base paste. The other is the catalyst paste. The base paste is usually available in different shades to facilitate a color match with the tooth being restored. However, the universal shade will be satisfactory for most (85%) patients.

An equal volume of each paste is dispensed on a small paper mixing pad. A dispensing spatula is supplied with the material to perform this task. One end of the spatula is used to stir and dispense the base material, and the other is used for the catalyst. This avoids contamination of the remaining material left in the jars. The two equal portions are kept separated on the mixing pad until the mixing procedure begins.

Once the cavity preparation is finished, the dental assistant uses either end of the dispensing spatula to mix the two pastes together for 20 to 30 seconds. The material can be delivered to the dentist on the mixing pad for incremental packing into the preparation with a Teflon filling instrument. Another choice is to load the mixed material into a composite syringe that the dentist uses to inject the material into the cavity preparation.

Light-accelerated systems

Another form in which composite materials are marketed are single-paste systems that are simply placed in a prepared cavity and hardened by the use of either ultraviolet or visible light (Fig. 17-2). No mixing is required when these materials are used. The assistant should not dispense the material on the paper pad until it is needed to avoid prolonged exposure to room light.

These materials can be placed in the cavity preparation by either incremental packing or by injection with a composite syringe.

Acid etching and enamel bonding
(Figs. 17-1 and 17-2)

Both of the systems just discussed also incorporate the use of the acid-etch technique in the restorative

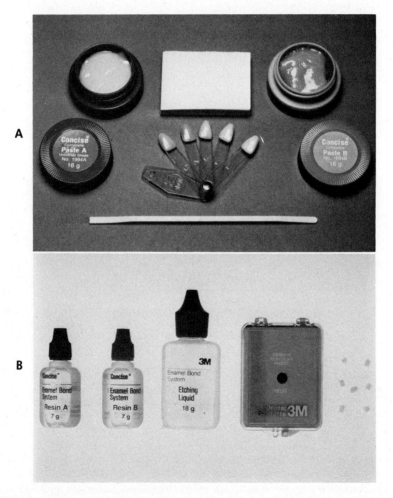

Fig. 17-1. Paste-paste composite material. **A,** Materials for mixing composite. **B,** Materials for etching and bonding procedures.

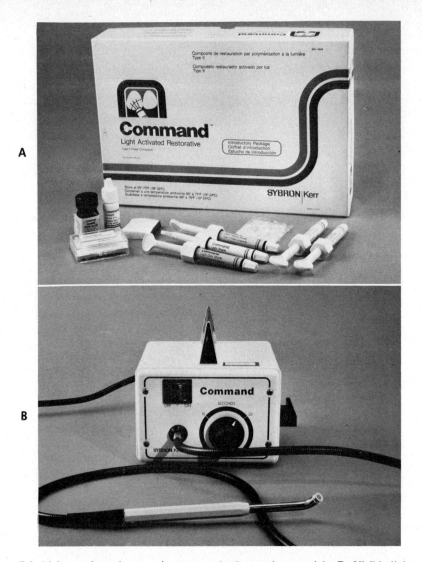

Fig. 17-2. Light-accelerated composite system. **A,** Composite materials. **B,** Visible light source.

procedure. The enamel margins of a prepared tooth are gently bathed with a mild acid (50% phosphoric acid) for 60 seconds. Cotton pliers and cotton pellets (or tiny sponges provided by the manufacturer) are used to apply the acid, which is rinsed away with the air-water syringe and oral evacuator for another 60 seconds, and the tooth is dried. The acid essentially roughens the enamel margins, which helps to bond the composite material when it is placed in the prepared cavity. Several manufacturers provide an enamel bonding agent that is painted on the etched enamel and allowed to set. The light-accelerated systems require application of the light to the bonding agent for approximately 10 to 15 seconds. The bonding agent simply improves the bonding between the composite restoration and the enamel margins.

• • •

Composite materials are also available as core materials for use in crown and bridge procedures. This will be discussed in greater detail in Chapter 20.

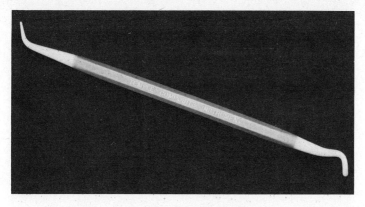

Fig. 17-3. Teflon-tipped filling instrument.

INSTRUMENTS AND SUPPLIES
Filling instrument (Fig. 17-3)

Plastic or Teflon-tipped filling instruments are used to place composite material in the cavity preparation when the bulk packing technique is used. This instrument does not stick to the composite, which simplifies the filling procedure. Metal filling instruments should not be used because they tend to discolor the composite material.

Composite syringe (Fig. 17-4)

One of the problems dentists often encounter in the fabrication of a composite restoration is the placement of the restorative material in the rather small preparation. The material is a thick, sticky paste. It tends to be pulled out of the preparation because it sticks to filling instruments. Because it is a thick paste, the material is also difficult to force into the retentive areas of the preparation to ensure adequate adaptation and retention of the restoration.

The composite syringe has solved both of these insertion problems. The syringe tip is filled with composite material and placed in the syringe. Then the material can be slowly injected into the preparation.

This is a great convenience to the dentist, but it requires the use of a little more composite material than is required when only a filling instrument is used.

Scalpel (Fig. 17-4)

The surgical scalpel is a popular instrument for finishing composite restorations. The 12B style blade

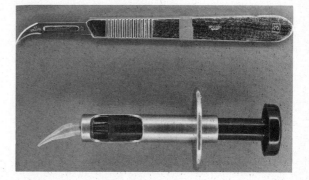

Fig. 17-4. Composite syringe and No. 12B scalpel.

is a common choice for this procedure because of its curved shape and the double cutting edge. The scalpel blade is disposable; therefore new blades ensure maximum instrument sharpness.

The scalpel blade is specifically used to trim away excess composite along the margins of the restoration after the matrix is removed.

Matrix strips (Fig. 17-5, *A*)

Matrix strips act in a similar fashion to the matrix bands used in amalgam restorations. They serve to shape the proximal aspect of the restoration.

Matrix strips are made of either clear plastic (Mylar) or celluloid. No retainer is required to hold them in place. The matrix is simply held in place by the contact of the adjacent teeth (Fig. 17-12). The use of an interproximal wedge is sometimes advisable to

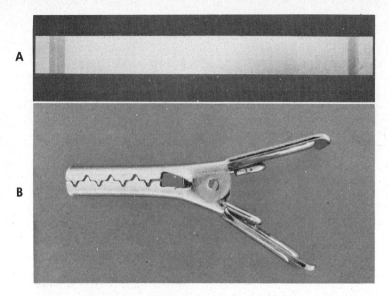

Fig. 17-5. A, Matrix strip. **B,** Matrix strip holder.

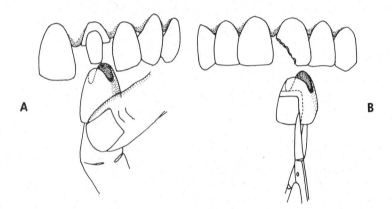

Fig. 17-6. A, Transparent celluloid crown trimmed and fitted to prepared tooth. **B,** Incisal angle of celluloid crown can be cut from the rest of crown and used as a form to shape restorative material in a Class IV restoration.

hold the matrix in place, prevent overhangs, and separate the teeth.

Matrix strip holder (Fig. 17-5, *B*)

The matrix strip holder is a clamplike device that can be used to hold the matrix in place after the composite material has been inserted into the cavity preparation and the matrix is wrapped around the tooth to form the proximal surface.

Celluloid crown forms

Celluloid crown forms are designed to act as molds to reconstruct a part of or the entire crown of a prepared tooth. The crown forms are available in various sizes of canines, lateral incisors, and central incisors. These crowns are fitted to the prepared teeth and filled with either acrylic or composite. The filled crown form is placed over the prepared tooth and allowed to harden (Fig. 17-6, *A*). Then the crown form is re-

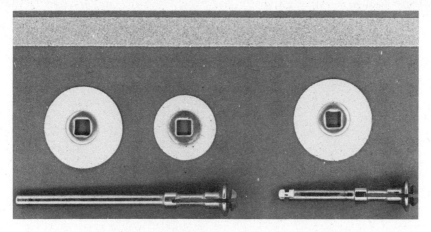

Fig. 17-7. Finishing strip and disks with mandrels.

moved and discarded, and the esthetic restorative material is left on the prepared tooth. This type of crown is also used as a temporary covering for a prepared tooth until a permanent crown can be made.

Portions of the celluloid crown form can be cut away and used to shape portions of teeth. It is common for dentists to use the incisal portion of a crown form to shape the incisal edge of a composite restoration or to use one half of a crown form to shape a Class IV composite restoration (Fig. 17-6, *B*).

Finishing stones (Fig. 5-6)

The best finish on a composite restoration is that which is left by the matrix strip. However, minor finishing is usually required to achieve smooth margins and proper occlusal contact.

Composite restorations can be finished nicely with fine diamond stones or fine green and fine white stones in a conventional-speed handpiece. Stones are available in both HP and RA types and in various shapes.

Finishing disks and strips (Fig. 17-7)

Finishing disks are small, abrasive disks of sandpaper that are used to contour and polish various restorations including composites. They are available with either paper or plastic backing. Disks vary in size from ½ to 1 inch in diameter. A variety of grits are offered by various manufacturers, ranging from coarse to extremely fine. They are used on the conventional-speed handpiece with a Moore's mandrel.

Polishing strips are used to contour the proximal surface of a composite restoration and to smooth margins that cannot be reached by a disk. Strips are available in various widths and grits.

Strips can be inserted interproximally by one of the following methods:

1. Some of the abrasive material is scraped away midway along the length of the strip; then it is inserted like dental floss into the interproximal area (Fig. 17-8, *A*). Some manufacturers provide strips with a smooth area already on the strip.
2. A long diagonal on the end of the strip is cut to create a point that can be threaded into the interproximal area from the facial aspect of the teeth (Fig. 17-8, *B*).

Water soluble lubricant (Fig. 17-9)

When rotary instruments such as burs and stones are used to grind composite materials, a water-soluble lubricant is recommended. The lubricant reduces frictional heat and prevents the instrument from being clogged with debris.

THE COMPOSITE RESTORATIVE PROCEDURE

Since the composite resin is the most common restorative material used in esthetic restorations today, this procedure will be described in detail.

Armamentarium

A suggested armamentarium for the esthetic (composite) restoration is shown in Fig. 17-10.

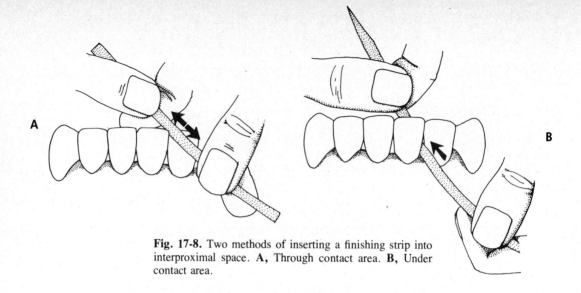

Fig. 17-8. Two methods of inserting a finishing strip into interproximal space. **A,** Through contact area. **B,** Under contact area.

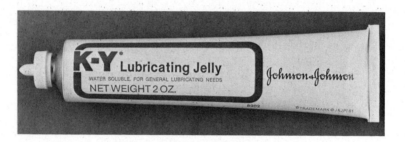

Fig. 17-9. Water soluble lubricant.

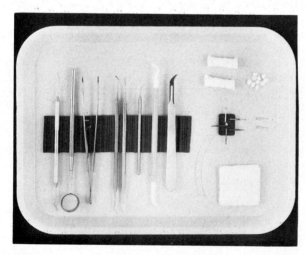

Preset tray

Cowhorn explorer, No. 3
Mouth mirror, No. 4
Cotton pliers
Spoon excavator
Wedelstaedt chisel
Liner applicator
Teflon filling instrument
Scalpel, No. 12B blade
Cotton rolls
Cotton pellets
Burs: FG No. $1/2$, No. 1, No. 2, and No. 34
Round finishing diamond
Wedges
Mylar matrix strip
Gauze sponges, 2x2 inch

Add-on items

Calcium hydroxide liner
Polishing strips and disks
Composite syringe (optional)
(Restorative material)
Cavity varnish
Water-soluble lubricant

Fig. 17-10. Esthetic restoration armamentarium.

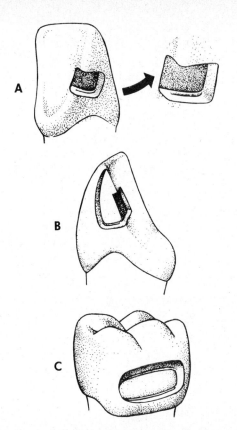

Fig. 17-11. Common preparations in which esthetic restorative materials are used. **A**, Class III. **B**, Class IV. **C**, Class V.

Esthetic cavity preparations

The restorations discussed here are indicated for use in Class III, IV, and V cavity preparations in which esthetics is a primary consideration. Whenever possible, the labial aspect of a tooth should be preserved to enhance the esthetic quality of the final restoration. It is for this reason that Class III restorations are usually prepared from a lingual approach. Class IV and V preparations should be kept as conservative as possible to improve the appearance of the final restoration.

The designs of cavity preparations for esthetic restorations are shown in Fig. 17-11.

Composite restoration: a Class III example

The Class III is the most common cavity preparation that is used for esthetic restorations. The fabrica-

tion of this restoration follows the scheme listed:
1. Anesthesia administration
2. Isolation of the operative field
3. Cavity preparation
4. Cavity medication
5. Matrix strip placement
6. Insertion phase
7. Finishing phase

Anesthesia administration. The infiltration method of local anesthesia is employed to anesthesize maxillary teeth and mandibular anterior teeth, which are the usual candidates for this restoration.

Isolation. Rubber dam isolation is considered the best isolation method for any restoration when it can be used. Careful use of cotton roll isolation is also acceptable.

Cavity preparation. The entire cavity preparation for a Class III composite restorative procedure can be accomplished with round burs and a Wedelstaedt chisel. The preparation is made from a lingual approach to maximize esthetics whenever possible.

Cavity medication. Cavity medication can be accomplished with calcium hydroxide liners. It is advisable to avoid the use of zinc oxide–eugenol as a cavity liner. Eugenol can interfere with the setting of the composite material that comes in contact with it.

Matrix placement. The matrix strip is placed through the contact area in a faciolingual direction. A wooden wedge can be placed cervically to adapt the strip against the tooth surface (Fig. 17-12, *A* and *B*).

Insertion. Once the matrix strip is in place, the composite is mixed according to the manufacturer's directions. These materials set rather quickly. It is advisable to be well organized, with proper instrumentation ready and the cavity preparation ready to receive the material.

After the material is mixed, it can be inserted into the cavity preparation. The method of insertion may be either incremental packing of the composite with a plastic filling instrument or injecting the material into the preparation with a composite syringe. The incremental packing method must be done with care to avoid entrapment of air in the restoration, which would cause air bubbles to show up later as opaque spots in the restoration. This is very noticeable in Class IV and V restorations. The injection technique is the method of choice for insertion. Its only disadvantage is a slight increase in cost because more material is required to fill the syringe than is actually used (Fig. 17-12, *C*).

After the material is inserted in the preparation, the

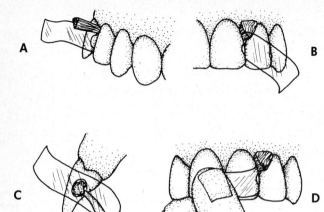

Fig. 17-12. Insertion of composite restorative materials. **A,** Matrix strip and wedge in place, lateral view. **B,** Matrix and wedge in place, anterior view. **C,** Injection of material into preparation. **D,** Strip pulled into position to form proximal surface of restoration.

matrix strip is pulled tightly around the tooth to form the proximal aspect of the restoration (Fig. 17-12, *D*). The strip is held in place until the material reaches its initial set. The dentist can determine this by holding a sample of the excess material in the hand to feel when it has achieved its initial hardness.

The strip and wedge are removed when the initial hardness is reached. The restoration can now be trimmed and polished during the finishing phase.

Finishing. Excessive material that squeezes out of the cavity preparation when the strip is pulled is called *flash*. Flash can be trimmed away from the cervical and facial margins with a scalpel (and polishing disks if needed). The lingual flash can be removed with a large round finishing bur or a fine-grain diamond stone that has been lubricated with water-soluble lubricant. The lingual contour of the restoration can also be formed with these cutting instruments. Polishing strips can be used to refine the proximal contour of the restoration if needed.

Many experts in composite materials believe that the restoration with the least amount of finishing required will resist staining to a greater degree than a restoration that requires a good deal of finishing.

Fabrication of a Class IV restoration

The Class IV restoration is used to restore teeth with missing incisal angles as a result of fracture or extensive caries (Fig. 17-13, *A*).

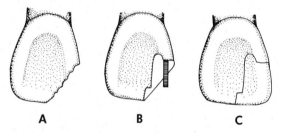

Fig. 17-13. Restoration of a Class IV cavity with an esthetic material. **A,** Fractured incisor. **B,** Prepared tooth with a retention pin. **C,** Finished restoration.

The armamentarium used for this procedure is the same as that used for the Class III restoration.

The fabrication of this restoration employs the following scheme:

1. Anesthesia administration
2. Isolation of the operative field
3. Cavity preparation
4. Cavity medication
5. Matrix placement
6. Insertion phase
7. Finishing phase

Anesthesia and isolation methods. Anesthesia and isolation methods are the same as those used for the Class III restoration.

Cavity preparation. After the outline form has been completed, the preparation is often so extensive that additional retention is needed to hold the restorative material in place. This can be accomplished using the following methods:

1. *Pin retention* (Fig. 17-13, *B*). The same types of pins that are used for the pin-retained amalgam can be used for this purpose.

2. *Adhesive composite resin materials.* A relatively new concept in composite restorative materials is to attach the material to the tooth structure by bonding. These special materials function much like the occlusal pit and fissure sealants (Chapter 1). The tooth structure is etched with a mild acid to enhance the adhesion of the material to the tooth. Some dentists prefer to use both adhesive materials and pins for maximum retention.

Cavity medication. Cavity medication follows the scheme outlined in Chapter 15, with the exception that preparations which are deeper than normal can be medicated with calcium hydroxide liners on the axial wall.

Matrix placement. Matrix strips can be used in less extensive cases to form the proximal aspect of the restoration. The operator can properly shape the incisal aspect, using a polishing disk to grind away the excess material.

In more extensive cases a celluloid crown form is trimmed with scissors so that the appropriate incisal angle is removed from the rest of the crown (Fig. 17-6). This celluloid ''incisal angle'' is used as a matrix to shape the proximal and incisal aspects of the restoration.

Insertion. When the celluloid crown method is used, the crown is filled with material while the dentist places some material in the retentive areas of the preparation with a plastic filling instrument or the composite syringe. The filled crown is then placed over the prepared cavity and held in place until the material reaches its initial set. The operator should punch a small hole in the incisal-angle portion of the crown to avoid air entrapment while filling the crown.

Finishing. After the material has reached its initial set, the crown is removed and the restoration is shaped and polished with polishing disks, strips, and large finishing burs lubricated with water-soluble lubricant.

Fabrication of a Class V composite restoration

The only difference in the fabrication of a Class V composite restoration is that a matrix band is not needed in the procedure. The restorative material can be easily inserted into the preparation and shaped with a plastic instrument. Finishing should be kept to a minimum, using a scalpel and polishing disks.

SUMMARY

Composite restorations are probably second only to the amalgam restoration in terms of the frequency that they are done in a general practice. Consequently the dental assistant must be very familiar with the specific materials that are used as well as the instruments and supplies that are needed for the procedure.

BIBLIOGRAPHY

Charbeneau, G.T., and others: Principles and practice of operative dentistry, ed. 2, Philadelphia, 1981, Lea & Febiger.

Craig, R.G., O'Brien, W.J., and Powers, J.M.: Dental materials: properties and manipulation, ed. 3, St. Louis, 1983, The C.V. Mosby Co.

CHAPTER 18

CAST GOLD INLAY
RESTORATIONS

Gold has been used continuously as a restorative material since the Etruscans first used it hundreds of years before Christ. Pure gold and alloys of gold have many properties that make them extremely desirable restorative materials.

The following are some of the principal properties that are desirable from a dental point of view:

1. Gold can be easily melted and accurately cast into various shapes.
2. Gold alloys are extremely strong and resist the crushing forces generated during the mastication of food far better than amalgam.
3. Gold has superb edge strength so that the margins of a gold restoration will not fracture, which often occurs with an amalgam restoration.
4. Gold does not corrode or discolor in the presence of oral fluids.

A gold inlay is a restoration that is made from gold alloy that has been cast to fit a cavity preparation made by the dentist. The term *inlay* implies that the bulk of the restoration is contained within the confines of a tapered cavity preparation. Various types of inlays are fabricated for Class I, II, III, IV, V, and VI preparations.

A modification of the cast gold inlay is the protected cusp or onlay restoration (Fig. 18-1). These restorations extend over the cusps of posterior teeth to prevent fracture of the teeth when biting forces are applied.

The procedure for the fabrication of either type of restoration is basically the same. Two separate appointments are required. During the first appointment the tooth is prepared, and impressions are taken from which models of the patient's teeth are made. The inlay is fabricated in the dental laboratory using these

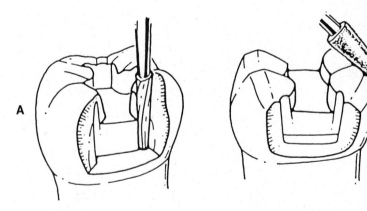

Fig. 18-1. Onlay preparation. **A,** Tapered fissure bur used to develop internal form. **B,** Diamond stone used to reduce cusp height.

models. The patient wears a temporary restoration while this laboratory procedure is accomplished. Upon return for the second appointment the temporary restoration is removed, and the inlay is fitted to the cavity preparation, the adjacent teeth, and the patient's occlusion. After all refinements are completed the inlay is cemented in place.

The following instruments and supplies are required for the "preparation" and the "seating" appointments.

COMMON INSTRUMENTS AND SUPPLIES
Items needed for the preparation appointment

Rotary and hand instruments. Most cast gold instrument setups consist of the common rotary and hand instruments discussed in Chapter 5. A sample armamentarium is shown in Fig. 18-2.

Occlusal clearance wax. Occlusal clearance wax is a thin sheet of wax with a 28-gauge thickness. When a 1½ × ½ inch strip is folded three times to form a ½-inch square, it can be used as a gauge to determine if the dentist has removed enough tooth structure from the occlusal surface in onlay and crown preparations (Fig. 20-4, *D*). The tooth structure removed from the occlusal surface will be replaced with gold.

After the ½-inch square is prepared, it is placed over the prepared tooth, and the patient is instructed to close the teeth together in his normal bite relationship. If there is proper clearance between the occlusal surfaces of the prepared tooth and the opposing teeth, there will be no indentations in the wax square. If there is inadequate clearance, more tooth structure will have to be removed.

Gingival retraction cord (Fig. 18-2). Gingival retraction cord is usually impregnated with a vasoconstrictor such as epinephrine. After the gold cavity preparation has been completed, a piece of this cord is tucked into the gingival sulcus along any cervical margins. The vasoconstrictor in the cord will cause temporary shrinkage of the gingiva away from the tooth and allow impression material to be easily injected into the gingival sulcus. This assures the dentist of a good impression of the cervical margin of the preparation, which is critical to the fabrication of a properly fitting gold restoration.

Hemostatic agents (Fig. 18-2). After the preparation of a tooth for a gold restoration, there is often some gingival bleeding caused by minor abrasion of the gingiva by preparation instruments. Control of gingival bleeding during impression taking is essential to obtain maximum accuracy. Hemorrhage is often halted by the vasoconstrictor in retraction cord. Control of bleeding can be enhanced by wetting the retraction cord with an astringent or hemostatic agent.

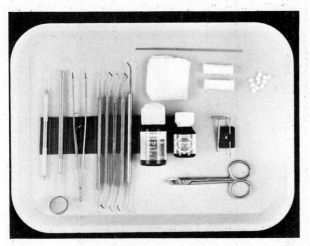

Preset tray

Cowhorn explorer, No. 3
Mouth mirror, No. 4
Cotton pliers
Spoon excavator
Enamel hatchet 8E
Gingival margin trimmers, No. 12 and No. 13
Plastic filling instrument, F.P. No. 1
Gingival retraction cord
Hemostatic agent
Gauze sponges, 2 × 2 inch
Lightning strip
Cotton rolls
Cotton pellets
Lightning disk
Burs, No. 171 and straight tapered diamond
Scissors (crown and collar)

Add-on items

Temporary cement
Final impression material setup
Impression trays
Alginate impression setup
Occlusal registration material

Fig. 18-2. Gold restoration armamentarium (preparation appointment).

These agents induce clotting of blood in the small capillaries of the gingiva.

Impression trays (Fig. 18-3). Impression-taking is a duplication process whereby accurate replicas of the teeth and surrounding tissues can be made. Accuracy is essential in duplicating a prepared tooth for a cast gold restoration. Since gold inlays are fabricated in the laboratory on a replica of the patient's tooth, called a die, it must be an exact copy of the real tooth.

An important step in the impression-taking proce-dure is the selection of impression trays that will fit the patient's dental arches. Various manufacturers make stock trays of different sizes. Perforated metal trays (Fig. 18-3, *A*) are used for alginate impression material. Perforated plastic trays (Fig. 18-3, *B*) can be used for either alginate or one of the impression materials used to make the die. These plastic trays are disposable.

Alginate impressions are used to make study mo-dels of the patient's teeth. This technique is described

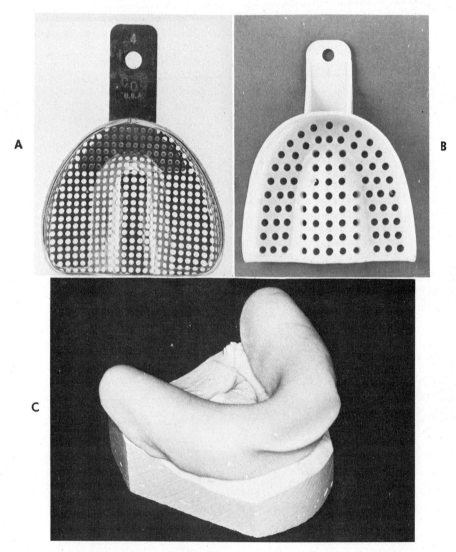

Fig. 18-3. Impression trays. **A,** Perforated metal. **B,** Perforated plastic. **C,** Custom acrylic.

in Chapter 24. Alginate is also used to take an impression of the teeth that oppose the tooth being restored.

The custom acrylic tray (Fig. 18-3, *C*) is made specifically for the patient being treated. A study model of the patient's teeth is used to make this custom impression tray. Since this tray fits the patient's arch more accurately, it is generally preferred over a stock tray for taking the impression of the dental arch that contains the tooth which has been prepared for the inlay restoration. Mercaptan (rubber base) or silicone impression materials are generally used in custom acrylic trays for the inlay impression procedure.

Regardless of which types of trays will be used, they must be a part of the setup during the preparation appointment.

Impression materials. There are three basic types of impression materials that can be used to take an impression of a prepared tooth. They are mercaptan (rubber base), silicone, and agar hydrocolloid. Each material is very accurate. The selection of the material to be used for impression-taking is a matter of the personal preference of the dentist. A text on dental materials should be consulted for the particular chemical and physical properties of these materials.

All three of these materials can be used in the syringe-tray technique of impression-taking discussed on page 237. These impression materials and the syringe-tray technique are routinely used in restorative procedures. The same basic impression-taking technique is used in the fabrication of inlays, crowns, and fixed bridges.

Another impression material that is often used in dentistry is alginate. Alginate is *not* used to make the replica of the prepared tooth (die). It is used to take preoperative study models and impressions of the opposing teeth that will be needed to create the proper occlusion on the gold restoration. Alginate impressions are taken with only an impression tray. The syringe-tray technique is not used for this impression material.

Alginate impressions. Alginate impressions require the use of the items shown in Fig. 18-4.

The mixing procedure is as follows:

1. Prepare the material by adding premeasured alginate powder to the rubber-mixing bowl, which contains a premeasured amount of water. Manufacturers provide the proper measuring devices with their product.
2. Mix the powder and water together with the wide-bladed spatula within 1 minute. The mix must be smooth and creamy. To accomplish this, press the alginate against the sides of the rubber bowl with the spatula while mixing.
3. Load the material in the tray and place in the patient's mouth. (A description of the alginate impression technique is presented on p. 331.) Setting times range from

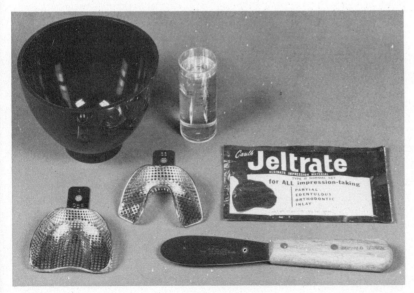

Rubber mixing bowl
Wide-bladed spatula
Water measure
Powder scoop (unless premeasured packets are used)
Alginate material
Alginate impression trays

Fig. 18-4. Alginate impression armamentarium.

1½ to 3 minutes, depending on whether regular-set or fast-set alginate is used. The temperature of the water also influences setting time. Most manufacturers recommend a temperature of 70° (21.1° C) for maximum accuracy and ample working time.

4. After the impression is removed from the patient's mouth, rinse it with lukewarm water and wrap it in a wet paper towel. For maximum accuracy, a model should be made from the impression within the first 30 minutes after removal.

A handy tip for the assistant is to use premeasured bags of alginate powder that are available from the manufacturer or to premeasure the alginate from a bulk container and store it in plastic sandwich bags. This is a good way to save valuable chairside time.

Mercaptan and silicone impressions. The items required for the preparation of mercaptan and silicone impression are shown in Figs. 18-5 and 18-6.

Both of these types of impression materials are available in different consistencies. There is a light-bodied, or thin, consistency that is loaded in an injection-type syringe, and a very heavy-bodied, or thick, consistency that is used to fill the impression tray. Both consistencies are used for impression taking in gold restorations.

The procedure that is commonly used to prepare these materials is as follows:

1. *Dispensing.* Dispense the mercaptan material on the mixing pads as shown in Fig. 18-7, *A*. Dispense the syringe material so that equal lengths of base and catalyst paste lie side by side on the mixing pad. Repeat the same for the tray material. Be careful not to allow the base material to contact the catalyst until the mixing process is ready to begin. The actual amount dispensed is determined by the number of teeth to be included in the impression. The dentist should be consulted to guide the assistant in this regard.
2. *Mixing the syringe material.* If you are going to mix both the syringe and tray material for the dentist without help, the syringe material should be mixed first. Mix the syringe base and catalyst rapidly, using the tip of the spatula with a circular movement (Fig. 18-7, *B*). After the mix is rather uniform in color, wipe the spatula clean with the paper towel. Continue the mixing process using the flat surface of the spatula blade (Fig. 18-7, *C*). This completes the blending of the materials and eliminates air bubbles in the mix.
3. *Loading the syringe.* The impression syringe consists of four parts: plunger, barrel, hub, and tip. To fill the syringe with impression material, the syringe tip must be in place and the plunger removed. Force the mixed material into the barrel by sliding the open end of the barrel

through the mix repeatedly (Fig. 18-7, *D*). After the syringe is loaded, insert the plunger into the barrel. The syringe is ready for use.

4. *Mixing the tray material* (Fig. 18-8, *A* to *C*). Prepare the tray material in the same manner as the syringe material. The only difference between the two procedures is that the tray material is physically more difficult to mix. The total amount of material used and the consistency both contribute to the difficulty in mixing.

   When the mix is complete, load the material into an impression tray (Fig. 18-8, *D*).
5. *Mixing time.* Although the mixing time can be varied somewhat, learn to be able to mix each component within 1 minute, to give the dentist adequate working time to take the impression.

The mixing scheme just outlined describes the technique for mixing mercaptan. However, although the silicone impression material is prepared in the same manner, the method of dispensing is different. Silicones are packaged so that both the syringe and tray material utilize tubes of base material, light-bodied for the syringe and heavy-bodied for the tray. The base is activated by adding drops of accelerator to the base. This differs from the mercaptan procedure, in which equal lengths of base and catalyst pastes are used. This difference is critical when estimating the amount of silicone base to be dispensed. Since only a few drops of silicone accelerator are used, it does not significantly increase the volume of material, as does the catalyst paste with the mercaptan materials.

Mixing techniques and the loading of the syringe and tray are the same for the silicones as they are for the mercaptan materials.

Impression trays that are used with these materials are either disposable plastic trays available in various sizes and shapes or custom acrylic trays that are made to fit the individual patient. Both types of trays are usually perforated to allow impression material to ooze out of the perforations. This provides mechanical retention of the impression material in the tray after it sets. A tray adhesive is also used to enhance this retention. The adhesive can be applied to the interior surface of the tray well in advance of the impression procedure. The retention of the impression material in the tray is critical to the achievement of an accurate impression. Considerable force is generated during removal of the impression from the patient's teeth. This force is in the form of a pull on the material and tends to pull it out of the tray. Tray perforation and tray adhesives prevent this from occurring.

Agar hydrocolloid impressions. These require

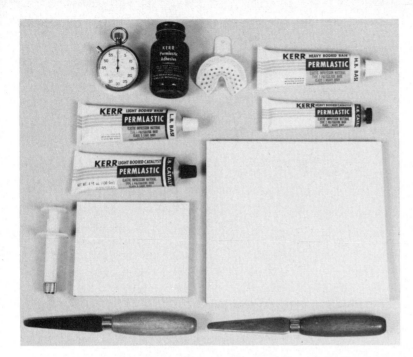

Two mixing pads
Two stiff-bladed spatulas
Two paper towels (not shown)
Injection syringe
Impression tray
Impression material (syringe and tray types)
Tray adhesive
Stopwatch

Fig. 18-5. Mercaptan (rubber base) impression armamentarium.

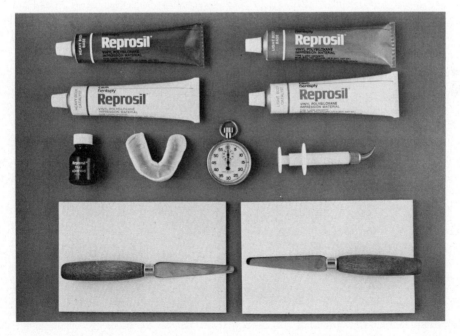

Fig. 18-6. Vinyl polysiloxane (silicone) impression armamentarium.

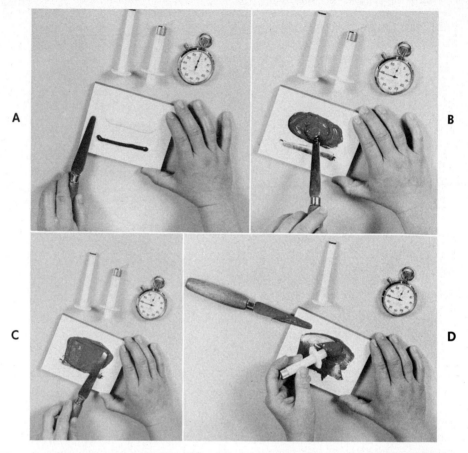

Fig. 18-7. Preparation of syringe mercaptan material. **A,** Dispense material in equal lengths. **B,** Initial mixing, using tip of spatula in circular motion. **C,** Final mixing, using flat surface of spatula blade. **D,** Loading the syringe. (NOTE: The assistant in this illustration is left-handed.)

more bulky and expensive equipment than any of the other impression taking systems. The required items are shown in Fig. 18-9.

Agar hydrocolloid is packaged in a gel state. A great deal of this material is water (up to 85%); therefore care must be exercised to store and handle it according to manufacturer's directions to prevent evaporation.

The basic method used to take a hydrocolloid impression is to convert the solid (gel) state to a semiliquid (sol) state by heating the material in a hot-water conditioner. Once the material is in a semiliquid form, it can be inserted in the patient's mouth via an injection syringe and a special impression tray and

then cooled to convert the material back to the solid state (gel). When the material is back in the solid state, the impression can be removed.

The conversion of the hydrocolloid from the gel to the sol state involves the use of three hot-water baths. The tray material is placed in all three baths during processing. The syringe material is placed only in the first two baths.

The preparation and technique of impression-taking with agar hydrocolloid are as follows (Fig. 18-10):

1. *Loading the syringe.* Insert one small stick of syringe hydrocolloid into the barrel of the syringe. It is advisable to remove the protective cap from the needle of the

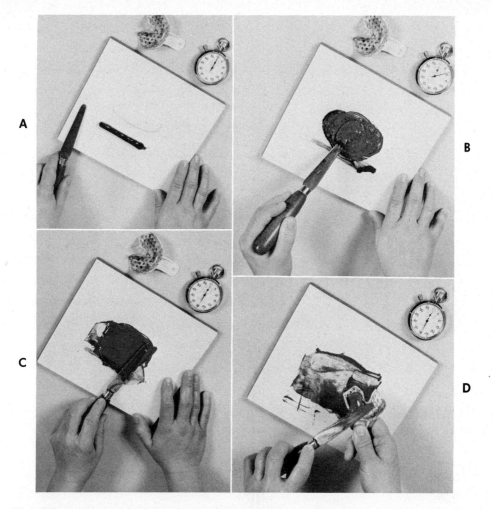

Fig. 18-8. Preparation of tray mercaptan material. **A,** Dispense material in equal lengths. **B,** Initial mixing with spatula tip. **C,** Final mixing with flat surface of spatula. **D,** Loading the tray. (NOTE: The assistant in this illustration is left-handed.)

syringe and insert the plunger into the syringe barrel, forcing out excess air around the hydrocolloid stick. Replace the cap over the needle. This prevents expansion of air in the syringe during the heating process, which could force the plunger out of the syringe and let the hydrocolloid escape into the water bath.
2. *Boiling bath* (212° F [100° C]). Place the loaded syringe and a tube of tray-type hydrocolloid in the boiling-water bath for 10 to 15 minutes. This converts the gel to the sol state.
3. *Storage bath* (149° F [65° C]). Both the syringe and tray materials can be transferred to this bath if the materials

are not going to be used immediately. They can remain in the storage bath for several hours before the material is used.
4. *Tempering bath* (113° F [39° C]). When the cavity preparation has been completed and the gingival retraction cord has been placed, remove the tube of tray material from the storage bath. Next, fill the hydrocolloid impression tray with the soft, semiliquid material. Place the filled tray in the tempering bath for 5 minutes. This cools the material within tolerable limits to avoid burning the patient. It also causes the tray material to thicken slightly.

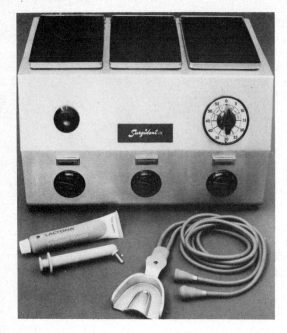

Agar hydrocolloid material (syringe and tray types)
Hydrocolloid conditioner
Injection syringe
Water-cooled trays
Water-coolant tubes

Fig. 18-9. Agar hydrocolloid conditioner armamentarium. *Left to right:* tray material (tube), syringe, impression tray, cooling tubes.

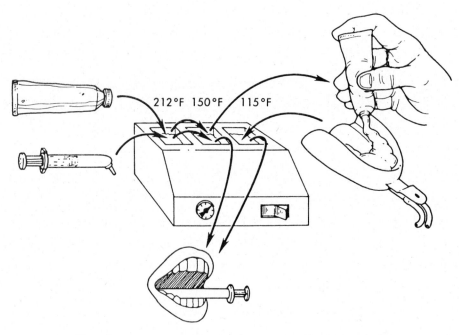

Fig. 18-10. Preparation of agar hydrocolloid impression material.

The syringe material is not tempered. Tempering would thicken the material inside the syringe so that it would be too thick to inject through the thin syringe needle.

5. *Impression procedure.* After removal of the retraction cord, the hydrocolloid syringe is removed from the storage bath and the needle cap is removed. The material is injected around the prepared tooth. Then the filled impression tray is removed from the tempering bath and the cooling tubes are attached quickly. The tray is placed in the patient's mouth over the prepared and adjacent teeth.

The impression tray contains small tubes that allow water to be circulated around the impression material to cool it, thus converting it back to the gel or solid state.

The coolant tubes that are attached to the tray provide the water supply and the exhaust for the circulating water. One tube can be connected to the air-water syringe for a water source. The patient can be instructed to activate the water button. The exhaust tube can be draped into a nearby sink or a large plastic container to collect the exhausted water.

Cooling usually requires from 3 to 5 mintues at a water temperature of 55° F (12.7° C).

6. *Pouring the model.* After the impression is in the solid state, it is carefully removed. Once removed, the model should be poured at once. Agar hydrocolloid is very delicate material. It loses its dimensional accuracy rapidly as a result of water loss. On the other hand, if it is placed in water for any length of time, it absorbs water and swells. Either condition must be prevented to ensure maximum accuracy. The impression should be gently wrapped in a moist paper towel while the die stone material is being prepared for pouring the model.

Agar hydrocolloid has diminished in popularity since the development of the mercaptan (rubber base) and silicone materials. However, it should not be overlooked, since it is a very accurate impression material if handled properly.

Bite registration material. After the impression-taking procedure is finished, some dentists prefer to fabricate a device to orient the upper and lower models in the proper bite relationship during the laboratory phase. This device is commonly referred to as a bite registration. A variety of materials are frequently used for this purpose. Some of the more common ones include pink baseplate wax, self-curing acrylic, and zinc oxide–eugenol bite registration paste.

The patient simply bites into the selected material while it is soft. After the bite registration material hardens it is removed from the teeth. The imprints of the biting surfaces of the teeth are then used as guides to orient the upper and lower laboratory models of the teeth together (Fig. 18-19).

Temporization materials. After the preparation and impression procedures have been completed, the prepared tooth must be protected (temporized) until the patient's next appointment.

There are several ways to temporize a prepared tooth. The specific method selected depends on the type of preparation and, to some extent, the personal preference of the dentist.

Inlay temporization is usually accomplished by filling the prepared cavity with a semisoft material that will be easy to remove at the next appointment, when the restoration is fitted to the tooth and cemented in place. Examples of such materials are Dura-Seal,* Ward's Tempak,† and Coe-Pak.‡ Dura-Seal is a plastic material that is painted into the preparation with a sable brush. The brush is dipped into the liquid component and then into the powder. The wetted powder is carried to the preparation and inserted with the brush. This is continued until the preparation is filled. Ward's Tempak and Coe-Pak are mixed to a thick consistency on a paper pad according to the manufacturer's directions. A few strands of cotton fibers from a cotton pellet can be incorporated in the mix for added strength. The material is placed in the preparation, and the patient is asked to bite down on the material. The excess filling material is carved away, and the material is allowed to harden before the patient is dismissed (Fig. 18-11).

Items needed for the seating appointment

Armamentarium. A suggested armamentarium for cementation of an inlay is shown in Fig. 18-12.

At the appointment for inserting the gold restoration (the seating appointment) a few instruments should be added to the armamentarium. Some of these instruments and devices are described here.

Inlay seating devices. To properly check the fit of a gold restoration, it must be seated completely on the tooth. A convenient way to accomplish this is to concentrate biting forces onto the occlusal surface of the restoration. This will drive the restoration to its final position on the tooth. Fig. 18-13 shows the use of the three most common devices for this purpose.

After all adjustments have been made on the res-

*Reliance Dental Manufacturing, Chicago.
†Westward Dental Products Co., San Francisco.
‡Coe Laboratories, Inc., Chicago.

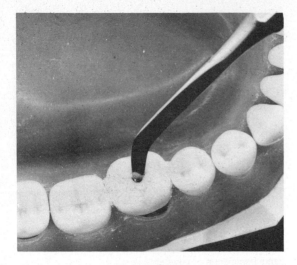

Fig. 18-11. Temporization of an inlay preparation with Ward's Tempak.

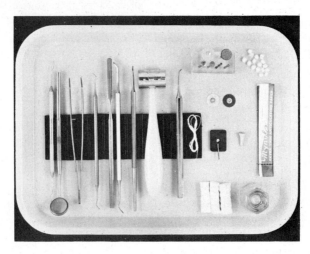

Fig. 18-12. Gold restoration cementation armamentarium.

Preset tray

Cowhorn explorer, No. 3
Mouth mirror, No. 4
Cotton pliers
Spoon excavator
Cement spatula, No. 324 or No. 24
Plastic filling instrument, F.P. No. 1
Gold foil condenser, straight
Gold foil mallet
Hand burnisher, 5S
Dental floss
Craytex polishing wheels
Moore's mandrels
Green stone, wheel shaped
Green stone, knife edge
Ball burnishers, H.P.
Cotton pellets
Moore's disks
Articulating paper
Bur, R.A. No. 4
Cooley peg
Cotton rolls
Dappen dish

Add-on items

Finel cement material
Cavity varnish
Isopropyl alcohol
Mixing slab or pad

toration, the final cement is prepared and placed on the tissue surface of the restoration. The restoration is placed on the tooth and initially seated with finger pressure. Then it is finally driven into place with one of the seating devices. Next, it is burnished, and any minor adjustments can be made.

Burnishers (Fig. 5-14). Burnishers are available in hand types and straight-handpiece types. They are used to bend the fine margins of a gold restoration down on the tooth surface immediately after cementa-

tion. The margins frequently are bent in the handling of the gold restoration. The burnisher is rubbed across the gold margin from the gold toward the tooth structure. This perfects the fit of the margin to the tooth structure.

Finishing stones, burs, and disks (Figs. 5-5, 5-6, and 5-7). A variety of shapes and styles of fine-grit grindstones and finishing burs are available to make minor adjustments on gold restorations. They are used to correct occlusion, finish margins, and reduce

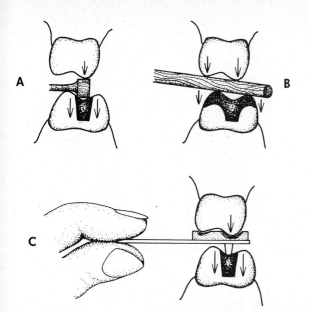

Fig. 18-13. Gold restoration seating devices. **A,** Cooley peg. **B,** Orangewood stick. **C,** Inlay seating device.

heavy contact between a gold restoration and an adjacent tooth. Sandpaper disks are used to finish proximal margins.

Dental cements for final cementation. There are basically three types of cement that are popular for use as final cementation agents for gold and porcelain restorations. These are zinc phosphate, polycarboxylate, and zinc oxide–eugenol. A text on dental materials should be consulted for the properties and characteristics of these cements.

Two critical characteristics of any dental cement are film thickness and strength. Cement must be rather thin so that it can ooze out between the tooth structure and the gold restoration when the crown is seated. A cement that is too thick can prevent the restoration from seating completely during cementation procedures. On the other hand, the strength of a cement is important to retain the restoration and to maintain a proper seal between the tooth and restoration. If the cement is mixed so that it is too thin, strength is markedly reduced.

Zinc phosphate cement. Zinc phosphate cement is one of the oldest cementation agents used in dentistry today. Proper mixing of this material is accomplished by mixing it to a specific consistency within a time limit. There are several methods used to achieve the proper consistency of zinc phosphate for use in the cementation of a gold restoration. The method as described uses the following materials (Fig. 18-14, *A*):

Zinc phosphate (powder and liquid)
Measuring stick
Glass slab
No. 324 cement spatula
Stopwatch

The mixing procedure is as follows:

1. *Dispensing the materials.* This cement produces heat when the powder and liquid components are combined. Therefore a glass slab is required as a mixing surface to absorb the heat and cool the mix. The measuring stick has a small cup on one end and a large cup on the other. Press the cups into the bottle of powder to pick up and measure the amount of powder being dispensed.

   The liquid:powder ratio that works well is 1 large cup and 1 small cup of powder to be mixed with 6 to 7 drops of liquid. After the powder is dispensed, divide all the powder into 6 equal-sized sections. Then dispense 6 to 7 drops of liquid onto the surface of the slab to the left of the divided powder (Fig. 18-14, *B*). A large cup of powder can be placed in the upper right-hand corner of the slab in case it is needed.

2. *Incremental mixing.* The object of this mixing technique is to slowly mix the powder and liquid together to minimize heat production. However, if the mixing time is excessive, the mix will begin to set. Trial mixes have demonstrated that a favorable mixing pace calls for adding and mixing 1 of the 6 sections of powder every 15 seconds. Thus it will take 90 seconds to mix all 6 sections into the liquid. However, all 6 sections may not be needed to reach the proper consistency for cementation. Add each section of powder to the liquid and spatulate it with broad strokes over an area the size of a silver dollar (Fig. 18-14, *C* and *D*).

3. *Testing the mix* (Fig. 18-14, *E*). After the addition and mixing of the fourth section, it is good to test the mix for proper consistency. Proper consistency is determined by gathering the mixed cement into a small puddle on the slab. Dip the broad surface of the spatula into the puddle and raise the spatula slowly from the slab. The cement should string out approximately 1 to 1½ inches between the slab and the spatula blade before it drops off the spatula back into the puddle. If it strings out longer than 1½ inches, the mix is too thick. If it is less than 1 inch, more powder must be added. Continue testing as the fifth and sixth sections of powder are added. Sometimes it is necessary to add some of the extra powder stored in the upper right-hand corner of the slab to achieve the proper consistency. *Consistency* is a key word. Mixing zinc phosphate cement is not just a matter of combining 6 to 7 drops of liquid with 1 large and 1 small cup of powder every time a mix is made. The temperature and

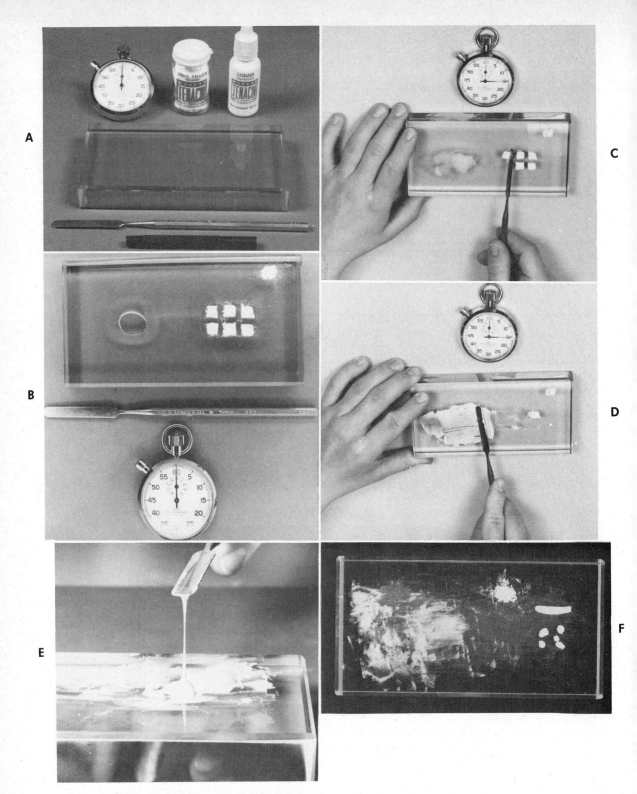

Fig. 18-14. Preparation of zinc phosphate cement. **A,** Armamentarium. **B,** Dispensed materials. **C** and **D,** Increment of powder added to liquid every 15 seconds and mixed, using broad spatulations. **E,** Testing the mix. **F,** Cement base consistency.

humidity of the day will influence how much powder can be added to the liquid before the ideal consistency is reached.

4. *Application of the cement.* When the proper consistency of the cement has been reached, cover the tissue surface of the restoration with a thin coat of cement. Deliver the restoration to the dentist on the slab, with the restoration resting on the coated surface. A filling instrument should accompany the delivery of the restoration so that the dentist can add some additional cement to the preparation before seating the restoration in place.

Zinc phosphate cement base. Zinc phosphate cement is not only used for final cementation purposes but also as a cement base under various restorations. A cement base is a strong dental cement that has been mixed to a doughlike consistency and used as artificial dentin in deep cavity preparations. (p. 192).

To prepare zinc phosphate cement for use as a cement base, the basic mixing technique just described is used, except that 2 to 3 scoops of powder are placed in the upper right-hand corner of the slab instead of the 1 scoop that is recommended for cementation purposes.

Once the cement is mixed to the consistency described for cementation, the extra powder from the upper right-hand corner of the slab is brought into the mix, ½ scoop or less at a time, until the cement is well blended into a thick, doughlike consistency. The fingers can be coated with powder from the slab, and the doughlike cement can be rolled into a rope. Small

pieces can be cut off the "rope" and delivered to the operator for use in the prepared cavity (Fig. 18-14, *F*). The entire mixing time should not exceed 2½ minutes to allow enough working time for the operator to place the cement base.

Polycarboxylate cement. This is a relatively new cement being used in dentistry. It possesses some of the desirable characteristics found in zinc phosphate cement, but does not cause the pulpal irritation produced by the acidic zinc phosphate. A big plus from the dental assistant's viewpoint is the ease of mixing compared with that of zinc phosphate cement. The following materials are needed to prepare polycarboxylate cement (Fig. 18-15):

Polycarboxylate cement (powder and liquid)
Paper mixing pad
Measuring scoop
Spatula
Stopwatch

Following is a description of the preparation of Durelon,* a brand of polycarboxylate cement:

1. *Dispensing the ingredients.* Place one scoop of powder in the center of the mixing pad. The special measuring scoop is provided by the manufacturer. Place three drops of the liquid component adjacent to the powder.
2. *Mixing technique.* Combine the liquid and powder all at one time. The powder must be completely wetted by the liquid. Use a folding action with the spatula to accom-

*Premier Dental Mgf., Philadelphia.

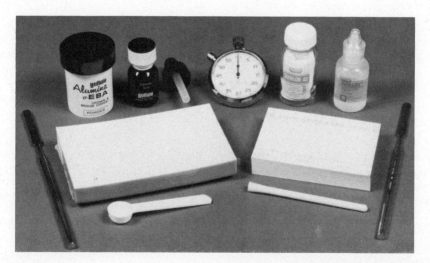

Fig. 18-15. Zinc oxide–eugenol *(left)* and polycarboxylate final cementation materials *(right).*

plish this. For a smooth mix, spread the mix over an area the size of a silver dollar with the broad surface of the spatula. The mixing should be completed within 30 seconds.

3. *Coating the restoration.* Place the cement on the restoration in the same manner as described for zinc phosphate cement. Durelon cement sets rather quickly so that care must be taken to avoid delay in delivering the restoration to the dentist.

Zinc oxide–eugeneol cements. These cements have been used in dentistry since the 1890s. Until recent years they have been used primarily as temporary cements and interim dressings. Manufacturers have developed new zinc oxide–eugenol cements that have adequate strength and film thickness to be used as a permanent cementation agent. Dentists prefer to use nonirritating substances in cements, such as zinc oxide–eugenol and polycarboxylate, as long as they meet strength and film thickness requirements.

The following materials are needed to prepare a typical zinc oxide–eugenol cement (Fig. 18-15):

Mixing pad
Zinc oxide–eugenol cement (powder and liquid)
Measuring scoop
No. 324 spatula
Stopwatch

Following is a description of the preparation of EBA with Alumina, a common brand of zinc oxide–eugenol cement:

1. *Dispensing the ingredients.* Dispense one level scoop of powder on the slab along with 4 drops of liquid.
2. *Mixing technique.* All the ingredients can be combined at once by a folding action of the spatula. Once the powder is completely wetted, press the mix against the pad with the broad surface of the spatula. Use repeated strokes over the mix with the spatula, in a barber's "stropping" motion, to produce proper film thickness in the mix. The mix should be completed within 30 to 45 seconds. The cement should string out 1 inch above the pad when being tested for consistency.

THE CAST GOLD INLAY PROCEDURE

Having completed an overview of the more common instruments and supplies used in the cast gold inlay procedure, the following is a step-by-step description of how it is accomplished. The MOD (Class VI) has been selected as an example.

Inlay-preparation appointment: Class VI (MOD) example

As mentioned previously, fabrication of an inlay usually requires two appointments. One appointment is devoted to the preparation of the tooth and impression taking. The second appointment is used for cementation of the finished restoration. The time between these two appointments must be sufficient to allow for the casting of the inlay in the laboratory. The patient wears a temporary dressing in the prepared tooth between the two appointments.

The sequence of events that takes place at the preparation appointment is as follows:

1. Anesthesia administration
2. Isolation
3. Cavity preparation and medication
4. Gingival retraction
5. Impression taking
6. Opposing model impression
7. Bite registration
8. Temporization

Anesthesia administration. See Chapter 7 for anesthetic techniques.

Isolation. Cotton roll isolation works very well during gold preparation procedures. If a rubber dam is used, it must be removed before gingival retraction and impression taking.

Cavity preparation. Gold inlays are fabricated for all classes of cavity preparations. All these cavity preparations have internal draw built in their design.

Draw is a term used to describe the relationship of the cavity walls from the floor of the cavity preparation to the cavosurface margins. The walls must be slightly tapered so that the gold restoration can slide into place (Fig. 18-16). Excessive taper would result in loss of retention of the restoration in the tooth. Dentists use tapered burs (No. 171) and straight tapered diamonds to establish the proper amount of taper.

Most dentists prefer to place small bevels on the cavosurface margins of the preparation. It is easier to fit gold castings to a beveled surface than to a butt joint. A flame-shaped diamond stone and gingival

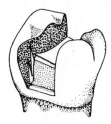

Fig. 18-16. Class VI inlay preparation.

margin trimmers are useful for this purpose.

Inlay preparations must have smooth cavity walls to achieve a proper fit of the inlay inside the tooth. Enamel hatchets are often used to plane the cavity walls.

Cement bases are placed at this time if they are needed (p. 192).

Gingival retraction. After the preparation is finished, the gingiva must be retracted away from the cervical margins of the preparation. The purpose is to create a space between the cervical portion of the tooth and the gingiva to allow impression material to accurately record the cervical margin.

This retraction is accomplished by gently tucking gingival retraction cord in the gingival crevice in the region of the cervical margin of the preparation (Fig. 18-17). The plastic filling instrument can be used for this purpose. A quite common practice is to place two strands of the cord to gain adequate retraction. The cord is treated with a vasoconstrictor, which causes temporary shrinkage of the gingiva. The cord must remain in place for 3 to 4 minutes. Hemostatic agents are sometimes used to stop gingival bleeding that may occur.

The impression material can be dispensed and mixed while the operator is waiting for the retraction to take place.

Impression-taking. Impression-taking is a method used by dentists to make a duplicate of the patient's teeth and surrounding tissues. The laboratory technician makes an exact model of the patient's teeth and the prepared cavity from this impression. The gold inlay is made on this model and returned to the dentist for cementation in the patient's prepared tooth.

The most common method of impression-taking employs the syringe-tray technique. This technique requires the use of two consistencies of the same impression material. One thinner consistency of material is mixed and loaded in a special injection syringe. A second, thicker material is mixed and loaded in an impression tray that will fit over the patient's teeth.

Following is the sequence of events in taking the impression:

1. The gingival retraction cord is removed.
2. The preparation is air dried.
3. The injection syringe is used to squirt impression material into the widened gingival crevice and into the cavity preparation (Fig. 18-18, *A*). The procedure eliminates entrapment of air bubbles in the impression.

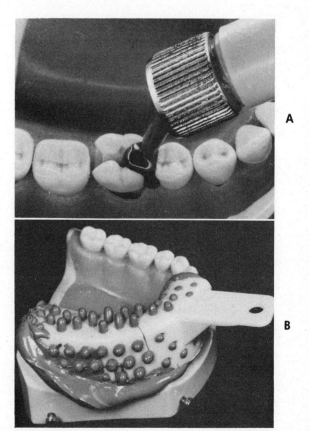

A

B

Fig. 18-18. A, Injection of syringe-consistency impression material into cavity preparation and gingival crevice. **B,** Impression tray with heavier, tray-consistency material in place.

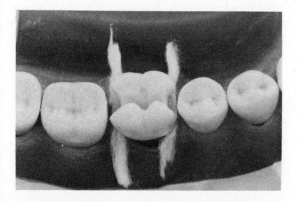

Fig. 18-17. Gingival retraction cord in place.

4. The tray filled with the thicker impression material is placed over the prepared tooth and the adjacent teeth (Fig. 18-18, *B*). This records the relationship of the prepared tooth to the adjacent teeth.
5. After the material reaches its final set, the impression is removed from the patient's mouth.

Three types of material can be used for this syringe-tray type of impression: (1) mercaptans (rubber base), (2) silicone, and (3) agar hydrocolloid. Each dentist has a personal preference for one material for impression taking. All the materials mentioned are extremely accurate.

Opposing model impression. A model of the opposing teeth is needed by the laboratory technician to fabricate the occlusal portion of the inlay. If an inlay is being made on a lower tooth, then a model of the upper teeth is needed to determine how the lower inlay fits the anatomy of the upper teeth when the patient closes his teeth together.

This model is made from an impression taken of the opposing teeth. An impression tray is filled with a rapid-setting impression material called alginate. The tray is placed over the opposing teeth and allowed to set. The impression is removed, and the opposing model can be made. The syringe-type technique is not necessary to make this impression.

Bite registration. For the fabrication of an inlay that will properly fit the bite of the patient, the laboratory technician must have four things:

1. A model of the opposing teeth.
2. The model containing the prepared tooth.
3. A registration of the patient's biting relationship, to guide the technician as to how the two opposing models fit together.
4. Some device to hold the models in the proper biting relationship and simulate the movement of the jaws. Such a device is called an articulator.

Bite registration can be accomplished in various ways. A popular method is to have the patient bite into a small wad of self-curing acrylic (Duralay) after it has reached a doughy consistency. Once the patient has closed the jaws completely together with the acrylic between the posterior teeth, the acrylic is allowed to harden. Then it can be carefully removed.

The opposing models can be fitted in the appropriate sides of the acrylic bite registration and then mounted on the articulator, with plaster used to hold them in place (Fig. 18-19).

Temporization. After cavity preparation, impression-taking, and bite registration are completed, a

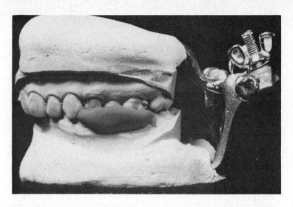

Fig. 18-19. Bite registration used to mount models on articulator. Plaster is used to fasten models to articulator.

temporary filling material is placed in the cavity preparation. This material is usually a temporary zinc oxide–eugenol cement or a flexible plastic filling material (Fig. 18-11).

The temporary restoration accomplishes the following function:

1. Prevents sensitivity in the prepared tooth
2. Aids in preventing fracture of the prepared tooth
3. Prevents the prepared tooth from drifting out of position between appointments

Inlay-cementation appointment: Class VI (MOD) example

After the preparation appointment the patient wears the temporary restoration while the inlay is fabricated in the laboratory. The patient then returns for a second appointment to have the inlay cemented in the prepared tooth.

The sequence of events in the completion of the inlay restorative procedure is as follows:

1. Anesthesia administration
2. Isolation
3. Removal of the temporary dressing
4. Contact adjustment
5. Occlusal adjustment
6. Polishing
7. Cementation
8. Margin finishing

Anesthesia. The same type of local anesthesia is administered as was required during the preparation appointment. It should be noted that some patients do not require anesthesia during seating appointments. In such instances it is desirable not to use anesthesia, since this may inhibit the patient's ability to bite normally.

Isolation. Cotton roll isolation is probably the most popular isolation method used for this procedure because the patient will be required to close the teeth together several times during the seating process. The rubber dam clamp would prevent the closure if a rubber dam were used for isolation.

Removal of the temporary restoration. The temporary filling material can be removed from the cavity preparation with the spoon excavator. Sometimes it is helpful to remove some of the filling material with a slow-speed round bur (No. 4). This must be done carefully so that the preparation is not damaged in the process. The cavity preparation must be absolutely free of any of the temporary material or other debris. Any debris left in the preparation will prevent the inlay from seating completely in the tooth. Cotton pellets are helpful in removing debris. A thorough rinsing of the preparation with the air-water syringe will complete the cleaning process.

Contact adjustment. The contact areas of an inlay are the areas on the inlay that contact the proximal surfaces of the adjacent teeth (Fig. 18-20). These areas are often excessively contoured by the laboratory technician. If this is the situation, the excessive gold is ground away until the inlay will seat completely in the tooth.

After the inlay is seated in the tooth, the amount of contact between the inlay and adjacent teeth can be checked by passing dental floss through the contact areas. The contacts must be snug but not so tight that it is difficult to pass floss between the inlay and the adjacent teeth. On the other hand, the floss should not pass through freely. A contact that is not tight enough will allow food to be forced in between the teeth, which can be damaging to the interproximal gingiva.

It is a good policy for the dental assistant to hold a filling instrument on the occlusal surface of the inlay during the check with the dental floss. This will prevent the inlay from being dislodged from the tooth, which could result in the patient swallowing or aspirating the restoration.

To check the contact fit of the inlay, it is necessary to have the inlay completely seated in the cavity preparation. The wooden Cooley peg is used to force the inlay all the way into the preparation.

After the contacts are checked and adjusted, the cervical areas are checked with the explorer to determine the fit of the inlay along the cervical margins. If the gold is too bulky in this area, the inlay is re-

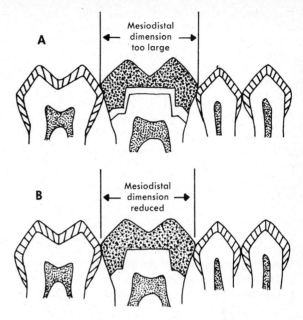

Fig. 18-20. Adjusting contact areas. **A,** Mesiodistal dimension is too large, and inlay will not seat completely. **B,** Corrected mesiodistal dimension allows inlay to seat completely.

moved, and the excessive gold is ground away with a finishing stone or disk until the fit is perfected.

If the inlay is difficult to remove from the preparation, a straight gold foil condenser can be tapped gently on a proximal surface of the inlay to drive it out of the preparation. The assistant must keep a finger on the inlay to prevent it from dropping out of the tooth.

Occlusal adjustment. After the inlay is completely seated, the fit of the occlusal surface of the inlay to the opposing teeth must be assessed. This is done by having the patient bring the teeth together on a piece of articulating paper. If the inlay is too high, or in hyperocclusion, heavy marks will show on the occlusal surface of the inlay when the paper is removed. In addition, the patient can usually sense even the slightest hyperocclusion in a restoration.

If the inlay is in hyperocclusion, the excessive gold on the occlusal surface is ground away until the inlay fits the occlusal surfaces of the opposing teeth and the hyperocclusion is eliminated. This often requires repeated try-ins and corrections until the occlusion is perfected.

A correct bite registration and mounting of the laboratory models during the fabrication of the inlay will greatly reduce or even eliminate the need for occlusal adjustment.

Polishing. When all corrections have been made on the inlay, the external surface of the inlay is polished with a fine abrasive rubber wheel (Craytex). It is then taken to the dental lathe and polished with various abrasive polishes to impart a high shine to its surface.

The inlay can be cleaned in an ultrasonic cleaner to remove all polish residue. It is then placed in a dappen dish filled with alcohol to disinfect it while the cement is being prepared.

Cementation. The inlay is now ready to be seated in the prepared tooth permanently with a final cement material. Figs. 18-14 and 18-15 show several of the popular brands available for this purpose. If zinc phosphate cement is used, it is necessary to varnish the dentin before the inlay is cemented in place. This is to prevent the acidic cement from irritating the prepared tooth. Varnish is not necessary if the other cements are used.

The prepared tooth is rinsed thoroughly and dried. The operative field must be well isolated and kept dry until the inlay is cemented in the preparation. The cavity varnish is applied at this time if it is needed. The inlay is removed from the alcohol and dried.

Zinc phosphate cement is mixed with the cement spatula on a mixing slab (Fig. 18-14), and the tissue surface of the inlay is coated with cement. The cement slab can be brought to the operative site with the inlay turned down on the slab. The operator can then coat the preparation with cement, using the plastic filling instrument. The inlay is placed in the preparation and seated with finger pressure. The Cooley peg is then placed over the inlay, and the patient is instructed to bite on the peg to drive the inlay to seat completely into the preparation. The patient is asked to maintain biting pressure until the cement reaches its initial set (Fig. 18-13, *A*).

Margin finishing. After the cement has reached its initial set, the peg is removed. Excessive cement can be removed from the site with a spoon excavator and explorer.

All margins can be checked for fit with the explorer. Any margins that are bulky on the occlusal and proximal surfaces can be polished with finishing stones or a disk in a conventional speed handpiece.

Next, the margins are burnished with ball burnishers in the straight handpiece and with the hand burnisher (Fig. 5-14). Burnishing is a procedure of pressing the malleable gold tightly against the tooth margin by slight stretching of the metal. This improves the seal of the inlay and smooths the junction between the tooth structure and the gold.

After the cement has reached the final set, the mouth can be rinsed, and the patient can be dismissed.

Dental assistant's role

In addition to the standard chairside duties, the dental assistant has many important tasks to perform during the fabrication of the gold inlay restoration. The preparation of impression materials, bite registration, temporization materials, and cementation agents is critical to the success of the procedure.

A skilled assistant can also perform many laboratory phases of the procedure, such as custom acrylic–impression tray fabrication, model and die construction, and polishing the finished inlay. Many assistants have even mastered the skills required to completely fabricate the inlay in the laboratory. Some state laws permit dental assistants to place temporary fillings.

Direct inlay procedure

A less popular inlay procedure called a direct inlay can be used instead of the indirect inlay method just described.

This procedure follows the same basic steps as the indirect method, except there is no impression taken of the prepared tooth. The wax pattern for the inlay is carved directly in the prepared tooth and not on a model of the tooth in the laboratory as with the indirect procedure.

This method is generally limited to less extensive inlays in the more accessible areas of the mouth.

SUMMARY

The armamentarium, dental materials and procedural steps described in this chapter are not applicable to only the cast gold inlay procedure. With very few modifications the information provided here applies to the fabrication of a wide variety of crown and bridge restorations to be discussed in Chapter 20.

BIBLIOGRAPHY

Charbeneau, G.T., and others: Principles and practice of operative dentistry, ed. 2, Philadelphia, 1981, Lea & Febiger.

Craig, R.G., O'Brien, W.J., and Powers, J.M.: Dental materials: properties and manipulation, ed. 3, St. Louis, 1983, The C.V. Mosby Co.

Howard, W.W., and Moller, R.C.: Atlas of operative dentistry, ed. 3, St. Louis, 1981, The C.V. Mosby Co.

CHAPTER 19

COHESIVE GOLD RESTORATIONS

The cohesive gold restoration is the only pure gold restoration used in dentistry. Pure gold is used because it will cohere, or weld to itself, at cool temperatures. Because it is malleable, it can easily be worked into different shapes.

A cohesive gold restoration is placed into a cavity preparation by condensing it into place in a similar fashion to that used in amalgam restorations. Many dentists consider the cohesive gold restoration to be superior to all other restorations if it is done properly and used in the proper types of cavity preparations. The finished restoration is extremely strong and has a better adaptation to cavity walls than a gold inlay. A well-fabricated cohesive gold restoration can last up to five times longer than similar amalgam and composite restorations.

Cohesive gold restorations have not enjoyed widespread popularity in dentistry despite their high quality. The reasons for this center primarily around objections to the time it takes to fabricate the restoration, the difficulty of the technique, and the cost to the patient.

COMMON COHESIVE GOLD INSTRUMENTS AND SUPPLIES
Armamentarium

A typical armamentarium for the fabrication of a Class I or Class V restoration is shown in Fig. 19-1.

Cohesive gold (Fig. 19-2)

Cohesive gold is pure gold that will stick to another piece of pure gold if they are pressed together. Cohesive gold is available in gold foil ropes, bars of mat gold, and powdered gold wrapped in gold foil to form small pellets. Since gold foil was the first form of gold available in dentistry, cohesive gold restorations are frequently referred to as "gold foil restorations."

All forms of these pure golds are usually purchased in a semicohesive state; that is, there is some surface contaminant on the gold to prevent it from sticking to itself in the container. The surface contaminant is usually a volatile substance such as ammonia that can be removed by heating the gold before its insertion in a prepared cavity. The removal of the surface contaminant is called annealing.

Hand cutting instruments (Fig. 19-3)

A wide variety of multiangled chisels and angle formers are available to prepare cohesive gold cavities. Generally these preparations are small and somewhat inaccessible to standard hand cutting instruments. The creation of special cutting instruments for cohesive gold allows the dentist to gain access to make the necessary preparation refinements achieved with hand instruments.

Cohesive gold condensers (Fig. 19-4)

Cohesive gold is inserted in a prepared cavity and condensed or pressed into position with a cohesive gold condenser. There are three basic types used for this purpose: hand condensers, spring-activated automatic condensers, and electric mallet condensers.

Cohesive gold must be condensed vigorously to ensure the coherence of one piece of gold to another and to strain-harden the gold. Hand condensing is usually limited to the first few additions of gold to control the initial insertion. The remainder of the gold is condensed with an electrical condenser or a spring-activated condenser. Both of these devices have an assortment of condenser points that can be attached to fit any area of the mouth. These automatic devices make condensation easier for the dentist and create a higher quality restoration for the patient.

Condenser points differ from amalgam condensers

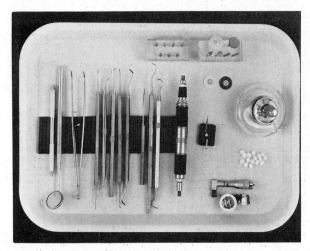

Fig. 19-1. Cohesive gold armamentarium.

Preset tray

Cowhorn explorer, No. 3
Mouth mirror, No. 4
Cotton pliers
Spoon excavator
Chisels, hoes, hatchets, and angle formers
Gold foil carrier
Holding instrument
Hand-type gold foil condenser
Automatic condenser
Assorted condenser points
Craytex polishing wheel
Green stone, wheel shaped
Moore's mandrels
Ball burnishers, HP
Moore's disks
Alcohol lamp
Burs, FG No. 33$\frac{1}{2}$, and FG No. $\frac{1}{2}$
Cotton pellets
Prophylaxis angle and rubber cup
Polishing paste

Add-on items

Cavity medications
Silex polish
Tin oxide paste
Matches
Stick compound
Cohesive gold

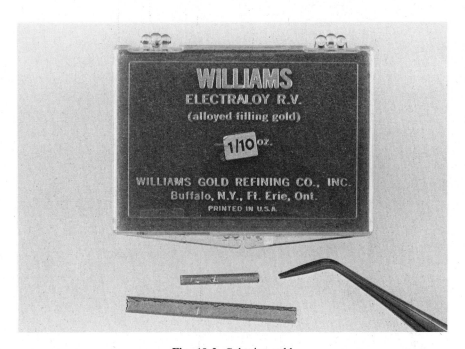

Fig. 19-2. Cohesive gold.

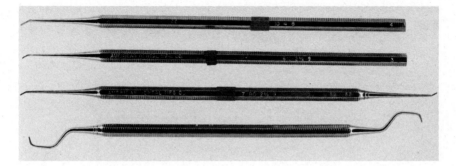

Fig. 19-3. Hand cutting instruments for preparing cohesive gold cavity preparations.

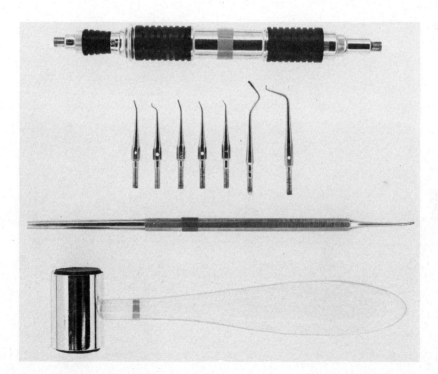

Fig. 19-4. Cohesive gold condensers. *Top,* Automatic condenser and assorted points. *Bottom,* Hand-held condenser and mallet.

in that the working tip of the instrument is serrated whereas the amalgam condenser is smooth. The serrated tip aids in attaching one piece of gold to another during the condensation procedure.

Annealing lamp (Fig. 19-5)

There are expensive electrical annealers available that can be used to remove the ammonia contaminant on semicohesive gold. However, a less expensive method is to use a simple alcohol lamp filled with acetone-free methyl alcohol.

Small pieces of cohesive gold are inserted in the alcohol flame with a sharp probe called a gold foil carrier. The gold is held in the flame until it is a cherry red, then quickly removed and delivered to the prepared tooth on the carrier.

Holding instrument (Fig. 19-6)

This hook-shaped instrument is used to hold the first few increments of gold in place in the cavity preparation until sufficient gold is added to retain itself in the retentive aspects of the preparation (Fig. 19-9, *A*).

Gold knife (Fig. 19-6)

This is a small-bladed knife used to remove excess overhanging gold in the cervical areas of Class III and IV cohesive gold restorations.

Rhein trimmer (Fig. 19-6)

This paddle-shaped instrument is used for initial contouring of a cohesive gold restoration. It is used with a pull motion to file away excess gold along the margins of a restoration.

COHESIVE GOLD RESTORATION PROCEDURE
Cohesive gold cavity preparations

Cohesive gold is usually limited to rather small cavity preparations such as Classes I and V. Conservative Class II, III, and even IV restorations are done less frequently.

These preparations require prominent retention areas in the cavity design to hold the gold in place.

Fabrication of a cohesive gold restoration: Class V example

Each class of cavity preparation that is used for a cohesive gold restoration has its own unique demands on the skill of the dentist. The technique that will be discussed here is not intented to ignore the special problems associated with the fabrication of the more difficult Class II, III, and IV restorations. Since the Class V restoration is one of the most common cohesive gold restorations in use today, it is a logical choice for an example of the cohesive gold technique.

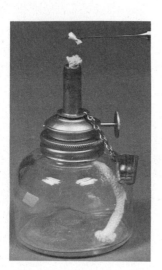

Fig. 19-5. Alcohol lamp for annealing cohesive gold held in gold foil carrier.

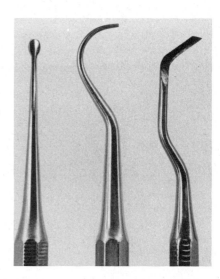

Fig. 19-6. Miscellaneous cohesive gold instruments. *Left to right:* Rhein trimmer, holding instrument, gold foil knife.

The following sequence is frequently used to construct this restoration:

1. Anesthesia administration
2. Isolation
3. Cavity preparation
4. Cavity medication
5. Insertion and condensation
6. Contouring and finishing

Anesthesia administration. The appropriate area is anesthetized with the standard anesthetic setup and technique described in Chapter 7.

Isolation. Without question, the rubber dam is the isolation method of choice in the fabrication of cohesive gold restorations. Gold will only cohere, or "stick to itself," if it is free of surface contaminants. Contamination of the gold with saliva, blood, or any other substance will render the material noncohesive and result in failure of the fabrication process.

The rubber dam is the most reliable method that dentists have available to ensure the operating team a clean, dry field in which to work.

Most other classes of restorations can be done with the standard rubber dam clamps described in Chapter 8. The Class V restoration requires the use of a special clamp designed to hold the dam in place while at the same time it retracts both the dam and the gingival tissue away from the operative site. This clamp is a No. 212 Ferrier type (Fig. 19-7). It is advisable to isolate two teeth mesial and distal to the tooth to be restored. Softened dental compound is attached to these adjacent teeth and the clamp to prevent it from slipping during the procedure.

Cavity preparation. Most cohesive gold preparations are very small and can be prepared with the smaller-sized burs such as a 33½ inverted-cone bur and the ½ round bur. The outline form can be established with the 33½ bur, and exaggerated retention grooves can be placed with the ½ round bur (Fig. 19-8).

Refinement of the outline form is accomplished with various small hand cutting instruments (hoes, hatchets, and chisels) specially designed for small preparations. The retentive grooves are enhanced with a special angle-forming instrument. This instrument also sharpens the internal design of the preparation (Fig. 19-8).

There is great emphasis on retentive design in all cohesive gold preparations, since the restoration depends entirely on mechanical lock in the preparation to hold it firmly in place.

Cavity medication. Cavity medication is discussed in detail in Chapter 15. If the caries has extended beyond the normal cavity preparation depth, cement bases are used. If cement bases are used, the cement must be completely set before the cohesive gold is placed in the preparation. Any cement that has not completely set can contaminate the cohesive gold.

Many dentists avoid placing cohesive gold restorations in teeth that have pulp exposures. The force that is required to condense cohesive gold into the cavity

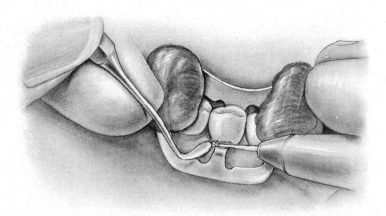

Fig. 19-7. Isolation of cervical area of tooth, using No. 212 clamp. (From Howard, W.W., and Moller, R.C.: Atlas of operative dentistry, ed. 3, St. Louis, 1981, The C.V. Mosby Co.)

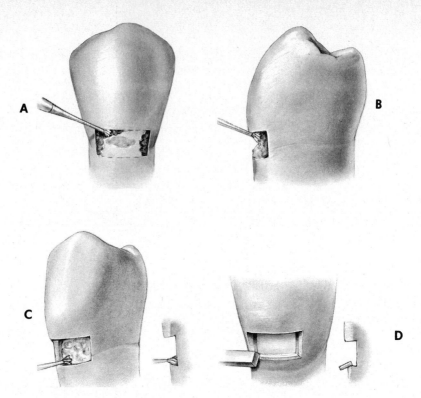

Fig. 19-8. Preparation of Class V cavity for cohesive gold. **A,** Opening preparation. **B** and **C,** Gaining cavity form. **D,** Cavity refinement. (From Howard, W.W., and Moller, R.C.: Atlas of operative dentistry, ed. 3, St. Louis, 1981, The C.V. Mosby Co.)

preparation is rather vigorous. Cavity medications can be driven into the pulp chamber as a result of this vigorous condensation. This will increase intrapulpal pressure, which results in significant postoperative discomfort.

Insertion and condensation. As mentioned previously, cohesive gold is marketed in three basic forms: gold foil, mat gold, and powdered gold. Each dentist prefers one form and finds it convenient to use. Manufacturers purposely contaminate all these forms to render them noncohesive so that they will not stick together in the containers during shipping, storage, and handling in the dental operatory. Ammonia is the most common agent used for this purpose. It also helps to prevent other contaminants from attaching permanently to the surface of the gold.

Before the gold is inserted into the preparation, it must first be annealed. Annealing is the process of

degassing or removing the ammonia and accumulated contaminants from the surface of the gold to make it pure and cohesive. Two popular methods of annealing are heating the gold on an electric annealer or over the open flame of a clean alcohol lamp. If the alcohol lamp is used, the wick must be clean and pure alcohol used as the fuel. Either pure ethyl alcohol or acetone-free methanol is acceptable. The piece of gold is held in the flame with a gold foil carrier until it glows slightly. It is immediately delivered to the cavity preparation for insertion and condensation. Each small increment is annealed in the same manner just before insertion (Fig. 19-5).

The gold is inserted in the cavity preparation in very small increments. Gold foil and mat gold can be cut into small increments with a gold knife. Powdered gold is available in various pellet sizes to meet the needs of the operator.

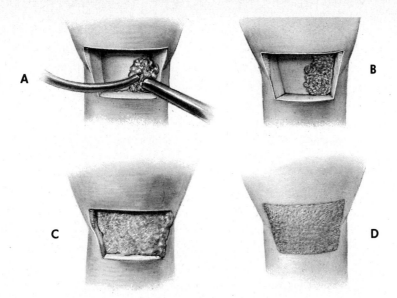

Fig. 19-9. Insertion and condensation of cohesive gold in prepared cavity. **A,** Small increment is placed and condensed, using both holding instrument and condenser. **B** to **D,** Continued additions of cohesive gold until preparation is filled. (From Howard, W.W., and Moller, R.C.: Atlas of operative dentistry, ed. 3, St. Louis, 1981, The C.V. Mosby Co.)

When the first increment of gold is inserted into the preparation, the dentist forces it into the retentive areas of one side of the preparation with a hand condenser. This increment is held in place with a holding instrument until subsequent increments are added and condensed on top of the first increment. The process is continued until a layer of gold extends from the retention of one side of the preparation to the other (Fig. 19-9). When the two retentive areas are united with a layer of gold, the gold layer will be mechanically locked into place. The holding instrument is no longer needed at this point to hold the gold in the preparation. Subsequent additions of gold will cohere to this initial layer of gold that is held in place by the retention area.

Once the base of the preparation is covered with gold, the dentist can begin using the spring-activated automatic condenser with assorted condenser points. This instrument delivers a sharp tap on the condenser point as it is depressed against the gold. Vigorous condensation is necessary to (1) adapt the gold tightly against cavity walls, (2) eliminate any voids in the gold mass and create a dense restoration, and (3) bend the pure gold increments into tiny "wads," which results in strain hardening.

Strain hardening is the process of distorting metals so that their crystal lattice is altered in such a way that the metal is made harder. This is desirable because pure gold is rather soft. Strain hardening improves the strength and hardness of the final restoration. The same principle is employed when a coat hanger is bent back and forth. The metal at the bend becomes harder. If the bending (distortion) continues, the metal will become brittle and will ultimately fracture.

Some dentists prefer to use a veneer method of filling the preparation. The base two thirds of the cavity is filled with either mat or powdered gold. Then the surface one third is covered with gold foil. Gold foil usually condenses more effectively than mat gold and gives a very dense gold surface to the restoration, which is easy to polish to a higher luster free of any voids. However, using gold foil alone to fill the preparation can be rather time-consuming. The use of mat gold to fill the bulk of the preparation expedites the filling process.

The operator always overfills the preparation with gold to be sure of an adequate quantity to work with in order to achieve a good marginal seal and desirable surface contour.

Contouring and finishing. The overfilled cavity preparation must now be reduced to a desirable surface contour with fine, smooth, well-sealed margins. One technique for accomplishing this is to grind away the excess gold with fine, carrot-shaped green stones and polishing disks. These instruments are turned in the direction from the gold toward the tooth margin, which improves the surface seal of the margin.

After the desired contour is produced by grinding the gold surface, the surface is strain hardened even more by spinning a ball burnisher on the surface with a straight handpiece. This also improves the strength of the margins of the gold.

Final polish of the restoration can be done with a prophylaxis angle and rubber cup filled with fine pumice paste. After polishing the gold with pumice, the operator uses a paste of even finer silex polish to improve the smoothness of the surface. A high luster can be placed on the gold by spinning a paste of tin oxide on the surface at a rather high speed with the rubber cup. The tin oxide paste should be dried with the air syringe as the rubber cup is spinning on the surface of the gold.

The polish can be rinsed away, the rubber dam removed, and the patient dismissed.

SUMMARY

The dental assistant is essential to efficient fabrication of all dental restorations. In addition to the standard chairside duties, the assistant must be proficient in the preparation and handling of many dental materials. A thorough knowledge of the basic operative procedures is mandatory before the assistant can effectively learn the individual dentist's method of doing a given dental restoration.

Knowledge generates efficiency.

BIBLIOGRAPHY

Charbeneau, G.T., and others: Principles and practice of operative dentistry, ed. 2, Philadelphia, 1981, Lea & Febiger.
Howard, W.W., and Moller, R.C.: Atlas of operative dentistry, ed. 3, St. Louis, 1981, The C.V. Mosby Co.
Howard, W.W.: Review of operative dentistry, St. Louis, 1973, The C.V. Mosby Co.

DENTAL SPECIALTIES

CHAPTER 20

CROWN AND BRIDGE PROSTHODONTICS

The area of crown and bridge prosthodontics involves extensive reconstruction of the crowns of teeth and/or replacement of missing teeth with a fixed bridge. The demand by the public for these services has increased markedly in recent years. This, plus the rather elaborate techniques that are used, have motivated many dentists to limit their practice to only extensive restorative dentistry.

The basic procedures used to fabricate a crown or a bridge are similar to those used for a gold inlay. To avoid repetition of some of the principles already described in Chapter 18, it is suggested that the reader review the discussions of the fabrication of a gold inlay, impression-taking procedures, and temporization methods before proceeding further. Having this information in mind will be helpful in simplifying the discussion of crown and bridge procedures.

No attempt will be made to discuss all restorative procedures, but rather a selection of a few representative restorations will be made to present the fundamentals of crown and bridge prosthodontics. The dentist's tasks vary considerably from one restorative procedure to another, but the assistant's role changes very little. Therefore the restorations that have been selected for discussion here should provide the assistant with enough background to assist the dentist regardless of which specific restorative procedure is being done. The cast gold crown, the esthetic crown, and the fixed bridge represent the basic spectrum of restorative dental services commonly done today. The fabrication of all three of these types of restorations involves the following basic steps:

Oral examination appointment
1. Fabrication of study models and shade selection (esthetic crowns and bridges only)

Preparation appointment
1. Anesthesia administration
2. Isolation of the operative field
3. Cavity preparation and medication
4. Gingival retraction
5. Impression taking
6. Opposing model impression
7. Bite registration
8. Temporization

Cementation appointment
1. Anesthesia administration
2. Isolation of the operative field
3. Removal of the temporary dressing
4. Contact adjustment
5. Occlusal adjustment
6. Final polishing
7. Cementation
8. Margin finishing

Not only are the basic steps in restorative procedures the same as those for the fabrication of the gold inlay, but also the armamentarium is very similar if not identical. It is common for dentists to have the preset trays organized so that one setup is used for gold preparation appointments (inlays, crowns, bridges) and another is used for the cementation appointment. See Chapter 18 for a review of the armamentaria needed for the cast gold preparation and cementation appointments. Any additions to these basic instrument setups will be given during the discussion on the specific restorative procedure.

RETENTION CORES AND POSTS

Most teeth that are restored with crowns are significantly altered as a result of fracture, extensive caries, or large, worn-out operative restorations. Before a preparation for a crown or bridge can be done, the dentist must make a judgment as to whether the remaining tooth structure is sufficient to retain the restoration after it is made. In cases in which the natural tooth structure is insufficient to work with, a retentive core must be made before preparing the tooth for a crown. A retentive core can be made of amalgam, composite material, or gold in the form of a post.

Composite and amalgam cores are fabricated with the pin-retained amalgam technique described in Chapter 16. Composite resin is popular for use as a core because it is strong, lacks thermoconductivity, and sets quickly. The composite core achieves maxi-

mum hardness so quickly that the crown preparation can be done immediately after placement of the composite. Amalgam cores often require a separate appointment for the construction of the core because of the slow setting time of the amalgam. These pin-retained cores are most often done on teeth that still have a live pulp (Fig. 20-1). If a tooth has had endodontic treatment, the dentist has the option of either using the pin-retained core or a cast gold post (Fig. 20-2). The cast gold post fits into the hollow root portion of the tooth and is cemented in place. After the retentive core or post is placed, the tooth is prepared as though the core were actually tooth structure.

The final restoration is then made to fit over the remaining tooth structure and the core.

CAST GOLD CROWN

The cast gold crown is one of the most common restorations done in restorative dentistry. The term *crown* implies that a substantial portion of the natural crown portion of the tooth is reconstructed with gold, porcelain, or a combination of both. Cast gold crowns are most often made either to rebuild three fourths of the crown portion of a tooth (a three-quarter crown) or to completely cover the entire crown of a tooth (a full crown) (Fig. 20-3).

If a three-quarter crown is done on a tooth, the facial aspect of the tooth is usually left intact. This

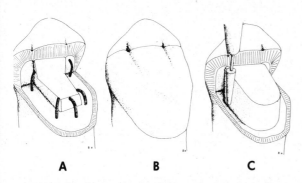

A　　　　**B**　　　　**C**

Fig. 20-1. Amalgam core. **A,** Pin placement. **B,** Amalgam in place. **C,** Forming crown preparation.

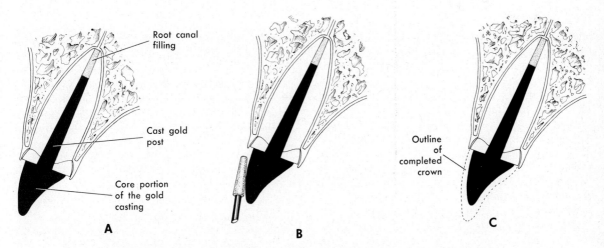

Fig. 20-2. Gold post and core cast to fit into prepared root canal of endodontically treated tooth. **A,** Gold post cemented in root canal. **B,** Final adjustments can be made on core portion of casting if necessary. **C,** Anterior crown can now be made to fit over cast post and core.

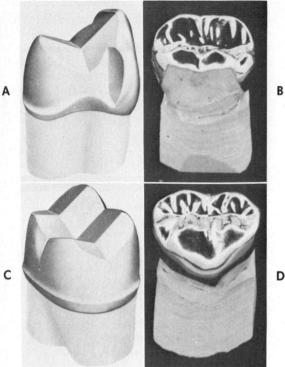

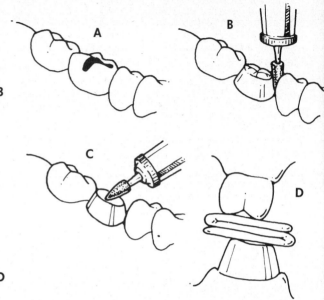

Fig. 20-4. Preparation of a tooth for a full cast gold crown. **A,** Before preparation begins. **B,** Reduction of circumference of tooth, creating "draw." **C,** Reduction of occlusal surface. **D,** Checking occlusal clearance with three thicknesses of 28-gauge green wax.

Fig. 20-3. Cast gold crowns. **A,** Three-quarter crown preparation. **B,** Cast three-quarter crown. **C,** Full crown preparation. **D,** Cast full crown. (**A** and **C** courtesy J.M. Ney Co., Hartford, Conn.; **B** and **D** courtesy Precision Dental Arts, Inc., Jackson, Mich.)

type of restoration provides the strength needed for proper function of the tooth and preserves the natural appearance of the facial surface for esthetics.

A full cast gold crown completely encases the remaining tooth structure to gain both maximum retention of the restoration on the tooth and strength to resist the forces created during mastication. Since these restorations are not as esthetically pleasing, they are usually placed on posterior teeth that are not as readily visible when the patient speaks or smiles.

Crown preparation

Crown preparations (Fig. 20-4, *A* and *B*) are done with the ultraspeed handpiece and either tapered fissure burs or diamond stones. These instruments permit rapid removal of tooth structure. Minor refinements can be made with the conventional-speed handpiece and fine grindstones and sandpaper disks.

The preparation for the full crown involves a reduction of the entire circumference of the tooth as well as its occlusal height (Fig. 20-4, *C*). The three-quarter crown is done in a similar fashion except that the facial surface is left intact.

The occlusal height of the tooth must be reduced enough to allow for adequate thickness of the gold crown on the occlusal surface. It is quite common for dentists to determine adequate occlusal clearance by having the patient bite into a ½-inch square of 28-gauge occlusal wax that has been folded into three thicknesses (Fig. 20-4, *D*). Adequate reduction is achieved when the clearance between the preparation and the opposing tooth equals the three thicknesses of wax.

The relationship of the vertical aspects of the prepared tooth is such that draw is established (Fig. 20-4, *B*). Excessive tapering of the vertical portion of the preparation must be avoided to prevent loss of the retention quality of the preparation.

After the preparation is completed, the gingiva is retracted, and an impression is made with mercaptan, silicone, or agar hydrocolloid impression material with the syringe-tray technique. The occlusal registration is taken at this time, and an alginate impression is made of the opposing teeth.

Posterior crown temporization methods

The prepared tooth can be covered with a temporary crown such as the aluminum shell type or with an acrylic crown made using the vacuum-adaptation technique.

Temporary crowns are usually cemented in place with a relatively weak zinc oxide–eugenol cement to facilitate easier removal at the cementation appointment.

Aluminum shell crown method. Stock aluminum shell crowns have been used for years as temporary crowns. They are available in either anatomical or nonanatomical forms and in a variety of sizes to fit molar and premolar teeth. They are all "a mile too long" and must be trimmed with crown-and-collar scissors to the proper length and cervical shape.

The cervical margin is smoothed with a fine green grinding stone. Proper crown contour can be achieved with contouring pliers. (The preparation of an aluminum shell crown is identical to that of the stainless steel crown, Fig. 23-6.) After the crown has been properly fitted to the tooth, it is filled with a zinc oxide–eugenol temporary cement and seated on the prepared tooth. Excess cement is removed, and the patient is dismissed.

Vacuum adaptation method. This is a relatively new method of making full-crown and three-quarter–crown temporary dressings for both anterior and posterior teeth. The procedure is as follows:

1. An alginate impression is taken of the area of the dentition to be treated. A plaster model is made from this impression.
2. The model is placed on the platform of the Omni-Vac* with the teeth upright (Fig. 20-5, *A*).
3. A sheet of plastic coping material is mounted in the holding frame.
4. The heating element is turned on, and the coping material is softened. When it sags in the middle approximately 1 to 1¼ inch (Fig. 20-5, *B*), the vacuum motor is turned on, and the holding frame is quickly lowered to place the softened material over the model (Fig. 20-5, *C*). The vacuum will draw the material onto the model and tightly adapt it to the shape of the teeth.
5. The machine is turned off after 15 seconds of adaptation, and the model is removed.

*Buffalo Dental Manufacturing Co., Brooklyn, N.Y.

6. The coping material can be cut away from the model with a scalpel blade (Fig. 20-5, *D*). The tooth to be prepared plus at least half of each adjacent tooth should remain intact to create the mold or matrix for the temporary dressing.
7. The plastic mold should be added to the gold preparation setup at the time of the preparation appointment after it has been placed in cold disinfectant solution and washed.
8. At the preparation appointment after the crown preparation has been completed and the necessary impressions obtained, the temporary crown can be made. The crown is made from self-curing acrylic such as Duralay. These materials are mixed into a thick paste and placed in the plastic mold (Fig. 20-5, *E*). The filled mold is placed over the prepared tooth, and the patient is instructed to bite down to hold it in place (Fig. 20-5, *F*). The mold should be removed and replaced repeatedly during the set of the acrylic to prevent it from locking on the teeth.
9. After the acrylic has hardened completely, the mold can be removed from the mouth. The acrylic is separated from the mold, and the excess acrylic is ground away.
10. The acrylic temporary crown is polished and seated temporarily with temporary cement (Fig. 20-5, *G*).

The vacuum adaptation method is gaining popularity because the same basic process can be used to make temporary bridges, bite splints, mouth guards, baseplates, and custom impression trays. The vacuum adaptation method is very convenient, and the result is excellent.

Cementation

The cementation appointment for placement of a crown involves the same procedure as for inlay cementation. The temporary crown is removed, and the preparation is cleaned thoroughly. The proximal contact, occlusion, and cervical margins must all be checked, and necessary adjustments made before the crown is cemented with a permanent cementation material. If zinc phosphate cement is used, the preparation must be coated with cavity varnish before cementation.

The assistant should not fill a crown completely with cement but rather place a coat of cement over the entire internal surface. Excessive cement makes it more difficult to seat the crown completely on the prepared tooth.

The crown can be delivered to the dentist on the mixing slab with its occlusal surface up. The dentist can then coat the prepared tooth with cement from the slab and easily grasp the upright crown for quick

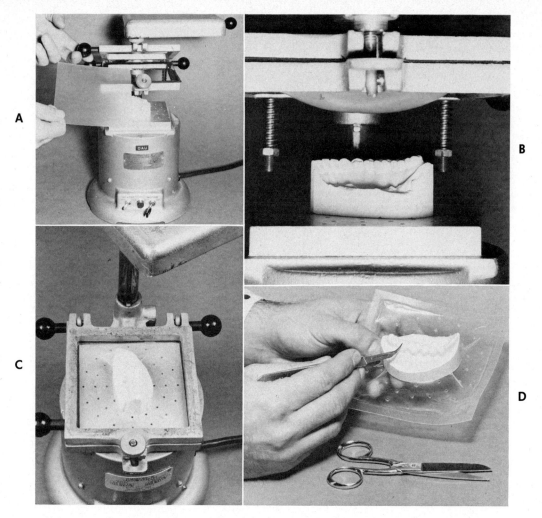

Fig. 20-5. Temporary crown construction using vacuum-adapted mold. **A,** Model positioned on Omnivac. **B,** Coping material sags 1 inch when softened enough to adapt. **C,** Holding frame drawn down over the model with vacuum turned on. **D,** Adapted coping material and model are removed from Omnivac. Mold is cut from model with scalpel and scissors. **E,** Filling the mold. **F,** Filled mold in place. **G,** Finished crown.

placement on the preparation. The crown is initially seated with hand pressure. Then the patient is instructed to bite on an orangewood stick or a Cooley peg that is placed over the crown to drive the crown into place (Fig. 20-6). This pressure is maintained until the cement sets. If any cervical burnishing is required, it is done with a hand burnisher after the cement reaches its initial set. Excess cement is removed, and the patient can be dismissed.

ESTHETIC CROWNS

Esthetics is a matter of personal preference of the individual patient. Some patients do not object to the appearance of gold in highly visible areas of the mouth, but others find it most objectionable. In fact, some patients even favor the appearance of ''gold teeth'' in their mouths. These preferences are based on the background of the individual with regard to ethnic differences, social habits, and occupational in-

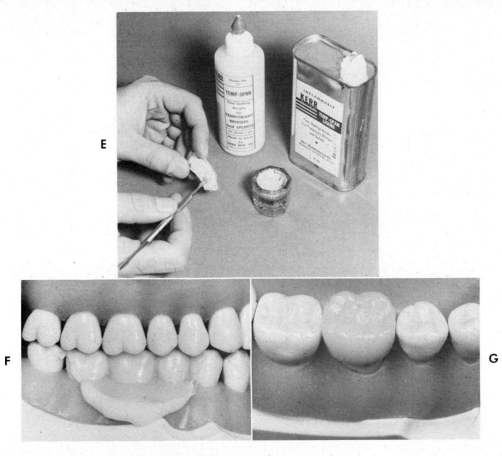

E

F

G

Fig. 20-5, cont'd. For legend see opposite page.

fluences. Beautiful models would probably not want their maxillary central incisors restored with full gold crowns, but there are some individuals who believe that this not only is attractive but also represents a sign of wealth. Of course, there are two extremes of esthetic preference, yet the dentist is frequently confronted with the choice of restoration that will meet the esthetic needs of the patient. Other influences in the choice are the strength requirements of the tooth to be restored and the economic situation of the patient.

An esthetic crown is defined as a full crown that has at least the facial aspect covered with a tooth-shaded material. There are two basic types of esthetic crowns: the all-porcelain jacket crown (Fig. 20-7, *A* and *B*) and the veneered gold crown (Fig. 20-7, *C* and *D*).

The porcelain jacket crown is made only for an-

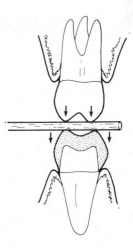

Fig. 20-6. Final seating of cast gold crown using orange-wood stick.

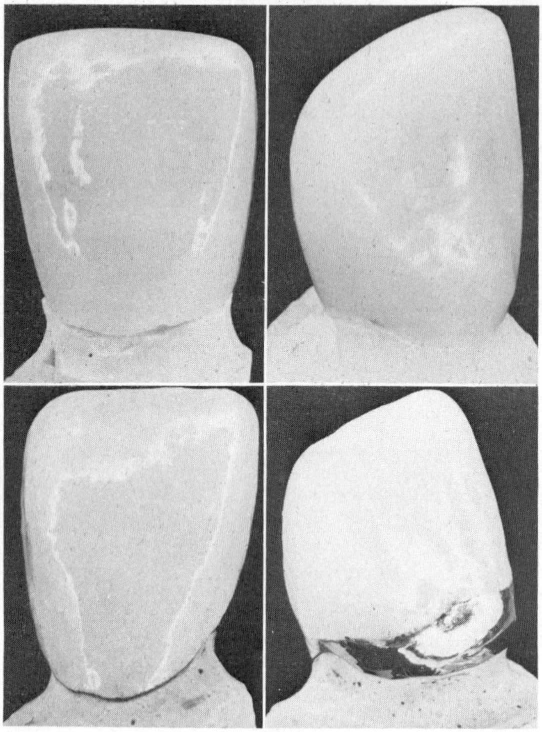

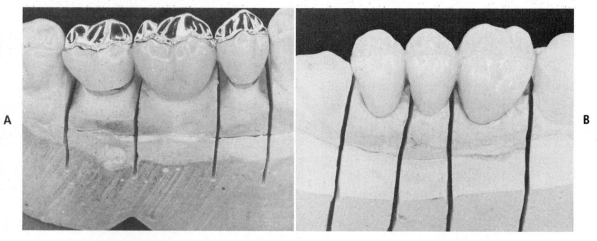

Fig. 20-7. Anterior esthetic crowns. A and B, Porcelain jacket crown. C and D, Porcelain fused to gold veneer crown. (Courtesy Precision Dental Arts, Inc., Jackson, Mich.)

Fig. 20-8. Posterior esthetic restorations. A, Acrylic veneered restorations. Acrylic is placed only on the facial surfaces. B, Porcelain veneered restorations. Porcelain is fused over the entire surface of the gold. (Courtesy Precision Dental Arts, Inc., Jackson, Mich.)

terior teeth. These crowns possess the most natural appearance of any crowns available. Porcelain completely surrounds the prepared tooth. Thus light can pass through the porcelain in much the same way that it passes through actual tooth structure, giving the restoration a very natural appearance. These restorations are limited to use on anterior teeth because of the brittle nature of porcelain. A complete porcelain crown on a posterior tooth would be vulnerable to fracture as a result of the extreme forces applied to it during mastication. These restorations will fracture even on anterior teeth if they are subjected to excessive force. Patients that have teeth restored with porcelain jacket crowns must exercise caution to prevent such an occurrence.

Even posterior teeth that are quite visible during

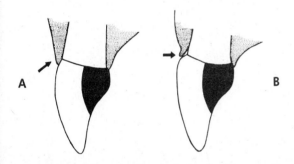

Fig. 20-9. Anterior veneered crown. **A,** Properly contoured crown. **B,** Poorly contoured crown.

normal oral functions demand the use of an esthetic restoration strong enough to resist fracture. Gold veneer crowns serve this purpose very well. These are gold crowns that completely cover the prepared tooth with a layer of gold. Then a layer of esthetic material is fused onto the surface of certain areas of the crown. If the esthetic material is a toothshaded acrylic, only the facial surface of the gold crown is covered (Fig. 20-8, *A*). If porcelain is fused to the gold to achieve esthetics, all surfaces of the gold crown can be covered with porcelain (Fig. 20-8, *B*). This is because the hard porcelain will resist wear on the occlusal surface, whereas the relatively soft acrylic will wear away too quickly. Porcelain is weak and brittle when used alone as a restorative material. However, when it is fused to a gold crown, its strength is greatly enhanced.

The porcelain-fused-to-gold veneer crowns are probably the most popular of the esthetic crowns in use today. Modern laboratory technology has created and improved this restoration so that it is now quite strong and attractive. It resists fracture, abrasion, and discoloration. It can be used in all areas of the mouth as a single restoration, or it can be joined with other restorations to form splints and bridges to replace missing teeth.

Esthetic crown preparations

Like cast gold crown preparations, the esthetic crown preparation is done principally with the ultraspeed handpiece and tapered fissure burs and diamond

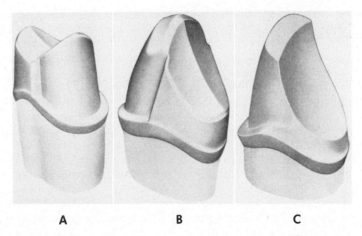

Fig. 20-10. Common esthetic crown preparations. **A,** Posterior veneer preparation. **B,** Anterior veneer preparation. **C,** Porcelain jacket preparation. (Courtesy J.M. Ney Co., Hartford, Conn.)

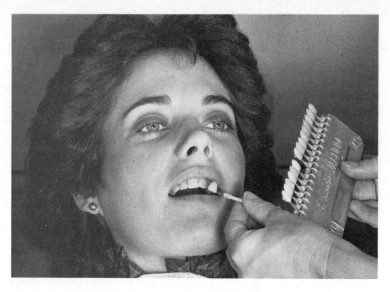

Fig. 20-11. Shade selection.

stones. Since these restorations involve full coverage of the prepared tooth, the entire circumference and vertical height of the tooth are reduced. The facial aspect of an esthetic crown preparation requires more reduction than the cast gold crown preparation. This additional reduction allows the necessary space to accommodate the thickness of gold and porcelain (or acrylic) on that surface. If additional reduction of tooth structure is not done, the finished restoration will be too bulky on the facial surface by the time a layer of gold and a layer of porcelain are added. This bulk detracts from the natural appearance of the restoration (Fig. 20-9). Fig. 20-10 illustrates some common crown preparations.

Before beginning an esthetic crown preparation, the dentist should select a shade so that the completed restoration matches the adjacent teeth. Shade is the combination of color and translucency of a tooth. The correct shade is obtained by comparing samples of various colors and translucencies, contained in a shade guide, with the tooth to be prepared and with adjacent teeth (Fig. 20-11). The shade guide must be added to the standard cast gold preparation setup when esthetic crowns are done. The shade samples are number coded so that the dentist can record the selection on the patient's record for future reference. Often teeth are combinations of shades, and the dentist will record these combinations. When the pa-

tient's models and dies are sent to the laboratory technician, the shade is included in the written instructions.

The shape of the tooth is also important to achieve proper esthetics. A preoperative study model is of considerable value to the technician in constructing the crown to a shape and contour that blend with the rest of the dentition. The impression for study models can be taken at the diagnostic appointment.

After the crown is prepared, an impression is taken with mercaptan, silicone, or agar hydrocolloid impression materials. Occlusal registration and an alginate impression are taken of the opposing teeth before a temporary crown is placed.

Temporization

Esthetic crown preparations require the use of a reasonably esthetic temporary crown. Therefore the aluminum shell crown is not frequently used.

Anterior teeth are temporized with either polycarbonate crowns (Fig. 20-12) or custom acrylic crowns made with the vacuum-molding technique. The custom acrylic crown has the advantage of a greater range of shade selection for the temporary crown. The polycarbonate crown is available in only one shade.

Anterior crown temporization has been made easier in recent years with the advent of the polycarbonate crown (Fig. 20-12), which is a very attractive crown.

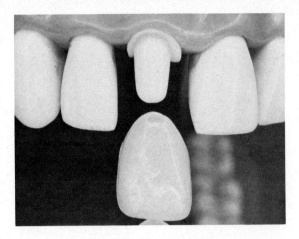

Fig. 20-12. Polycarbonate crown.

Various sizes of each anterior tooth are available in kit form. Some companies even offer maxillary premolar crowns. Polycarbonate crowns can be fitted to a prepared tooth by limited grinding with a green stone to contour the cervical area.

The crown can be filled with a temporary cement and seated on the tooth. If extensive alteration of the crown is anticipated, it is filled with a self-curing acrylic and placed on the prepared tooth. As the acrylic hardens, the crown should be removed and seated repeatedly to prevent the acrylic from adhering to the preparation. After the acrylic is completely hard, any alterations necessary to fit the crown properly can be made by grinding the filled crown. The crown can be polished and temporarily cemented to the prepared tooth with a thin layer of temporary cement.

Posterior teeth are generally temporized with a custom acrylic crown. Some manufacturers provide polycarbonate crowns for premolars, which are helpful. The advent of the vacuum-molding process has made fabrication of suitable esthetic temporary crowns much easier.

Cementation of esthetic crowns

Cementation of the porcelain jacket crown. The temporary crown is removed, and the preparation is cleaned thoroughly. The crown is placed on the preparation, and proximal contacts, occlusion, and cervical margins are checked and adjusted as needed. If adjustments are necessary, they are done with special porcelain grinding wheels (Dedeco). Various sizes

and grits are available. Any area that has been ground should be smoothed by a fine-grit Dedeco wheel on a conventional-speed handpiece and then polished with levigated alumina paste on the laboratory lathe. Porcelain jackets have a glaze on the outer surface that creates the fine finish on the crown and protects the restoration from staining. If extensive grinding is done during the adjustments, the crown should be reglazed before final cementation.

The porcelain jacket crown allows light to pass through the restoration. Therefore the shade of the finished restoration can be influenced to some degree by the color of the cement used to attach the restoration to the tooth. This is of some advantage to the dentist because slight alterations in the shade of the final restoration can be made by simply combining various colors of cement. Zinc phosphate cement is available in various colors of the powder component. The color of the powder selected can be mixed with glycerin and water to test the chosen color inside the porcelain crown when it is placed on the tooth. The mix will not set, so that there is no time limit on this color test. After the color of the cement is chosen, the test mix is completely washed off the preparation and the porcelain crown. The preparation is coated with cavity varnish, and the cement is mixed. Both the preparation and internal surfaces of the crown are covered with cement, and the crown is seated with hand pressure only. Pressure must be maintained until the cement is set. After the excess cement is removed, the patient can be dismissed.

Cementation of the gold veneer crown. The technique for cementation of the veneer crown is identical to that for cementation of the all-gold crown, except that any adjustments on porcelain must be done with porcelain grinding wheels. In addition, care must be exercised in seating crowns with porcelain fused to them so that excessive force is not placed on the porcelain by the Cooley peg. Some dentists prefer to drive the crown into place by having the patient bite firmly on a cotton roll that is placed over the restoration.

FIXED BRIDGE

A fixed bridge is a restoration that is used to replace missing teeth. The term *fixed* means that the restoration is cemented in place and therefore not removable by the patient. The term *bridge* has been adopted to designate this restoration because of its similarity in design to a bridge that spans a river (Fig. 20-13). The supports at the ends of the bridge are called *abut-*

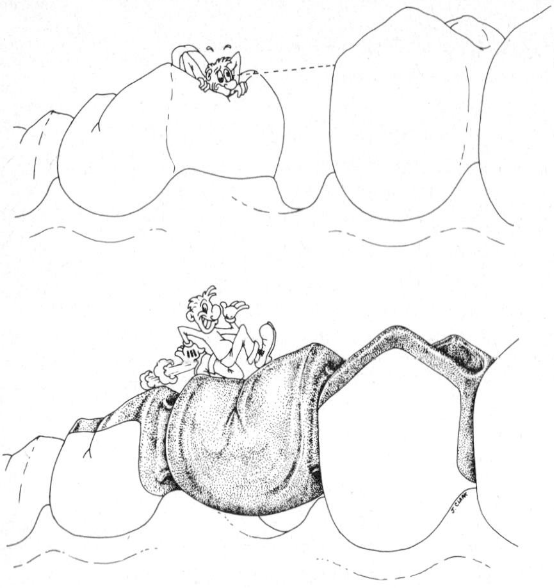

Fig. 20-13. Fixed bridge.

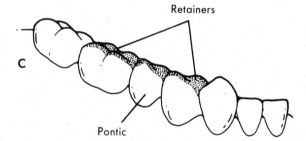

Fig. 20-14. Preparation of a three-unit fixed bridge. **A,** Edentulous space. **B,** Full crown preparations that "draw" with each other. **C,** Seated acrylic veneered bridge.

ments, as are the teeth that support the fixed bridge at each end. Whereas the river bridge spans the river, the fixed bridge spans edentulous spaces that were once occupied by teeth.

The basic parts of a fixed bridge are the retainers and the pontic. Retainers are restorations that connect the bridge to the abutment (supporting) teeth. The pontic is the artificial tooth that replaces the missing natural tooth (Fig. 20-14, *C*). Each individual retainer or pontic is commonly referred to as a unit of the bridge. The bridge shown in Fig. 20-14, *C* is an example of a three-unit bridge (two retainers and one pontic). Other bridges are designed to replace several missing teeth; therefore more units are joined to form these bridges. For example, if the four maxillary incisors are missing and a fixed bridge is fabricated to replace them, the bridge is six units long. There are four pontics to replace the missing teeth and two retainers to attach the bridge to the two canines.

Bridge retainers not only attach the bridge to the abutment teeth but may serve to restore the crown of an abutment at the same time. It is not uncommon for a patient to have abutment teeth that are in need of extensive restoration as well as needing a bridge to replace a missing tooth between them. Thus the retainers serve two functions at the same time. Re-

tainers usually are either three-quarter crowns or full crowns. Depending on the esthetic demands of the patient, full-crown retainers are either all gold or gold veneer crowns.

Pontics are either all gold or gold veneers. The pontic is connected to the retainers by gold joints on the proximal surfaces.

Need for a fixed bridge

The fixed bridge is usually the most favorable way to replace missing teeth if the abutment teeth are strong and well supported by alveolar bone. These restorations are far more comfortable and esthetic than a removable partial denture that could be used

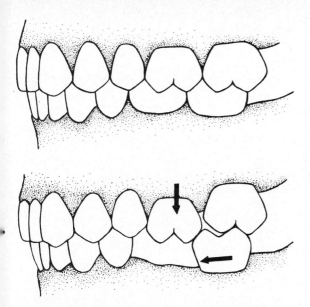

Fig. 20-15. Effects of loss of mandibular first molar. **A,** Dentition before loss. **B,** Changes that can occur after loss of tooth.

for the same purpose. Aside from esthetics, the need for a bridge is based on the fact that most of the teeth in the mouth depend on the presence of adjacent and opposing teeth to maintain their proper position in the dentition (Fig. 20-15). When a tooth is lost, the surrounding teeth can drift out of position, and the tooth opposing the empty space can overerupt (extrude) into the space. The result of this phenomenon is that teeth are tipped out of position, with the following undesirable effects:

1. The patient not only loses the biting function of the missing tooth, but also the abutment teeth are less efficient in chewing because they do not contact the opposing teeth properly.
2. The biting relationship of the teeth is changed to abnormal chewing patterns, which can result in injury to the temporomandibular joint.
3. The malaligned teeth can trigger clenching and tooth-grinding habits (bruxism). These habits can injure the temporomandibular joint and cause muscle spasms in the muscles of mastication.
4. Teeth that are tipped cannot resist the forces placed on them as well as they could when they were upright. Biting forces on a tipped tooth usually cause it to tip farther.

5. Abnormal force applied to tipped teeth often causes loss of the bone support of the tooth, resulting in its eventual loss.
6. Extrusion or overeruption of an opposing tooth over the edentulous space can create an interference in the normal biting pattern, which can result in temporomandibular joint damage.
7. Drifting and tipping of teeth cause contacts between teeth to open, which allows food to become trapped between the teeth. This food impaction is injurious to the gingiva.

Despite the negative effects of losing a tooth or teeth, not all patients are candidates for treatment for fixed bridges. Some are better treated with a removable partial denture. Still others may be better off with no treatment under certain circumstances. The best time to fabricate a bridge for a patient is as soon as healing is complete after an extraction and before drifting occurs. The supporting teeth must be reasonably sound with favorable bone support before this type of treatment is pursued.

Fabrication of a three-unit mandibular posterior bridge

Although specific designs of fixed bridges vary considerably according to the individual needs of the patient, the basic format used to construct the bridge is the same. The mandibular three-unit posterior bridge has been selected as an example because it is a rather common restoration in general dental practice. This example will demonstrate the replacement of a missing mandibular right second premolar with the bridge.

For discussion purposes, the bridge design used in this example will have a full crown retainer on the first molar. The premolar retainer will also be a full crown. This retainer and the pontic will be veneered with acrylic fused to gold for esthetic reasons.

Treatment planning. This is a major part of bridge construction. The dentist must have the essential information provided by the patient history, oral examination, radiographs, and study models to plan the appropriate treatment. All this information can be obtained in one diagnostic appointment and analyzed before the patient returns for treatment. The diagnostic information will guide the dentist's decision as to whether or not a fixed bridge is an appropriate form of treatment. If a bridge is appropriate, the information will be helpful for the dentist in designing the restoration to meet the patient's esthetic and functional needs.

Preparation of the abutment teeth. The abutment teeth are prepared for the full crown in a similar manner to that described previously. The exception to this is that these preparations must not only have draw within each preparation but they must draw with each other (Fig. 20-14, *B*). The finished bridge has to slide onto the prepared abutments and be cemented into place. Establishing draw between individual preparations for a bridge is one of the more difficult tasks for the dentist, and especially so in bridge designs that involve more than two abutments.

Taking the impression. After the preparations are finished and draw has been established between them, the gingiva is retracted, and an impression is taken, using the syringe-tray technique. A bite registration is needed, along with an alginate impression of the opposing teeth. Full arch impressions are more favor-

able than quadrant-sized impressions because the occlusion of the patient can be more accurately determined during the laboratory phase of the bridge fabrication.

Temporization. This is a very important part of bridge construction. A temporary bridge has to be constructed so that the abutment teeth cannot shift position in any direction. The opposing teeth must

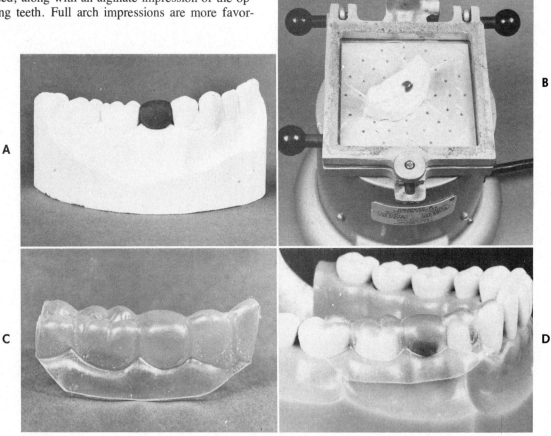

Fig. 20-16. Fabrication of temporary bridge by vacuum-adaptation mold technique. **A,** Clay pontic is placed in edentulous space on a preoperative study model. **B,** Coping material is adapted to model. **C,** Mold of area of bridge is cut away from rest of coping material. **D,** Mold and its relationship to prepared teeth. **E,** Filling mold with acrylic. **F,** Placement of filled mold over prepared teeth. **G,** Trimming temporary bridge. **H,** Finished bridge.

contact the temporary bridge when the jaws are closed to prevent extrusion. Any shifting of teeth during the interim laboratory phase will result in loss of fit of the permanent bridge on the abutment teeth and in improper occlusion. Patients should be instructed to contact the dentist immediately if a temporary bridge becomes dislodged or fractured. If a patient has to wear the temporary bridge for more than 2 weeks, it is wise to have the patient return periodically to check on the occlusal wear of the bridge.

An exceptionally favorable way to construct a temporary bridge is with the vacuum-adaptation method (Fig. 20-16). The technique is similar to that used to fabricate a temporary crown.

1. The edentulous space is filled with either a denture tooth that has been ground to fit or with a special high-heat clay material that can be formed into the shape of a tooth. This will represent the pontic in the temporary bridge (Fig. 20-16, *A*).
2. The study model with the pontic attached to it is placed in the Omnivac, and the coping material is vacuum-adapted to it to form the mold for the bridge.
3. The coping material is cut away from the model and trimmed.
4. After the preparations are finished, the mold is filled with temporary acrylic and placed on the preparations. The patient is instructed to bite on the filled mold to hold it in place.
5. After the initial set of the acrylic, the filled mold is

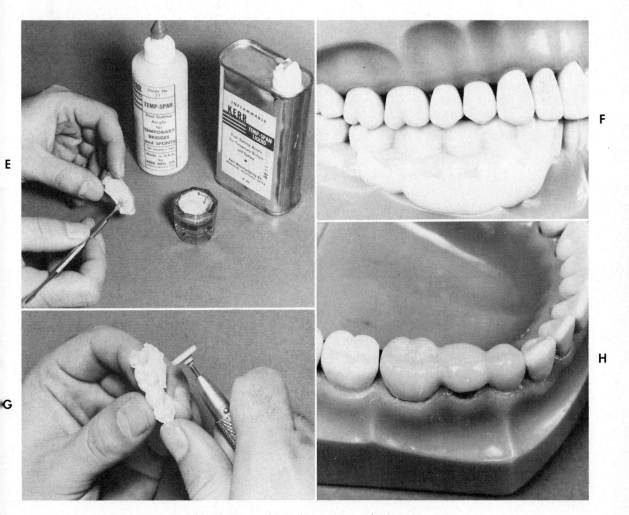

Fig. 20-16, cont'd. For legend see opposite page.

removed and the excess acrylic is trimmed away. The bridge is returned to the mouth for final setting. (The bridge should be lifted off the preparations periodically as the material hardens, to avoid fusion to the preparations.)

6. When the bridge has completely hardened, it can be trimmed, polished, and cemented with a temporary cement (Fig. 20-16, *G* and *H*).

Cementation. The basic procedure used for the cementation of a fixed bridge is the same as that for the gold crown and inlay. However, since the bridge spans a greater part of the occlusion than does a single crown, it is not at all uncommon to find more time spent on refining the biting relationship of the bridge to the opposing teeth. An additional consideration in the cementation of the bridge is the adjustment of the relationship of the pontic to the edentulous ridge. The pontic has to permit easy cleaning under the bridge during oral hygiene procedures. It must also contact the ridge so that it looks like a natural tooth in cases in which esthetics is a major concern.

Fixed bridges are cemented with any of the final cementing materials discussed previously (Fig. 15-6). After the cement has set, the excess is removed with a spoon excavator and explorer from around the retainers and under the pontic. The patient should be instructed to clean the bridge using normal toothbrushing techniques and dental floss with a floss threader (Chapter 2).

SPLINTS

Splinting teeth is a joining of two or more teeth together using gold restorations that are connected together at the contact area. There is no pontic between the joined teeth as there is in a fixed bridge.

Splinting is done to increase the retention of crowns on teeth when necessary and to increase the resistance of teeth to biting forces. Teeth that lack proper support from alveolar bone as a result of periodontal disease may benefit from a splinting procedure. Individual mobility of teeth is usually reduced when teeth are splinted together. Long-span fixed bridges often require the splinting of two or more teeth at each end of the bridge to achieve adequate retention and support.

SUMMARY

No attempt has been made to completely discuss the complex area of crown and bridge prosthodontics. The introduction to some of the fundamental procedures discussed should be viewed as a foundation on which to build the assistant's knowledge and skills in the more sophisticated restorative procedures being done in dentistry today and in the future.

BIBLIOGRAPHY

Johnston, J.F., et al.: Modern practice in crown and bridge prosthodontics, ed. 2, Philadelphia, 1965, W.B. Saunders Co.

CHAPTER 21

PERIODONTICS

Periodontics is the branch of dentistry that deals with the diagnosis and treatment of diseases that destroy the supporting tissues of the teeth. These supporting tissues are collectively referred to as the periodontium (Fig. 21-1). Diseases that damage the periodontium are called periodontal diseases.

Periodontal disease is the major reason for the extraction of teeth in patients 30 years old or over. In fact, studies have shown that as many as four fifths of the extractions in patients over the age of 30 are related to periodontal disease. It is estimated that nearly 100% of the population will have some degree of chronic destructive periodontal disease by the age of 45. These figures indicate the enormous impact that periodontal disease has on oral health. Although chronic destructive periodontal disease is uncommon in young people before puberty, it is not at all uncommon for children to have significant inflammation of the gingiva.

Dental caries and periodontal disease together are the most common conditions that the dentist must deal with in practice. The prevention and treatment of these diseases can ensure that patients will be able to preserve their teeth for an entire lifetime. The two most common periodontal diseases, gingivitis and periodontitis, will be discussed in this chapter.

ETIOLOGY OF PERIODONTAL DISEASE

Investigators have often described periodontal disease as a reaction of the periodontium to injury. The two major considerations in studying the development of periodontal disease, then, are (1) the causes of injury to the periodontium and (2) the degree of reaction to the injury, or the severity of the disease. Injury to the periodontium is primarily as a result of local irritants. These irritants initiate periodontal disease. The reaction to these injurious irritants varies depending on the influence of several contributing factors within each individual patient.

Local irritants

Local irritants are substances and materials that irritate periodontal tissues when the two come in contact for a prolonged period of time. Although there is some disagreement as to the exact mechanism involved, investigators theorize that both chemical and mechanical irritation of soft tissue are at work. Some of the most common local irritants and their possible mechanisms of action on the soft gingival tissue are listed in Table 21-1.

Regardless of the specific mechanisms involved, local irritants do cause injury to the gingiva. Once injury occurs, the disease process begins. Therefore the first step in the prevention of periodontal disease is to eliminate local irritants. Replacement of faulty dental restorations to eliminate open contacts or overhangs and to provide proper contours to deflect food away from the gingiva is certainly indicated. Periodic

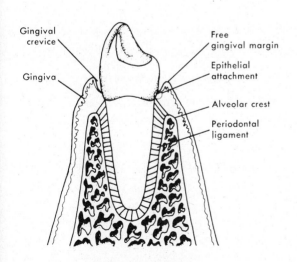

Gingival crevice

Gingiva

Free gingival margin

Epithelial attachment

Alveolar crest

Periodontal ligament

Fig. 21-1. Periodontium.

Table 21-1. Local irritants

Irritant	Possible mechanism of action
Dental plaque	Chemical irritation caused by bacterial toxins, enzymes, and breakdown products of epithelial cells
Calculus	Mechanical irritation caused by the soft tissues rubbing on the coarse surface of the calculus, in addition to the chemical irritation of the calculus itself, which contains bacteria that produce toxic products
Overhanging restoration margins and porous filling materials	Mechanical rubbing of the soft tissue plus being an ideal place for bacterial plaque to form and chemically irritate the soft tissue
Food debris	Chemical irritation caused by breakdown products of putrefying food and bacterial growth
Trauma from food	Mechanical irritation caused by food being forced onto the delicate gingiva as a result of open contacts between teeth and poor contours of restorations
Mouth breathing	Excessive drying of soft mucosal tissue, resulting in dehydration of the cells and chronic irritation

dental prophylaxis, toothbrushing and dental flossing are all designed to remove accumulations of irritating debris from the teeth.

Factors contributing to the progress of disease

The reaction of the periodontium to injury varies with the individual. It is quite possible for one person to have extensive tissue reaction to the smallest amount of local irritant but for another patient to have an abundance of local irritant contacting the gingiva with very little tissue reaction. This variability among patients results from one or more of the following factors:

Systemic factors of the patient
Nutritional status
Hormone balance
Drugs
Allergy
Systemic disease
Heredity
General resistance to disease

Dysfunctional factors
Traumatic occlusion
Bruxism (clenching and grinding of teeth)
Missing teeth
Malposed teeth
Unilateral chewing

The factors that influence the reaction of the periodontium to local irritation are divided into two categories: systemic and dysfunctional. Systemic factors relate to the makeup of the individual in a biological sense. These factors deal with the various biochemical phenomena that make the patient a true individual. Heredity, nutritional status, metabolic diseases, and hormonal functions all influence the patient's resistance to disease. Dysfunctional factors are defects in the chewing mechanism. The effect of these discrepancies results in excessive forces being applied to teeth during the mastication of food and the clenching of the teeth. Biting forces applied to malposed and malformed teeth can cause damage to both the periodontal ligament and the surrounding bone. These damaging forces, coupled with the injurious effects of a local irritant, can lead to profound periodontal disease.

The basic rationale of periodontal therapy is to remove local irritants, to correct defects in the dentition through orthodontic, restorative, and surgical procedures, and to eliminate as many systemic factors as possible to establish favorable periodontal health.

Progress of periodontal disease

The most common cause of irritation to the gingiva is the accumulation of dental plaque and calculus around the cervical areas of the teeth. The gingiva reacts to these irritants by becoming inflamed. Inflammation is an attempt by the body to ward off physical and chemical injury and bacterial invasion of the tissues. The injured area becomes engorged with blood to provide an abundance of nutrients, oxygen, and white blood cells. The white blood cells destroy invading bacteria and remove debris from the site of injury. The accumulation and congestion of blood in

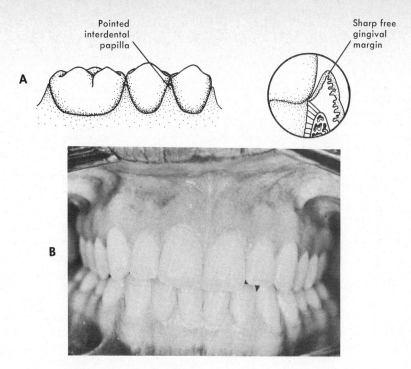

Fig. 21-2. Normal gingiva. **A**, Sketches. **B**, Photograph.

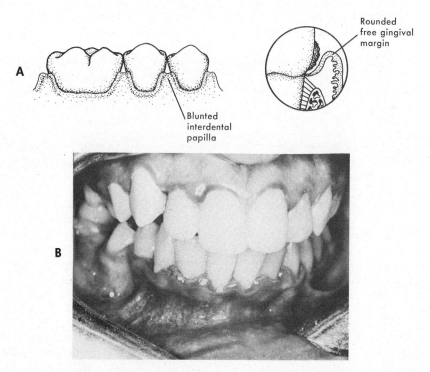

Fig. 21-3. Changes in gingival form associated with gingivitis. **A**, Sketches. **B**, Photograph.

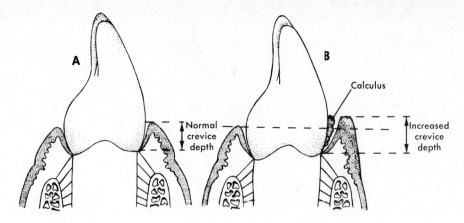

Fig. 21-4. A, Normal gingival crevice depth. **B,** Deepened gingival crevice resulting from swelling.

the injured tissue result in a change in color, shape, and texture of the gingival tissue.

Inflammation of the gingiva, or gingivitis, is diagnosed by examining the gingiva for changes in color, form, and density (texture). Normal gingiva is a firm, pale pink tissue with sharp, free gingival margins and pointed interdental papillae (Fig. 21-2). Inflamed gingiva has a reddish color, with rounded swollen gingival margins and blunt interdental papillae (Fig. 21-3). The density changes from firm to a spongy texture. The tissue may bleed readily when it is pressed or during toothbrushing. The gingival crevice may deepen slightly as a result of swelling of the gingiva (Fig. 21-4). The extent of these changes depends on the severity of the inflammatory process.

The treatment for gingivitis is a thorough dental prophylaxis coupled with meticulous home oral hygiene procedures. Dental restorations that are contributing to local irritation should be replaced. Once the local irritants are removed and prevented from recurring, the gingiva will return to normal.

If gingivitis is not treated, the inflammation will extend from the gingival margin deeper into the periodontium. The effects of this extension are destructive to the epithelial attachment, the periodontal ligament, and the alveolar bone. Inflammation of the deeper structures of the periodontium is called periodontitis. Periodontitis represents the most severe and destructive form of periodontal disease. It is rather common for dentists to use the terms *periodontitis* and *severe periodontal disease* interchangeably. Periodontitis can lead to tooth mobility and eventual loss of teeth.

During the gingivitis stage of periodontal disease, the delicate lining of the gingival crevice ruptures or ulcerates, which permits the invasion of bacteria, destructive enzymes, and bacterial toxins into the gingival tissues. The tissue reaction becomes more extensive and spreads deeper into the periodontium. This in turn stimulates the cells of the epithelial attachment to become repositioned apically on the root surface (Fig. 21-5). The result is a deeper gingival crevice. When the gingival crevice deepens because of enlargement of the gingiva as in gingivitis, the deepened crevice is called a gingival pocket, or a pseudopocket. The epithelial attachment remains stationary. Deepening of the gingival crevice resulting from migration of the attachment apically is called a periodontal pocket (Fig. 21-5).

Unfortunately, once a periodontal pocket is formed, the accumulation of irritants in the deep gingival crevice is more difficult if not impossible for the patient to remove. Thus the destructive process continues. As the inflammation reaches the alveolar bone, it stimulates cells called *osteoclasts* to increase resorption of bone. Bone resorption is also stimulated by occlusal trauma on the tooth. It is normal for bone to be continually formed and removed (resorbed) by cells located on the surface of bone throughout life. Inflammation and occlusal trauma together simply accelerate bone resorption at a rate faster than it can be reformed. As a result, there is a net loss of bone around the root of the tooth, and the tooth becomes hypermobile. If the periodontitis continues to destroy sufficient bone, the tooth will eventually be lost.

The treatment of periodontitis depends on the se-

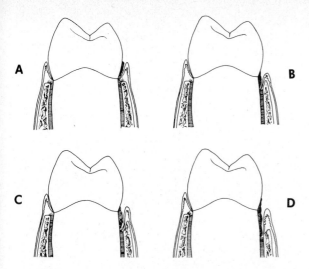

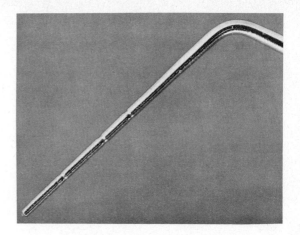

Fig. 21-6. O-style periodontal probe.

Fig. 21-5. Migration of epithelial attachment and destruction of alveolar bone, resulting in periodontal pocket. **A,** Accumulation of irritants. **B,** Apical migration of epithelial attachment in response to irritant. **C** and **D,** Continued migration of attachment and accumulation of irritant on root surface.

verity of the disease. One of the principal steps in treatment is the thorough removal of all local irritants from the periodontal pockets and around the teeth. This extensive scaling procedure is often called a periodontal scaling, to differentiate it from the routine dental prophylaxis that does not involve the scaling of deep periodontal pockets. Additional procedures may include the following:

1. Surgery—to eliminate periodontal pockets (gingivectomy)
2. Root planing—to smooth rough root surfaces
3. Occlusal adjustment—to eliminate excessive occlusal trauma
4. Restorative procedures (splints, bridges, and crowns)—to establish proper contacts, occlusion, and contours of teeth

PERIODONTAL DIAGNOSTIC PROCEDURES

The same diagnostic procedures as described in Chapter 3 are used in periodontics. The specific information the dentist is looking for with regard to periodontal status will be discussed here.

Medical-dental history

The patient's medical-dental history should reveal systemic conditions such as chronic illness, nutritional deficiencies, and personal habits that may influence the progress of periodontal disease or its treatment.

The dental portion of the history provides valuable information regarding the dental status of the patient. The frequency of brushing, flossing, and dental prophylaxis procedures is a good indication of the patient's effort to prevent periodontal disease. Knowledge of missing teeth, dates of extractions, orthodontic treatment, and restorative procedures is of value to the dentist.

The history should also reveal the patient's all-important attitude toward the preservation of his teeth. Successful periodontal treatment depends greatly on a positive attitude by the patient.

Oral examination

A visual inspection of the gingiva is essential to detect the changes that are associated with the inflammatory process. Changes in the color and shape of the gingival tissue are critical to the diagnosis. Palpation of the gingiva with the side of an explorer will reveal the texture, or density, of the tissue.

Periodontal probing is essential to diagnose the existence of periodontal pockets. The probe is a thin dipstick-like device that is used to measure the depth of the gingival crevice and to determine the relationship of the epithelial attachment to the cementoenamel junction. The O-style probe (Fig. 21-6) is marked in increments of 3, 6, and 8 mm from the tip toward the shank of the instrument. Probing is often done at six points on a tooth, three on the buccal aspect and three on the lingual (Fig. 21-7). The probe

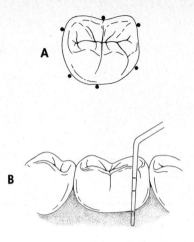

Fig. 21-7. Common sites for measuring the gingival crevice.

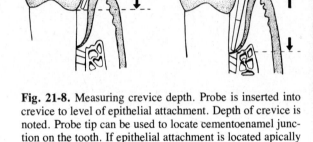

Fig. 21-8. Measuring crevice depth. Probe is inserted into crevice to level of epithelial attachment. Depth of crevice is noted. Probe tip can be used to locate cementoenamel junction on the tooth. If epithelial attachment is located apically to junction, periodontal pocket exists.

is inserted in the gingival crevice to the depth of the epithelial attachment. The distance between the attachment and the gingival margin is recorded (Fig. 21-8). If apical migration of the attachment is suspected, the probe tip can be used to locate the cementoenamel junction. The distance from here to the gingival margin is recorded. The two recordings can be compared to determine the amount of apical migration, or true periodontal pocket formation.

Accumulation of plaque, stains, and calculus on the teeth should be noted and recorded. This is helpful in correlating areas of tissue damage with the areas of accumulation of local irritants. A general assessment of the patient's oral hygiene should also be noted. Use of disclosing agents is a valuable method of detecting the more subtle accumulations of plaque.

Each tooth should be tested for mobility by pushing it in a buccolingual direction and pressing on the occlusal or incisal surface. A simple scale of 1-2-3 is often used to describe mobility: 1, slight mobility; 2, moderate mobility; and 3, extensive mobility in all directions. These figures can be recorded on the dental chart for future reference. Drifted teeth, missing teeth, malposed teeth, and open contacts should all be recorded, since they make up the dysfunctional factors in the progress of periodontal disease.

An assessment of existing restorations and prosthetic devices should be done to determine their possible contribution to periodontal problems.

Analysis of the patient's occlusion, or bite, is an integral part of a periodontal examination. It is well known that improper contacting of upper and lower teeth when the jaws are closed can create undesirable traumatic forces on teeth, which can contribute to the progress of periodontal destruction.

Study models and photographs

Diagnostic study models and photographs are useful to document oral findings. Models provide the dentist with a three-dimensional view of the patient's teeth, jaws, and gingiva. Malposed teeth, undesirable occlusal relationships, and poor gingival contours can be examined thoroughly on the models. Excessive wear areas (facets) on teeth are easily detected on the study models. These are often good indications of excessive occlusal forces on a tooth.

Photographs provide a color recording of the gingiva and plaque and calculus accumulation for future reference. Models and photographs should be kept as permanent records to document the progress of periodontal treatment. The dates on which study model impressions and photographs are taken should be recorded in the patient's record, the models, and the photographs.

Radiographs

Radiographs are useful in determining the degree of periodontal involvement. The loss of bone around teeth can be seen on the radiograph, although it cannot be relied on completely (Fig. 21-9). Periodontal

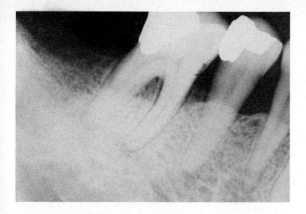

Fig. 21-9. Radiograph revealing extensive loss of alveolar bone resulting from periodontitis.

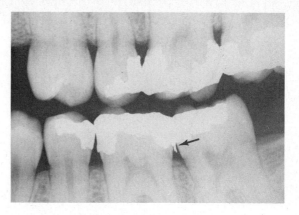

Fig. 21-10. Bite-wing radiograph demonstrating existence of cervical overhang of amalgam restoration.

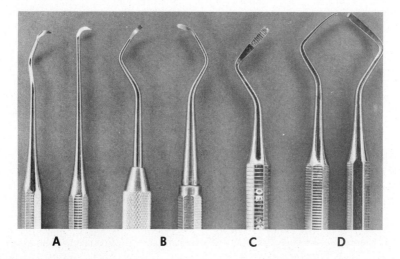

Fig. 21-11. Common periodontal hand instruments. **A,** Sickle scalers. **B,** Curette scalers. **C,** Periodontal file. **D,** Hoe scalers.

probing is the most accurate method of assessing the location and extent of bone loss. Overhangs on restorations are readily seen on bite-wing radiographs (Fig. 21-10).

COMMON PERIODONTAL INSTRUMENTS

Scalers. Scalers are hand instruments used to remove local irritants from the tooth surface and to plane roughened root surfaces. They are available in a variety of shapes and styles. Most styles fit into one of three basic categories: sickles, curettes, and hoes.

Sickle scalers derive their name from their sickle-like shape (Fig. 6-8, *A*). The narrow, tapering tip of the instrument makes it convenient for use in scaling proximal surfaces of teeth. They are especially useful in scaling proximal surfaces of anterior teeth because of the limited size of the interproximal space. Sickles are available in straight or modified (Jacquette) designs (Fig. 21-11, *A*).

Curette scalers (Fig. 21-11, *B*) are available in a number of designs. Each design seems to vary the relationship of the blade to the handle of the instrument. The basic design features in all of them are (1) a rounded tip, (2) a rounded back of the blade, and (3) a cutting edge along two of the edges of the blade. Curette scalers are used to scale all surfaces of the teeth. They are particularly favorable instruments for removing subgingival calculus without damaging the root surface. Root planing and subgingival curettage can also be done with the curette scaler.

Hoe scalers (Fig. 21-11, *D*) are less popular than the sickle and curette types. The sharp corners on the cutting edge create a risk in using it for subgingival scaling. The corners of the blade can gouge grooves in the soft root if the instrument is not handled carefully. Hoe scalers are most frequently used to remove very heavy accumulations of supragingival calculus on the buccal and lingual surfaces of teeth.

Periodontal files (Fig. 21-11, *C*). Periodontal files are miniature-size files that can be inserted into interproximal areas and periodontal pockets. They are used with a pull motion to remove small residual calculus particles after scaling and to smooth roughened tooth surfaces. The periodontal file and curette scaler are often used together in root planing procedures.

Periodontal probe (Fig. 21-6). The periodontal probe is a measuring device that is used to determine the depth of the gingival crevice. The O-style probe has markings on the instrument that serve as references to determine pocket depth.

The marks on the instrument are located at distances of 3, 6, and 8 mm from the tip. Crevice depth is determined by inserting the instrument subgingivally to the depth of the epithelial attachment. The depth is read from the reference marks on the instrument at the level of the free gingival margin. Fig. 21-8 demonstrates a crevice depth of approximately 6 mm.

The use of the periodontal probe is the most accurate method available to determine the degree of bone loss in periodontitis. From the six points of probing shown in Fig. 21-7, the level of the epithelial attachment can be compared with the level of the cementoenamel junction to determine the presence of bone loss around a tooth.

Although several styles of periodontal probes are available, the O-style probe is one of the most popular. It has a very thin working end, which permits easier insertion of the probe into a narrow pocket with minimal discomfort to the patient.

Scalpels. The surgical scalpel is commonly used for oral surgical procedures, including the gingivectomy. A standard scalpel handle is used with replace-

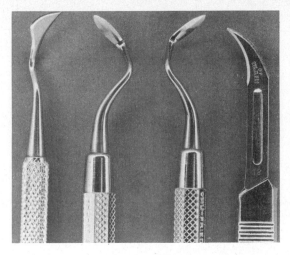

Fig. 21-12. Periodontal surgical knives. *Left to right:* Kirkland knife, No. 1 and No. 2 Orban knives, and No. 12B scalpel.

able blades of various shapes (Fig. 21-12). The Bard-Parker No. 12B blade is a convenient blade for removing gingival tissue on the facial aspect of the alveolar process. Because of its double cutting edge, it can cut with both pulling and pushing motions. The sharp tip of the blade is used to remove interproximal soft tissue.

Periodontal knives (Fig. 21-12). Gingival surgery involves not only the removal of unwanted gingiva but also the contouring of remaining soft tissue, which is necessary to reestablish the normal function of the gingiva. Periodontal knives were developed to give the operator access to areas of the mouth that could not be reached with standard scalpel blades. The lingual aspect of the alveolar process is a typical area that is inaccessible for gingivectomy procedures using a scalpel blade.

Periodontal knives have the necessary angles in the shank of the instrument, making it convenient to use in resecting and contouring the gingiva. The Orban No. 1 and No. 2 style knives are excellent choices for removing interproximal soft tissue because of their narrow blade design. The disadvantage of periodontal knives is that they require precise sharpening after each use to keep them functional.

Electrosurgery setup (Fig. 21-13). Electrosurgery is a useful surgical method that employs the use of a tiny arc of electrical current to make the incision in

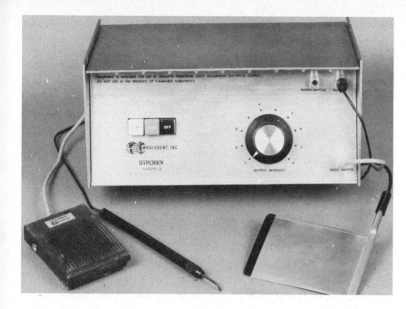

Fig. 21-13. Electrosurgery unit.

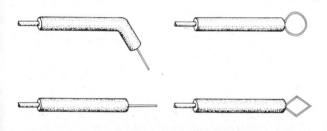

Fig. 21-14. Various cutting tips for electrosurgery unit.

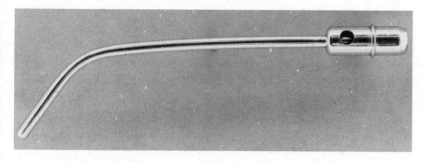

Fig. 21-15. Surgical evacuator tip.

the gingiva. In electrosurgery not only is soft tissue cut but also blood is coagulated, which limits bleeding during the procedure.

The device consists of a control box, a foot-operated on-off switch, and two terminals. One terminal is held by the patient or placed in contact with him in some fashion. Some manufacturers utilize as one terminal a metal plate that the patient sits on during the surgical procedure. The other terminal is held in the dentist's hand. This terminal is in the form of a probe with a wire end.

When the dentist touches the patient's gingiva with the tip of the probe and activates the foot switch, current flows through the wire tip and burns the incision in the gingiva. The assistant must keep the oral evacuator near the surgical site to remove the odor of burning tissue. A word of caution is in order at this point. It is wise to use nonmetal evacuator tips and mouth mirrors during electrosurgery procedures in case the cutting probe inadvertently contacts these instruments. Various cutting tips are available for better access to difficult working areas of the mouth (Fig. 21-14).

Evacuator tip (Fig. 21-15). Oral surgical procedures require constant removal of blood from the surgical site to maintain visibility for the operator. The smaller surgical suction tips are better for this purpose. They remove the small quantities of blood from the incision effectively, since the smaller tip can be directed specifically to smaller areas in the surgical field.

The tip should be dipped in sterile saline solution occasionally during the surgery, to aspirate some fluid through the tip and hose. This clears away clotted blood that accumulates in the tip and evacuation hose.

COMMON PERIODONTAL TREATMENT PROCEDURES
Scaling and root planing

Scaling procedures eliminate plaque and calculus from the surfaces of the teeth. The armamentarium for a periodontal scaling procedure is identical to that used for the dental prophylaxis (Fig. 2-1).

Periodontal scaling and the dental prophylaxis share the same ultimate goal: remove irritants to prevent periodontal injury. The difference is in the location of the irritants to be removed. The routine prophylaxis usually involves removal of irritants such as calculus above the gingival margin (supragingival calculus) or located just below the gingival margin (subgingival calculus) (Fig. 21-16). Periodontal scaling implies more extensive scaling procedures to remove subgingival calculus located in periodontal pockets.

Scaling must be done with sharp scalers to ensure complete removal of the very adherent calculus. Once calculus is removed from a root surface, the underlying cementum is often rough from the damaging effects of the calculus. This roughness must be removed to prevent the gingiva from being continually irritated. Voids in the cementum become ideal areas for the rapid accumulation of plaque and subsequent calculus formation all over again. These voids are re-

moved by root planing. This is a process of planing or shaving the root surface with a scaler or a small periodontal file to remove surface roughness (Fig. 21-17).

Subgingival curettage

One method of eliminating minor pocket formation is through the use of curettage. This procedure involves the removal of the delicate lining (epithelium) of the periodontal pocket. Not only is the lining removed but also damaged tissue as well (Fig. 21-18, *A*).

Once the calculus and other debris have been removed and the pocket lining curettaged, the periodontal ligament may reattach to the root surface, thus eliminating the pocket (Fig. 21-18, *B*). The entire procedure can be accomplished with standard curette scalers. The success of subgingival curettage depends on the extent of pocket formation and the healing capabilities of the patient.

Gingivectomy

Once periodontal pockets are formed, they must be eliminated, for they have the following undesirable effects on the patient:

1. They accumulate assorted debris and bacteria, which can lead to local and systemic infection.
2. Root caries can develop quickly as a result of debris accumulation in the pocket.
3. Putrefaction of pocket debris can create bad tastes and foul mouth odors.
4. Untreated pockets continually collect debris, which results in a deepening of the pocket as alveolar bone is destroyed. This results in hypermobility and eventual loss of the tooth.

One method of eliminating severe periodontal pockets is by surgically removing the diseased gingival tissue. This procedure is called a gingivectomy. Besides eliminating the ill effects of periodontal pockets listed previously, the gingivectomy procedure benefits the patient in the following ways:

1. Diseased gingival tissue is removed.
2. Favorable gingival contour can be reestablished, within limits.
3. The surgical removal of the wall of the pocket gives the operator direct access to remove calculus (Fig. 21-19) and plane rough root surfaces.
4. The patient gains access to clean the root surfaces previously inaccessible because of the existence of the pocket.

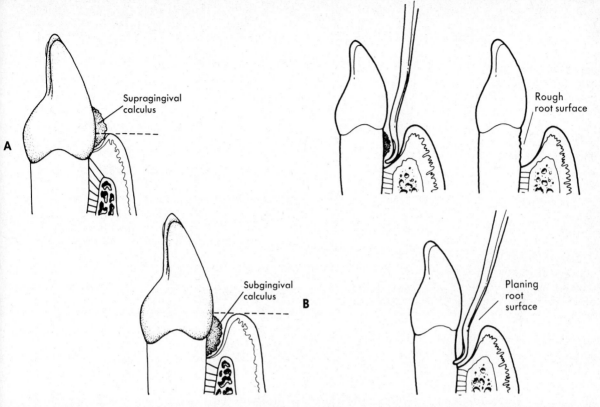

Fig. 21-16. Location of calculus. **A,** Supragingival. **B,** Subgingival.

Fig. 21-17. Exaggerated sketch of scaling and root planing.

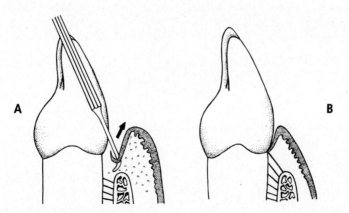

Fig. 21-18. A, Subgingival curettage of lining of gingival crevice. **B,** Reattachment of gingiva to root surface.

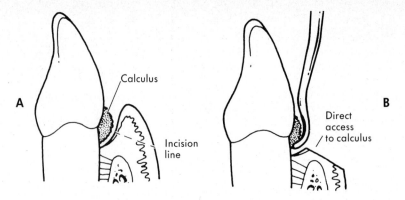

Fig. 21-19. Surgical elimination of periodontal pocket, **A,** gives direct access to subgingival calculus, **B.**

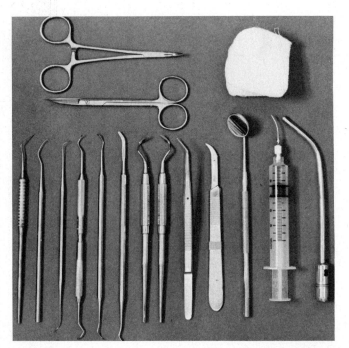

Hemostat
Suture scissors
Sterile gauze sponges, 2 × 2 inch
Periodontal probe
Explorers, No. 17 and No. 3
Curette scalers, Columbia No. 13 and No. 14
Sickle scaler, Jacquette
Plastic filling instrument, F.P. No. 1
Periodontal knives, Orban No. 1, No. 2
Cotton pliers
Bard-Parker scalpel handle
Bard-Parker scalpel, No. 12B blade
Mouth mirror
Irrigation syringe (for sterile saline solution)
Surgical suction tip

Add-on items

Sterile cup of saline solution
Surgical gloves for operator and assistant
Periodontal dressing
Cotton tip applicator
Iodine lotion
Mixing pads, paper
Cement spatula, No. 336
Petroleum jelly
Anesthesia setup

Fig. 21-20. Gingivectomy armamentarium.

Armamentarium for a gingivectomy (Fig. 21-20). Gingivectomy procedures are usually done with a scalpel, periodontal knives, surgical scissors, or electrosurgery. The choice is made according to the preference of the dentist.

Gingivectomy procedure: a sample method. There is some difference of opinion as to whether a patient requiring gingival surgery should have a peri-odontal scaling done before the surgery. Dentists who wish to prescale before surgery will schedule a separate appointment for that purpose. A typical appointment scheme is shown in Table 21-2.

At the surgery appointment the patient is premedicated if necessary and anesthetized with local anesthesia. The following is a step-by-step description of the surgical procedure.

Table 21-2. An appointment schedule for the gingivectomy patient

Appointment	Treatment
1	Prescale the teeth
2	a. Gingivectomy (pocket elimination) b. Residual calculus removal c. Root-plane rough surfaces d. Placement of the surgical dressing
3	a. Remove surgical dressing after 1 week b. Rinse area of surgery with hydrogen peroxide c. Gently polish the teeth with a soft rubber cup and dental floss d. Rinse thoroughly with warm water e. Place a new surgical dressing
4	a. Remove final surgical dressing 1 week after placement b. Repeat rinsing and polishing procedures c. Patient home care instructions given
5	Recall patient 6 weeks after surgery to evaluate healing and home care effectiveness

1. The area to be operated on may be swabbed with iodine lotion to reduce bacterial contamination in the surgical field.
2. The field is isolated with sterile 2 × 2 inch gauze sponges.
3. Pockets are marked on the facial and lingual gingiva by measuring the pocket depth with a periodontal probe and puncturing the gingiva with the probe tip at the level of the base of the pocket (Fig. 21-21).
4. After all the pocket depths are marked on the facial and lingual aspects of the alveolar process, the resulting blood spots from the punctures will outline the contour of the incision.
5. Using either a scalpel or a periodontal knife, the dentist incises the gingiva just apical to the puncture marks (Fig. 21-22, *A*). The blade of the instrument is positioned so that a bevel is created along the incised gingiva. This reestablishes the normal tapered contour of the free gingival margin.
6. The interdental papillae are incised with a narrow-bladed periodontal knife (Orban, No. 1 or No. 2).
7. After the incision is made, the detached gingiva is removed with a curette scaler and tissue forceps (Fig. 21-22, *B*).
8. After the diseased gingiva is removed, the operator has direct access to any residual calculus not eliminated during the prescaling appointment. Once the calculus is removed, root surfaces can be planed with periodontal files and curettes as needed.

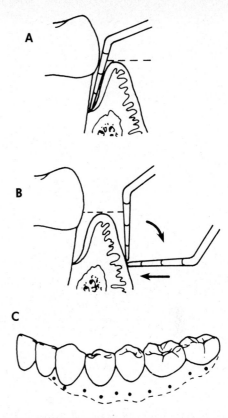

Fig. 21-21. Marking periodontal pockets for gingivectomy procedure. **A,** Measuring depth of pocket. **B,** Transposing measured depth to gingival surface. Gingiva is marked by puncturing mucosa at level of pocket depth. **C,** Incision is made just apical to puncture marks.

9. The surgical field is thoroughly rinsed and inspected for complete pocket elimination and proper contour. Refinements are then made if they are needed.
10. The periodontal surgical dressing is prepared and placed over the entire surgical area. The dressing is held in place by the mechanical lock of the dressing that is forced into the interproximal spaces (Fig. 21-22, *C*).
11. The patient should be given postoperative instructions in written form before being dismissed.

Fig. 21-23 illustrates the preoperative and postoperative appearance of a periodontitis patient.

Assistant's role in gingivectomy procedures. The assistant's role in the gingivectomy centers on effective retraction and evacuation in addition to the other standard chairside duties. Evacuation is of extreme

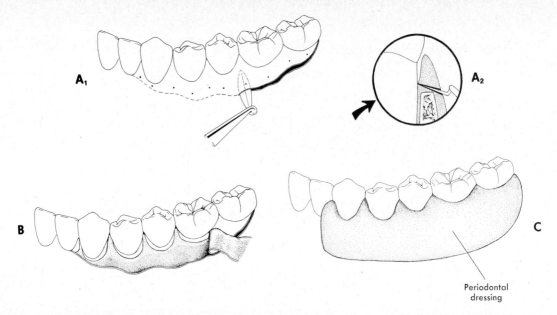

Fig. 21-22. A, Incision and resection of gingiva during gingivectomy. **B,** Removal of excised gingiva with tissue forceps. **C,** Periodontal dressing in place.

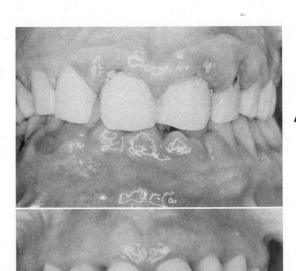

Fig. 21-23. A, Severe periodontitis before surgery. **B,** View of same patient 6 weeks after surgery. (Courtesy Dr. Raul D. Caffesse, Ann Arbor, Mich.)

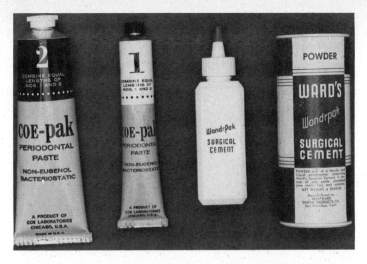

Fig. 21-24. Two popular brands of periodontal surgical dressing material.

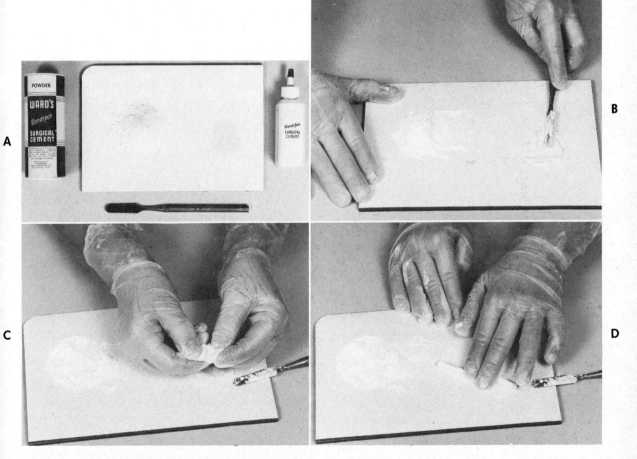

Fig. 21-25. Preparation of Ward's Wondrpak periodontal dressing. **A,** Dispensing the material. **B,** Initial mixing using heavy-bladed spatula. **C,** Kneading dressing. **D,** Rolling dressing.

importance in maintaining the operator's visibility and the patient's comfort.

The assistant prepares the periodontal dressing to be placed over the operative area. There are several preferred formulas used to make a periodontal surgical dressing. Two popular commercial brands (Fig. 21-24) are prepared as follows:

Ward's Wondrpak (zinc oxide–eugenol)

1. Dispense 15 drops of liquid and approximately 1½ tablespoons of powder on a parchment mixing pad (Fig. 21-25, *A*).
2. Incorporate a teaspoon of powder into the liquid and mix thoroughly (Fig. 21-25, *B*).
3. Continued additions of powder should be made until the mix is too thick to handle with the spatula.
4. Apply powder to the surgical gloves and pick up the mix with the fingers. Knead the mix like dough, working in as much powder as possible (Fig. 21-25, *C*). This strengthens the pack.
5. Once the pack is very heavy, yet still can be molded, roll it into a rope on the mixing pad using a rolling motion with the fingers (Fig. 21-25, *D*). A 1-inch piece of the material should be cut off the rope for use in packing the interproximal areas.

Coe-Pak

1. Extrude equal lengths of material from the tubes onto the mixing pad (½ to 1 inch are usually sufficient for a quadrant).
2. Spatulate with a 336 spatula or a disposable tongue blade for 45 seconds.
3. Wait 1 to 3 minutes before handling, until material loses its tackiness.
4. Moisten the surgical gloves with saline solution; then the material can be picked up and shaped. The moistened gloves will not stick to the packing material.
5. The Coe-Pak can be applied to the area of surgery in the same manner as that used for Ward's Wondrpak.

Modified Widman flap

Another surgical technique designed to eliminate periodontal pockets is the modified Widman flap procedure. The patient is prepared for surgery with a thorough periodontal scaling, overhang removal, and instruction in oral hygiene procedures. After a 3- to 4-week period of maintaining a high level of oral hygiene, the surgery is performed.

The Widman procedure involves the removal of the lining of the periodontal pocket and some adjacent marginal gingiva (Fig. 21-26). During the surgery a conservative flap is retracted on both the buccal and lingual aspects of the involved teeth. The flap retraction allows the dentist to gain access to the roots of

the teeth and the surrounding alveolar bone. The damaged tissue is removed after being incised. Curettes are used to remove the incised tissue (Fig. 21-27). The roots of the teeth are planed, and alveolar bone is recontoured as needed. The surgical site is flushed thoroughly with sterile saline solution, the flap is repositioned and sutured in place, and a conventional periodontal dressing is placed.

One week after surgery, the dressing and sutures are removed and the teeth are polished. Home care instructions are reviewed again with the patient.

The chairside assistant's tasks during this procedure include the following:

1. Operatory preparation
2. Patient preparation
3. Retraction of soft tissue
4. Evacuation of oral fluids
5. Debridement of the surgical site
6. Delivery of instruments and materials to the operator
7. Trimming suture material after placement

A sample armamentarium for the Widman flap procedure is shown in Fig. 21-28. The procedure is outlined as follows, using the four-handed dentistry technique.

Patient preparation. The patient is prepared for surgery according to the personal philosophy of the operator. The use of head wraps and patient drapes, as well as surgical gloves for both operator and assistant, is helpful in maintaining a sterile field.

The mandibular left posterior segment will serve as an example of an area of the mouth to be treated. The patient is placed in either a supine position with the operator in the 10 to 11 o'clock position, or the chair back is elevated and the base lowered to the maximum to place the patient's oral cavity at the elbow height of the operator. If the latter position is used, the operator assumes a 9 o'clock position. Anesthetic is administered in the usual manner with the hidden syringe transfer.

Procedure

1. A test for anesthesia is made by probing the gingiva throughout the surgical site with a periodontal probe.
2. The operator retracts the tongue with a mouth mirror in the left hand, and the assistant retracts the cheek with the evacuator in the right hand. The assistant's left hand can also be used for additional retraction as needed. The assistant transfers the No. 12B scalpel to the operator in exchange for the periodontal probe. The pickup-and-delivery instrument transfer can be used.

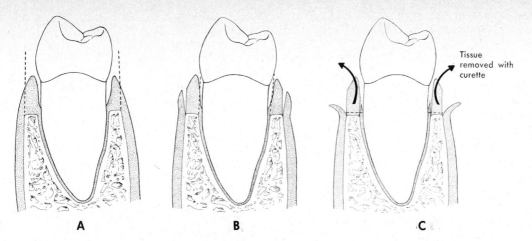

Fig. 21-26. Incisions required for modified Widman flap procedure. **A,** First incision at least 0.5 to 1 mm away from free gingival margin. **B,** Second incision extends from bottom of gingival crevice to alveolar crest. **C,** Third incision releases damaged tissue, which can then be removed with curette scaler.

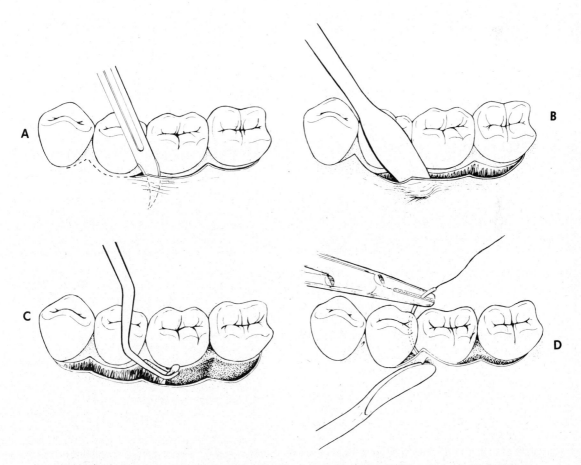

Fig. 21-27. Flap procedure performed with aid of chairside assistant (buccal view). **A,** Incising buccal gingiva. **B,** Flap reflection with periosteal elevator. **C,** Use of curette to remove granulomatous tissue and accretions. **D,** Chairside assistant can support buccal gingiva with periosteal elevator to facilitate penetration with suture needle.

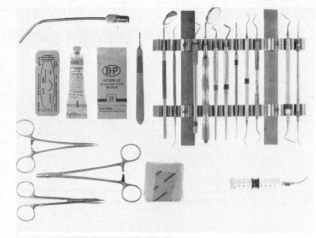

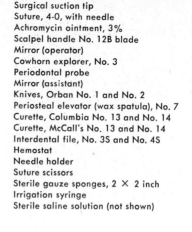

Surgical suction tip
Suture, 4-0, with needle
Achromycin ointment, 3%
Scalpel handle No. 12B blade
Mirror (operator)
Cowhorn explorer, No. 3
Periodontal probe
Mirror (assistant)
Knives, Orban No. 1 and No. 2
Periosteal elevator (wax spatula), No. 7
Curette, Columbia No. 13 and No. 14
Curette, McCall's No. 13 and No. 14
Interdental file, No. 3S and No. 4S
Hemostat
Needle holder
Suture scissors
Sterile gauze sponges, 2 × 2 inch
Irrigation syringe
Sterile saline solution (not shown)

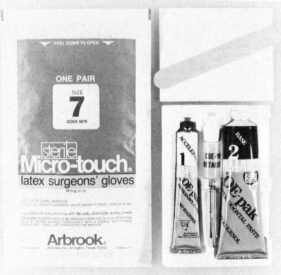

Surgical gloves (2 pair)
Mixing pad
Tongue depressor (spatula)
Periodontal dressing

Fig. 21-28. Armamentarium for Widman flap procedure.

3. The incision is made around the area to be treated. The patient's head is turned toward the assistant when the lingual gingiva is incised and toward the operator when the buccal gingiva is incised (Fig. 21-27, *A*). The assistant evacuates as needed along the incision using a surgical tip.
4. A periosteal elevator is transferred to the operator in exchange for the scalpel. The periosteal elevator is used to reflect the mucoperiosteal flap from the alveolar bone (Fig. 21-27, *B*).
5. A No. 13 or No. 14 curette is delivered to the operator in exchange for the periosteal elevator. The curette is used to remove the incised tissue from around the teeth (Fig. 21-27, *C*). The roots can be planed as needed.

The assistant continues to evacuate as necessary with the right hand. A 2 × 2 inch gauze sponge is held in the left hand to wipe the tip of the curette as debris is removed from the surgical site.
6. The surgical site is flushed with sterile saline solution from an irrigating syringe as the assistant evacuates the fluid. The surgical site is inspected.
7. Bone contouring can be accomplished at this point if required. The surgical site is rinsed again.
8. The suture needle is transferred in the needle holder in proper orientation for insertion from the lingual toward the buccal gingiva through the interproximal space. As the needle is passed through the interproximal space, the assistant can support the buccal flap with the back

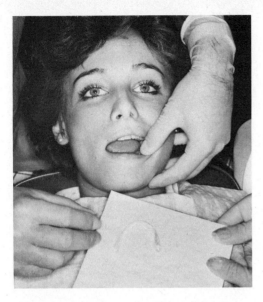

Fig. 21-29. Delivery of periodontal dressing.

of the large end of the periosteal elevator (Fig. 21-27, *D*). This holds the buccal flap in position so that the needle can penetrate the tissue without moving it out of position.

9. While the operator is securing the knot in the suture, the assistant retrieves the surgical scissors. The operator holds the strands of the suture material taut with the needle holder as the assistant cuts the material at approximately ⅛ inch above the knot. Suturing continues until the wound is closed, with the tissue held firmly to the alveolar bone. The surgical site is rinsed.
10. A 2 × 2 inch gauze compress moistened with saline solution is placed over the surgical site for the patient to bite on while the periodontal dressing is prepared by the assistant.
11. Saline solution is placed on the fingertips of the operator's gloves to prevent them from adhering to the periodontal dressing. A 3% tetracycline (Achromycin) ointment is placed over the sutures to help prevent infection and to prevent the sutures from being trapped in the periodontal dressing.
12. The periodontal dressing is rolled into a rope and delivered to the operator on the mixing pad (Fig. 21-29). The gauze compress is removed, and the dressing is placed.
13. The assistant can retract the cheek with a mouth mirror, using the right hand. The left hand delivers a filling instrument (FP No. 1) to the operator. The filling instrument is used to shape and trim the periodontal dressing. The assistant's left hand can be used to wipe

the tip of the filling instrument with a 2 × 2 inch gauze sponge as portions of the dressing are trimmed away.
14. After the periodontal dressing is in place, a complete mouth rinse is completed in the usual manner with the air-water syringe and a universal evacuator tip. The patient's face is cleaned, and postoperative instructions are given before dismissal.

Note that whenever a surgical tip is used to evacuate blood, it is good to periodically aspirate sterile water or saline solution from a container into the tip during a procedure to prevent clogging of the lumen of the tip with clotted blood.

•　•　•

The advantages of the Widman flap procedure compared with the gingivectomy procedure include the following:
1. Optimal coverage of root surfaces with soft tissue after healing, which facilitates oral hygiene and improves esthetics.
2. Less exposure of root surfaces, which may help to minimize root sensitivity and root caries.

Occlusal equilibration

The health of the periodontium depends not only on the constant elimination of local irritants and favorable nutrition but also on favorable forces being applied to the teeth. A healthy periodontium requires the stimulation of some occlusal force, yet excessive force can be severely damaging. A delicate balance exists between adequate forces needed for periodontal stimulation and excessive forces that cause injury. Each individual will vary in resistance to excessive occlusal forces.

The periodontium is designed to tolerate forces applied to a tooth in the direction of its long axis. Any force that tends to tip teeth out of position is potentially traumatic to the periodontal tissues. Teeth that are rotated, tipped, or drifted out of position are the most vulnerable. Opposing teeth that do not "mesh" properly are also subject to damaging forces (Fig. 21-30, *A* and *B*). Any occlusal arrangement that results in trauma to the periodontium is called traumatic occlusion.

It is generally agreed that traumatic occlusion does not cause periodontal pocket formation. Traumatic occlusal forces act to accelerate pocket formation in the presence of inflammation caused by local irritants. Traumatic occlusion alone can cause hypersensitivity and hypermobility, even in the absence of periodontal pocket formation.

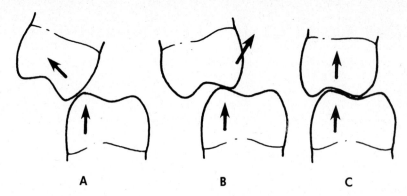

Fig. 21-30. A and **B,** Traumatic occlusion. **C,** Favorable biting relationship between opposing teeth.

It should be noted that some oral habits have traumatic effects on the periodontium of the teeth. Such chronic habits as pipe smoking, tongue thrust, pencil biting, clenching, and bruxism all create excessive forces on teeth that can traumatize the periodontium. These habits must be controlled to eliminate their resultant traumatic effect.

Discrepancies in a patient's occlusion are injurious not only to periodontal tissues but also to the temporomandibular joint and the muscles of mastication. Occlusal interferences and oral habits can cause a deflection of the mandible out of its normal position when the upper and lower teeth are brought together. This chronic shifting of the mandible during oral functions is traumatic to the joint, and muscle spasms are frequently associated with undesirable occlusion.

Favorable occlusion is an important key to periodontal health as well as the health of the entire chewing mechanism. Therefore the establishment and preservation of a favorable occlusion is an important goal in periodontal, orthodontic, restorative, and prosthetic procedures.

A periodontal treatment plan will include efforts to eliminate inflammation and periodontal pockets as well as efforts to eliminate traumatic occlusion. These efforts may include orthodontic treatment, extensive restorative dentistry, extraction of teeth, and selective grinding procedures. All these corrective procedures are directed toward the elimination of occlusal forces that tend to tip teeth and toward the distribution of occlusal forces as evenly as possible over several teeth. Any occlusal interferences that tend to force teeth out of contact with each other or deflect the mandible out of position when the jaws are closed

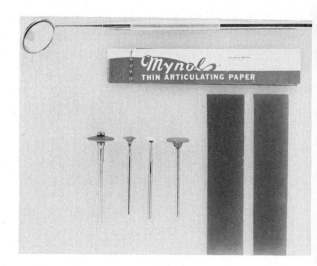

Fig. 21-31. Occlusal equilibration armamentarium.

must be eliminated. The biting surfaces of the teeth must mesh in such a manner as to allow movement of the mandible in all directions without locking on a few teeth, which would result in damaging forces on those teeth. The elimination of all occlusal interferences and establishing favorable occlusal forces on the teeth is called occlusal equilibration. The armamentarium for this procedure is shown in Fig. 21-31.

Procedure. Occlusal equilibration is most often accomplished by determining the location of occlusal interferences with articulating paper and occlusal wax and then removing them by selectively grinding the teeth. The grinding can be done with either the high-speed or conventional handpiece. Diamond stones are used in the high-speed handpiece, and various shapes of gem stones are used in the conventional handpiece. Once the grinding is complete, the ground surfaces are polished with abrasive rubber wheels. If occlusal interferences cannot be removed by selective grinding, alteration of the biting relationship must be accomplished by restorative procedures or orthodontic movement of the teeth. In some cases, it is necessary to extract some undesirably positioned teeth to eliminate interferences.

ORAL HYGIENE

The success of all periodontal treatment depends on the patient's ability to maintain a high level of oral hygiene. Rigorous home care efforts coupled with routine recall visits to the dentist are absolutely mandatory.

The oral hygiene procedures and devices discussed in Chapter 2 play an important role in home care for the patient. Patients who do not meet this responsibility are vulnerable to recurrence of periodontal disease. Patient education via plaque-control programs assists periodontal patients in achieving oral hygiene skills and sustaining the necessary motivation to preserve their teeth.

BIBLIOGRAPHY

Glickman, I.: Clinical periodontology, ed. 3, Philadelphia, 1968, W.B. Saunders Co.
Goldman, H.N., and Cohen, D.W.: Periodontal therapy, ed. 6, St. Louis, 1980, The C.V. Mosby Co.
Stone, S., and Kalis, P.: Dental auxiliary practice. Module 6. Periodontics, Baltimore, 1975, The Williams & Wilkins Co.
Ramfjord, S., and Nissle, R.: The modified Widman flap, J. Periodontal. **48:**601-607.
Ward, H.L., and Simring, M.: Manual of clinical periodontics, ed. 2, St. Louis, 1978, The C.V. Mosby Co.

CHAPTER 22

ENDODONTICS

One of the great strides forward in modern dentistry has been in the treatment of diseases of the dental pulp and the periapical tissues. The specialty that is concerned primarily with these diseases is called endodontics.

Before major advances in endodontics, many teeth were needlessly extracted. The demand by the public to preserve their teeth has been met in part by the dentist's ability to successfully treat injured or infected pulpal and periapical tissue. To lead the assistant to appreciate the need for endodontic therapy, the following topics will be presented in this chapter:

1. Causes of pulp injury or pulp death
2. Common diseases of the pulp and periapical tissues
3. Diagnostic methods used in endodontics
4. Treatment of pulpal and periapical disease

CAUSES OF PULP INJURY OR PULP DEATH

The dental pulp can be injured in several ways. Some injured pulp can be treated and returned to normal. On the other hand, some injured pulpal tissue dies after the injury. Whether a pulp survives an injury or not depends on many factors; among them are the following:

1. *Age of the patient at the time of injury*. Younger patients, generally speaking, have a greater ability to recover from any injury than older patients. The blood supply to the teeth is greater in a young patient.

2. *Extent of the injury*. A tooth that receives a mild blow will have a greater chance to survive than a tooth that has its crown completely fractured by a severe blow to the mouth.

3. *Period that the tooth is left untreated after exposure to the injurious agent*. Caries that invade the pulp and remain for a long time before being treated will cause the tooth to have less chance of surviving than a tooth that is treated immediately.

4. *Method of treatment*. There are many methods of treating an injured pulp. Some methods are more successful in certain patients than in others. Also, the skill of the dentist and the cooperativeness of the patient must be considered in any treatment method.

Many circumstances will contribute to the survival or death of a dental pulp that has been injured, but most of them will fit into the list of factors just mentioned.

The dental pulp is living tissue. Any living tissue

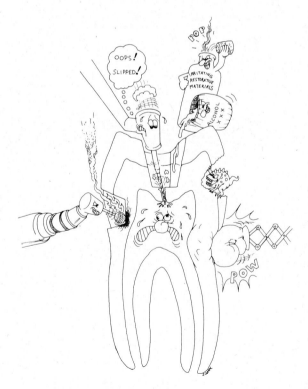

Fig. 22-1. Common causes of injury to pulp.

can die or, in other words, undergo necrosis after the slightest injury. Following are some of the most common causes of injury to the pulp (Fig. 22-1):

Traumatic blows to the teeth
Extensive dental caries
Mechanical pulp exposure
Chemical irritation
Thermal irritation
Galvanic shock

Traumatic blows to the teeth

All dental patients are subject to the hazards of everyday living that can result in unexpected injury to the facial area and specifically to the teeth. These hazards range from common household accidents, auto collisions, and athletic injuries to the most bizarre causes of facial injuries, such as those acquired in combat (both international in nature and with the kid next door).

This type of injury varies in extent from fracture of an entire jaw to a small fracture of one tooth. Any injury that disrupts the blood supply to the tooth or exposes the pulp to the environment outside the confines of the tooth can result in pulp death.

A sharp blow to one or more teeth can result in the fracture of either the crown or the root of those teeth, causing exposure or possible tearing of the pulp.

Even if the crown is only slightly fractured, or not fractured at all, as a result of a blow to the tooth, the pulp can still undergo necrosis. The reason is that the tooth is loosened in the surrounding alveolus enough to tear the blood vessels that enter the tooth through the apical foramen. These are the vessels that carry

the nourishing blood to keep the pulp alive. If this pipeline is permanently damaged, the pulp cannot receive the blood supply it needs to survive (Fig. 22-2).

Mild trauma to the pulp can result from a dental restoration being in hyperocclusion, in other words, a "high filling." This can result from inadequate carving of restorative materials during operative procedures. Such a pulpal trauma is easily corrected by recontouring the problem restoration.

Extensive dental caries

Untreated dental caries usually continues to increase in size in a tooth until treatment is accomplished or until the tooth is totally destroyed. When the size of the caries increases to the point at which it invades the pulp, this delicate tissue is severely threatened.

Dental caries is a combination of a variety of bacteria, the toxins and acids they produce, and caustic breakdown products of the destroyed dentin. The invading caries exposes the delicate pulpal tissue to these harmful substances, which destroy the cells of the pulp. If the process is not intercepted by treatment in time, the pulp will die.

Whether a pulp survives carious invasion, or a pulp exposure, depends largely on the size of the exposure and the age of the patient. The larger the exposure, the less chance the pulp has to recover. A massive exposure of the pulp to the caustic caries would simply overwhelm the defense mechanism of the pulp. Younger patients will have a greater chance to recover from pulp exposure because of the greater blood supply to young teeth. A more abundant blood supply to the pulp increases the defensive and reparative functions of the pulp.

The reason young teeth have a greater blood supply has to do with the large apical foramen present in such teeth. This large opening in the end of the root permits an abundant flow of blood to the pulp. The foramen gets progressively smaller with age, and thus the blood supply to the pulp also decreases with age. A small pulp exposure in a teenage patient would be expected to heal readily, whereas the same exposure in a 40-year-old patient would probably result in pulp death.

Carious exposure of the dental pulp occurs when the invasion of caries into the dentin progresses at a rapid rate. A rapidly advancing carious lesion surpasses the defensive response of the pulp to produce peritubular dentin and reparative dentin. A slowly advancing carious lesion has less chance of exposing the

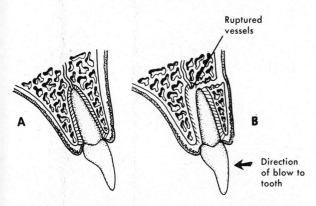

Fig. 22-2. A, Normal tooth and its apical blood vessels. **B,** Rupture of apical blood vessels as result of trauma to tooth.

pulp, since the pulp has time to produce these defensive barriers against the progressive decay.

Mechanical pulp exposure

In addition to dental caries, the pulp can be exposed by other means. These exposures are usually a result of dental procedures that inadvertently invade the pulp. Poor cavity preparation methods and improper pin placement procedures are two common causes of mechanical exposure (Fig. 22-1). As unfortunate as this situation is for the patient, it does occur and must be recognized. The same principles of size of the exposure and age of the patient apply to pulp recovery after mechanical exposures. However, mechanical exposures tend to heal more favorably than carious exposures because there are no toxic substances associated with them.

Chemical irritation

The health status of the pulp can be greatly influenced by certain chemical substances that come in contact with the dentin. Past clinical experience has clearly shown that patients can experience pulp injury or pulp death after the placement of certain chemical substances commonly used in restorative procedures. This is caused by permeability of the dentin layer, created by the presence of the dentinal tubules (Fig. 22-3, *A* and *B*). Any injurious substance that is applied to the dentin can harm or destroy the dentinoblastic processes in the tubules. In addition, it can penetrate the tubules and enter the pulp. This is particularly true when such a substance is placed on dentin deep in the tooth near the pulp.

There are several materials used in dentistry to restore teeth that can harm them if not handled properly. A classic example is the anterior restorative material, silicate. Silicate has many favorable characteristics that make it desirable as a restorative material. However, one of the principal disadvantages of this material is that it is acidic at the time of placement in the tooth. The acid from the material can penetrate the dentin and injure or even destroy the pulp. To use a material of this type in a tooth and, at the same time, prevent insult to the pulp, the tooth must be properly prepared for the potentially injurious material. Proper preparation places acceptable dental varnishes and base materials between the pulp and the silicate to prevent penetration into the pulp (Fig. 22-3, *C*).

Other chemical substances commonly used in the restoration of teeth that can damage the pulp if not properly handled include restorative acrylics and

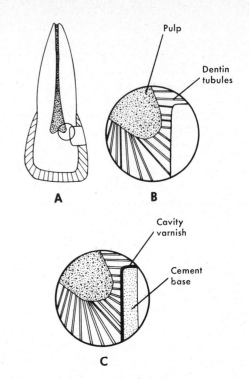

Fig. 22-3. A, Enlargement of Class III cavity preparation to show its relationship to dental pulp. **B,** Dentin tubules that form tiny passageways between cavity preparation and pulp. **C,** Open tubules sealed by cavity varnish and cement base.

acidic dental cements. The key to successful use of any irritating substances in restoring a tooth is proper mixing of these materials and proper usage of bases and cavity liners between the irritating material and the dentin nearest the pulp.

Another clinical situation that can result in chemical irritation of the pulp is a faulty restoration that allows leakage of oral fluids, juices, and beverages between the restoration and the dentin. This variety of fluids can irritate the pulp. Proper replacement of such a faulty restoration easily solves this problem.

Thermal irritation

The dental pulp, like many other tissues of the body, functions best at normal body temperature. If the temperature of the pulp varies significantly from body temperature, the patient will experience discomfort, and pulpal injury can occur. A common example of this occurs in cold climates where "stuffy noses" force individuals to breathe through their mouth. The cold air that is inhaled can cool the teeth substantially. This change in temperature is mildly irritating to the pulp. A pulpal hyperemia can result, and the patient will experience discomfort until its subsides. Hyperemia will be discussed later in this chapter.

Another frequent cause of thermal irritation to the pulp results from the placement of metallic restorative materials too close to the pulp. Metals such as dental amalgam and gold are excellent thermal conductors. In other words, metals transfer temperature change readily. A metal spoon in a hot cup of coffee transfers the heat from the coffee to the fingers through the handle of the spoon. The same phenomenon occurs when metal restorations are cooled. A patient with a metal restoration deep in the tooth can experience pulpal irritation because extreme temperature changes in the mouth are readily transferred through the metal to the pulp. A healthy drink of a cold beverage or a tasty bite of ice cream can be a painful experience for the patient.

Since the depth of cavity preparations is often determined by the size of the carious lesion being treated, dentists cannot control cavity preparation depth in every instance. However, the depth at which the restorative metal is placed can be controlled. This is accomplished by the use of cement base materials. These cement bases are nonmetals. Nonmetals do not transfer heat from one point to another very well. They function in the same manner as a hot pad used by cooks to handle hot cooking utensils. In other words, cement bases act as an insulating material between a metal restoration and the dentin nearest the pulp. Once again, proper use of bases between the restoration and the dentin covering the pulp protects this delicate tissue.

A third common source of thermal irritation to the pulp can occur during the preparation of a tooth with high-speed rotary instruments. Dental burs in a modern high-speed handpiece spin at range of 400,000 to 450,000 revolutions per minute. This creates an effective cutting instrument to quickly remove enamel and dentin. However, in the process of quickly cutting hard tooth structure, a great deal of frictional heat is generated between the bur and the tooth. If this heat is not minimized, significant heat is transferred to the pulp, and damage can result. This heat is controlled by the use of water-spray devices attached to the head of the handpiece. These water-spray devices direct water toward the cutting end of the bur to keep it cool during the cutting process. One of the chief duties of a dental assistant is to continually remove this water coolant from the patient's mouth as it sprays into the tooth being prepared. Although water-coolant sprays can be a nuisance at times because they tend to impair visiblity, they are essential to protect the pulp from becoming overheated during cavity preparation. Effective utilization of the dental assistant to control the water coolant has greatly reduced the inconvenience of this necessary technique.

Galvanic shock

Although galvanic shock is an unusual cause of pulpal damage, it is worthy of a brief explanation since it can be a temporary source of pulpal pain. Galvanism is the flow of electrical current between two different metals through an electrolyte. An electrolyte is a solution containing atomic substances that allow current to flow through the solution.

If a patient has two different metals present in his mouth and these metals contact each other, an electrical "battery" is created, and current will flow through the electrolyte (saliva) to complete the electrical circuit. The current that flows can be of sufficient magnitude to "shock" the pulp. The two metals can be entirely different, such as gold and silver amalgam, or simply different compositions of the same metal alloys. (Different manufacturers use different compositions in their silver and gold alloys.)

It is fairly common to have a patient complain of a "shock" when the teeth are closed after a new amalgam restoration has been placed in a tooth. This is especially true if the tooth contacts a different metal, such as gold, when the teeth are brought in contact during jaw closure. Another common example of this phenomenon is the accidental contact of an eating utensil with a metal dental restoration. The patient will respond by saying, "I got a shock when my fork touched my filling!" Many foods are wrapped in aluminum foil. Frequently patients may carelessly bite into a morsel of food that was not completely unwrapped and bring the foil in contact with a metal restoration. Galvanic shock results again, due to two different metals contacting in the presence of saliva (the electrolyte).

The pain the patient feels in the tooth is due to the fact that electrical current is an excellent stimulant to pulpal nerve fibers. Electrical stimulation of pulpal nerve fibers is actually used to test the vitality of a pulp. This matter will be discussed in conjunction with diagnostic methods used in endodontics.

COMMON DISEASES OF THE PULP
AND PERIAPICAL AREA
Hyperemia

Hyperemia means that an excessive amount of blood has collected in the blood vessels of any body part. The pulp is no exception. The first response of the pulp to injury is the dilation of the arterioles in the pulp. As these vessels dilate, they become engorged with blood.

Since the soft pulp is enclosed in a hard chamber of dentin, the enlargement of the vessels creates mild pressure within the pulp. This increase in pressure squeezes the nerve fibers of the pulp. The pressure only makes the nerve fibers more sensitive to added stimuli that may be added to the tooth. The tooth will not be painful unless it is further stimulated by either heat or cold. Cold temperatures elicit a painful response more often than heat. The pain will begin when the stimulus is applied and cease when it is removed.

The magnitude of hyperemia depends on the degree of injury to the tooth. Since hyperemia is not actually a disease itself, but rather the first stage of the inflammatory defensive process, it can be reversed if the injury is not too severe. Common causes of injury to the pulp have already been discussed.

Pulpitis

Pulpitis is the inflammation of pulpal tissue. Any of the causes of injury mentioned previously can result in pulpitis. Many dentists differentiate between degrees of pulpitis, using descriptive terms such as acute, subacute, chronic, and suppurative. This differentiation between the various degrees of pulpitis is helpful to the dentist in determining the status of the pulp and the appropriate treatment.

The degree of pulpitis present in a tooth is totally dependent on the type of injurious agent, its intensity, and the time of exposure to the pulp. Except for the most mild degree of pulpitis resulting from minimal insult to the pulp, pulpitis usually has to be treated by removing the entire pulp or at least a portion of it. Mild pulpitis will often recover by simply removing the insulting agent.

Necrosis

Necrosis is the death of previously living tissue. Pulpal necrosis is the result of severe pulpitis. It is this fact that is the rationale behind treatment of severe pulpitis by removing a portion or all of the pulp

in an injured tooth. Pulpal necrosis also occurs when the blood supply is halted because of traumatic injury to the tooth.

A tooth with a necrotic pulp cannot remain untreated. Dead tissue undergoes a series of chemical changes that result in a highly irritating end product. The process is called decomposition, or putrefaction. The decomposed end product consists of various toxins and other irritating substances created by the breakdown of the dead fleshy pulp. This foul-smelling mixture of irritating substances seeps out of the apical foramen and irritates the periapical tissues.

A patient with a necrotic pulp experiences pain from a "dead tooth" because of the painful irritation of the periapical tissue by the caustic decomposition products of the dead pulp. However, a patient can experience pulp death and subsequent periapical tissue destruction with little or no pain. On the other hand, this same process can be accompanied by excruciating pain. The variation seems to be related primarily to the rate at which these changes take place. A slower necrotic process tends to be less painful than a rapid one. Patients have been known to experience pulpal necrosis and extensive periapical destruction over several years without a trace of discomfort.

The term *gangrenous pulp* is a specific term that has been used to describe pulp death caused by the invasion of bacteria. This invasion is usually via extensive dental caries.

Apical periodontitis

Apical periodontitis is an inflammation of the periodontal tissues near the apex of a tooth with a nonvital (dead) pulp. The inflammatory response of the periodontal tissue is caused by contaminants from the pulp canal. These contaminants can be the caustic breakdown product of the necrotic pulp, bacteria that have entered the tooth via dental caries, or excessive endodontic medications used to treat the nonvital tooth. The inflammatory response begins with dilation of the blood vessels of the periodontal ligament in the apical region, and edema results. This creates pressure between the alveolar bone and the tooth. Two things result from this pressure. First, the tooth can be pushed slightly away from the apical part of the alveolus. The tooth will be "high" to the patient's bite, and pain will result when biting forces are placed on it. Second, the nerve receptors located in the periodontal ligament are squeezed as a result of the increase in pressure, so that even the slightest additional

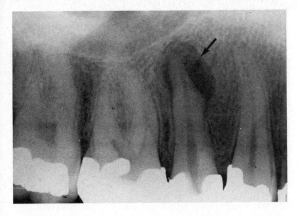

Fig. 22-4. Periapical bone loss resulting from formation of a granuloma *(arrow).*

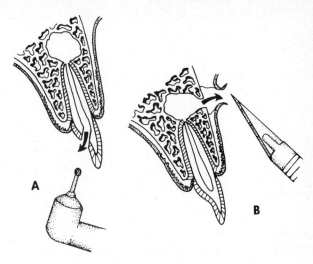

Fig. 22-5. Establishment of drainage for periapical abscess. **A,** Via crown of tooth. **B,** Via incision in mucosa.

force placed on the tooth will elicit a painful response. Thus tapping on a tooth is a common test for the presence of apical periodontitis.

The pain associated with apical periodontitis is usually less than the pain associated with pulpitis, since the pulp canal is far more confining to swollen tissue than the space between the tooth and alveolar bone. The degree of pain experienced in apical periodontitis may range from none at all to moderate. This is related in part to the amount of inflammation present.

Loss of bone around the apex of the tooth can occur if the inflammation is not eliminated. The pressure created by inflammation stimulates cells that are present in the surface of the alveolar bone to resorb (destroy) the surrounding bone. These bone-resorbing cells are called osteoclasts. As long as the pressure from the inflammation persists, bone resorption will continue (Fig. 22-4). It is possible for significant bone loss to occur with little or no pain.

Periapical abscess

If the apical periodontitis is extensive and left untreated, it may progress to a more profound stage of inflammation. Severe inflammation results in stagnation of blood in the dilated vessels, edema, and a massive invasion of white blood cells into the area. The reduced blood flow decreases the oxygen supply to tissues, which causes death of tissue cells. White blood cells die in the process of engulfing pulpal canal contaminants, dead cells, and bacteria. The tissue

fluid, dead tissue cells, and dead white blood cells creates a mixture called pus. The accumulation of pus continues to cause increased pressure in the tissue. This condition is called a periapical abscess.

The increasing pressure causes severe pain. The pus can be forced through the open marrow spaces in the bone and result in widespread swelling and pain. Bone resorption can accompany this increase in pressure so that the thin facial aspect of alveolar bone can be resorbed and the pus can "balloon out" through the thin alveolar mucosa. If the thin mucosa ruptures, the pus can escape into the oral cavity, and the pressure is immediately relieved.

One of the emergency treatment measures that is commonly used to treat a periapical abscess is to establish drainage of pus from the periapical area. This can be accomplished by making an opening into the pulp chamber through the crown with a dental bur (Fig. 22-5, *A*). Such an opening allows the pus to escape from the periapical area through the pulp canal to the oral cavity. Another method is to make an incision through the alveolar mucosa over the apex of the involved tooth (Fig. 22-5, *B*). This allows direct drainage from the periapical region to the oral cavity. Some cases may require the use of both drainage methods.

The process of periapical abscess can occur so quickly that it often surpasses the bone resorption process. Thus it is possible to have an extensive periapical abscess without any radiographic evidence of periapical bone loss.

Periapical granuloma

A granuloma is a collection of active white blood cells (defensive cells) and histiocytes (reparative cells). It occurs in the periapical region in response to chronic seepage of decomposition products of the dead pulp tissue through the apical foramen. The granuloma usually occupies the space where bone has been resorbed in the periapical area (Fig. 22-4). Researchers who have studied this process have described the granuloma as an army of defensive and reparative cells lying in wait at the periapex to destroy an invader from the pulp canal. This invader can be bacteria or decomposition products of the dead pulp. If the invaders become too abundant and overwhelm the defensive army, or granuloma, a periapical abscess can occur.

If all bacteria and decomposition products can be eliminated from the pulp canal and the apical foramen can be sealed, the granuloma can perform its second function—repair of damaged tissue. The essence of endodontic treatment is to accomplish that very task.

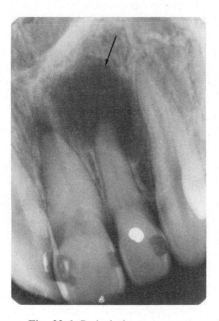

Fig. 22-6. Periapical cyst *(arrow)*.

Periapical cyst

A cyst is a fluid-filled cavity lined by epithelial cells. Some granulomas undergo a change from their original form to that of a cyst. It is believed that these cysts arise as a result of growth of residual parts of Hertwig's root sheath that have remained dormant after root formation has ended. The sudden active growth of these previously dormant cells results from irritation from pulpal contaminants. These epithelial cells are located in the granuloma and multiply in great numbers. They depend on their blood supply from the surrounding healthy tissue. After the granuloma reaches a size in which the cells in the center of the growing mass are too far from the surrounding blood supply, the central cells die and decompose to form a part of the fluid center of the cyst. Other fluid from the granuloma migrates to the center of the cyst to complete the cyst cavity. The bordering epithelial cells form the cyst lining (Fig. 22-6).

Periapical cysts can expand to considerable size. The pressure from their expansion can stimulate significant bone resorption and even cause teeth to move out of their normal position.

DIAGNOSTIC METHODS USED IN ENDODONTICS

Several mechanisms have been devised to assist the dentist in the diagnostic evaluation of the pulp and periapical tissues. Following are some of the most common diagnostic tools:

Patient history	Percussion
Radiographs	Selective anesthesia
Thermal tests	Test cavity preparation
Electrical pulp test	Transillumination
Clinical examination	

Patient history

A thorough medical and dental history is mandatory before any type of treatment is begun for a patient. The medical history reveals the patient's general health status so that precautions can be taken if necessary to prevent serious complications during dental treatment. Besides patient protection, the dental operating team must be considered in terms of possible spread of disease from the patient to the team members. It should be noted that there are virtually no medical reasons that would contraindicate endodontic treatment for a patient.

The medical history is a helpful guide for the dentist in the treatment regimen. The choice of pain-relieving drugs, antibiotics, and root canal medications is often dictated by the patient's history of allergies, cardiovascular condition, and numerous other conditions, including pregnancy.

The patient's dental history is a valuable aid to the dentist in that the patient can communicate a step-by-step account of signs and symptoms to the dentist. It is in this phase of history taking that patients often reveal valuable information regarding previous injuries to the teeth, even though they may have occurred many years previously. Following is an example of how important information can be obtained by conversation with a patient:

Doctor: "How long has this tooth bothered you?"

Patient: "I have never experienced pain in this tooth until 4 days ago. It started as a mild toothache, and it has grown worse. The tooth throbs periodically through the day. Aspirin doesn't even faze the pain!"

Doctor: "Are you bothered by any extreme changes in temperature on the tooth?"

Patient: "I took a drink of hot coffee yesterday and just about went through the ceiling!"

Doctor: "Does coldness seem to cause an increase in pain?"

Patient: "No, I haven't noticed that cold bothers it at all. The tooth hurts for several minutes after I drink something hot, but not cold."

Doctor: "There is no evidence of decay or a previous deep filling in the tooth. Have you ever been injured in or near the mouth?"

Patient: "Gee, not since my automobile accident eight years ago."

Doctor: "Were any teeth loosened at that time?"

Patient: "Yes, but they tightened back up after a few days, and I never had any problems since except this painful tooth got a little darker color afterward."

This mock dialogue is very typical of how a wealth of diagnostic information can be obtained by simply asking the patient a few pertinent questions during history taking. There is a well-known quote among physicians and dentists with regard to history taking: "Listen to your patient, and he will tell you what is wrong with him!" It cannot be overemphasized how true this is in so many ways!

Radiographs

Radiographs, or x-ray films, of the teeth and bone are perhaps the most valuable diagnostic tool the dentist has to evaluate the structures that cannot be seen by clinical observation, that is, the pulp and periapical tissues.

The presence of bone loss in the periapical area in response to a necrotic pulp can be detected on a radiograph. Bone loss, or resorption, appears as a dark area surrounding the apex of the root (Fig. 22-4). The presence of this dark area, or radiolucency, on a dental radiograph is one of the most important features used to diagnose pulp and periapical disease. Periapical cysts, granulomas, and abscesses all ap-

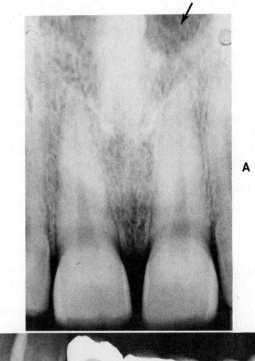

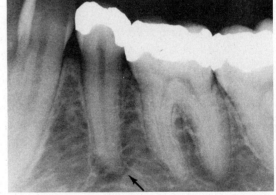

Fig. 22-7. Normal anatomical radiolucencies superimposed on apices of roots *(arrow).* **A,** Nostril spots. **B,** Mental foramen.

pear as radiolucencies on a radiograph. The differentiation between diseases as to which is actually represented by the bone resorption requires additional information that must be acquired by other diagnostic methods.

The dentist is often confronted with radiolucencies caused by normal structures being located near the apex of teeth. Two common instances are the maxillary anterior and the mandibular premolar areas. Often, when a radiograph is taken of the maxillary anterior area, the image of the nasal passages is superimposed over the apices of the roots of the central incisors. Such "nostril spots" can easily be confused with periapical disease (Fig. 22-7, *A*). Careful radiographic technique can eliminate this confusion. The second area involves the mental foramen, which is located near the roots of the mandibular premolars. If the image of the mental foramen is superimposed over the root apex of one of these teeth, it can be misinterpreted as periapical disease (Fig. 22-7, *B*). These two examples emphasize the need for other information besides radiolucencies on a radiograph to make a sound diagnosis of periapical disease.

Radiographs are helpful in other ways besides detecting radiolucencies. They can demonstrate possible causes of pulpal injury before bone resorption occurs. Root fracture, deep caries, and previous pulp exposures are a few examples of possible causes of pulpal injury that can be detected on radiographs.

Root length, abnormal root curvature, and abnormal calcification can be demonstrated in an accurate radiograph. This information is helpful in determining whether the tooth can be treated endodontically. If it is determined that it can be treated, such information as extreme root curvature is helpful to the dentist in planning treatment.

One outstanding feature of the dental radiograph is its permanent nature. A properly exposed and processed radiograph can last forever. Thus it becomes a permanent record of the condition of the patient that can be used for future reference. Comparison of initial radiographs with postoperative films is a valuable index to determine the success or failure of treatment. It should be noted that radiographs are valuable pieces of information that should be preserved for medico-legal reasons.

Thermal tests

Subjecting a tooth to extremes in temperature is an accurate method of identifying an offending tooth as well as determining the status of its pulp.

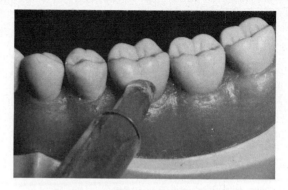

Fig. 22-8. Cold test using "ice pencil."

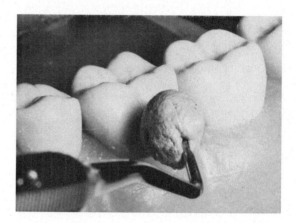

Fig. 22-9. Hot test using hot gutta-percha.

Cold tests can be done rather easily by making an "ice pencil." Used anesthetic cartridges or disposable needle covers are filled with water and frozen. These narrow sticks of ice are handy ways of applying cold to a tooth without using a bulky ice cube (Fig. 22-8). The suspected tooth is isolated and dried; the ice pencil is then applied to the tooth at the cervical area. A hyperemic pulp will respond readily to the decrease in temperature. If a freezer is not available, a cotton pellet can be sprayed with ethyl chloride until it frosts. The pellet is then applied to the cervical area of the suspect tooth.

Heat tests begin with isolating the suspect tooth and applying a thin film of lubricant at the cervical area. Out of the patient's line of sight, a piece of gutta-percha (⅛-inch diameter ball) is heated in a Bunsen burner while being held by a hand ball burnisher. The heating is continued until just before the gutta-percha begins to smoke, and then the material is applied to the cervical area. The lubricant keeps it from sticking to the tooth (Fig. 22-9).

Typical reactions to the heat stimulus and what they indicate are as follows:

Condition	Response
Hyperemia	Less painful than a cold test; pain disappears when heat is removed
Pulpitis	Painful response that lingers a few moments after the heat is removed
Abscess	Violent pain reaction to heat; relieved by application of cold
Necrotic pulp	No response to heat or cold

Teeth with extensive metal restorations on them often do not respond because sufficient heat is not generated by the warm gutta-percha. It has been suggested that a rubber polishing wheel or cup be spun on the surface of the metal restoration to create frictional heat to stimulate the tooth.

Electrical pulp test

Electrical current can be used to stimulate nerve fibers in the pulp via the dentin layer. If the current is applied at the cervical area of a tooth where the enamel is thin, the sensitive dentin layer is more accessible and stimulation is more effective. An instrument has been developed to accomplish this task, called simply an electrical pulp tester; the Vitalometer is an example. It is available as a battery-powered device or in a wall-plug style. The instrument has a rheostat switch that permits control of the intensity of stimulation delivered to the tooth. The current is delivered to the tooth through a probe that is attached to the rheostat switch.

The primary objective of the electrical pulp test is to determine whether a pulp is alive (vital) or necrotic (nonvital). A necrotic pulp will not respond to even the most intense stimulation by the instrument. A dying pulp can produce a variety of responses depending on the state of the pulp at the time of the test.

Many endodontists caution against the use of the electrical pulp tests to accurately determine the degree of vitality of a pulp. However, some general guidelines as to the status of the pulp can be obtained by comparing the response of a suspect tooth with that of a normal tooth of the same type on the opposite side of the mouth. For example, if the maxillary right canine is the suspect tooth, its test results should be compared with the test results of the maxillary left canine. The left canine becomes the control because it

is normal. If the suspect tooth requires less current to stimulate it than the control, probably the suspect tooth is hypersensitive as a result of pulpitis or hyperemia. Comparative tests should be repeated two or three times to validate the results. Since the amount of current delivered to a tooth is indicated by a scale from 1 to 10 on most instruments, it is a simple matter to compare test results.

To obtain the most accurate reading from electrical pulp tests, a specific procedure must be followed. First, the tooth to be tested must be isolated with cotton rolls and dried thoroughly. To ensure good electrical contact with the tooth, a material capable of conducting electricity should be placed on the end of the probe. Toothpaste works very well for this purpose. The probe is then applied to the cervical area of the tooth, the rheostat switch is turned to the number 1 setting, and the tooth is tested at that setting. The procedure is repeated, gradually increasing the current flow to the tooth by moving the rheostat from 1 toward 10 on the scale. When the patient senses heat or a tingling sensation in the tooth, stimulation of the nerves of the pulp has occurred. The number setting on the scale is then recorded as the test result. Newer electronic models as shown in Fig. 22-10 provide a numerical reading on a digital display. The intensity of the electrical stimulus is increased automatically at a rate that is selected by the operator.

Moisture on the tooth or directly touching the gingiva will result in stimulation of the nerves in the gingiva and produce a false reading.

Electrical pulp testing is a useful tool, but it has many shortcomings that reduce its value as an absolute "magical diagnostic wand." The current delivered by the instrument may differ because of variation in electrical current available in a given operatory. Batteries may wear out in battery-operated models. Teeth with extensive restorations vary widely in their response to pulp testing. Molars with several root canals baffle the dentist when one canal may contain necrotic pulp tissue. Control teeth may not be as "normal" as expected, and the test comparisons may be of little value.

The electrical pulp test is helpful in endodontic diagnosis, but it must be supported by other diagnostic findings.

Clinical examination

As in any diagnostic procedure, the value of the operator's hands and eyes cannot be underestimated.

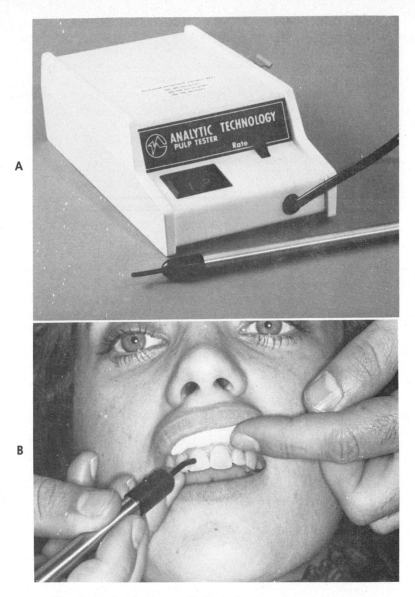

Fig. 22-10. A, Vitalometer. **B,** Probe in place on tooth being tested.

Clues to the nature of a patient's problems often lie in what the dentist can see and feel in the patient's mouth. Such clinical signs as discoloration of teeth, crown fracture, gross caries, swelling, abnormal soft tissue, and draining abscesses can be found in a clinical examination.

Clinical signs coupled with symptoms that the pa-tient describes during the dental history are of considerable value in arriving at an accurate diagnosis.

Percussion

Gentle tapping on the crown of a tooth with the end of a mirror handle is a simple test to determine the presence of acute periapical periodontitis. If a patient has an acute inflammation at the apex of the root, gentle tapping, or percussion, will squeeze the already inflamed area and pain will result. Several normal teeth should be checked for comparison.

Selective anesthesia

If a patient cannot accurately determine which teeth are the source of discomfort, the process of selective anesthesia can be of assistance. If other diagnostic tests have narrowed the choice down to two teeth, one of them can be anesthetized to see if the pain disappears. If the pain does not disappear until the second tooth is anesthetized, the second tooth is the probable offender. Selective anesthesia is best accomplished when the choice is between a maxillary and a mandibular tooth. The selective anesthesia process in the maxilla is reliable only when the two suspected teeth are at least two teeth apart. This method cannot be used to differentiate between two suspected mandibular teeth.

This process is often used in combination with hot and cold tests to increase the stimulus to the nonanesthetized tooth.

Test cavity preparation

If all other diagnostic tests fail to determine the vitality of a highly suspected tooth, the test cavity can be used as a last resort. The test consists of cutting a hole into the dentin layer of the tooth without anesthesia or water coolant, using the high-speed handpiece. The patient will readily respond if the tooth is vital. The test opening should be small and placed on a tooth surface that will minimize the disruption of the esthetic quality of the tooth.

Transillumination

Until the development of fiber optic lighting, transillumination has not been of any significant value in endodontic diagnosis. Fiber optics allow an intense concentrated light to pass through the tooth from the lingual to the facial aspect. This is done most effectively on anterior teeth.

Necrotic pulps cause the outline of the pulp chamber to appear darker than the surrounding tooth structure. Normal teeth do not demonstrate a difference between the tooth structure and the pulp chamber.

• • •

Endodontic diagnosis is a result of the utilization of several of the aids just discussed. Skillful use and interpretation of these diagnostic methods are essential for successful endodontic practice.

ENDODONTIC TREATMENT PROCEDURES

Although humans have been endowed with a living pulp in each tooth, it has been found that the pulp is not absolutely necessary to preserve the tooth once it is completely formed. Most dentists would agree that for a number of technical reasons, they prefer that teeth retain their vitality. Dentists also know that a tooth with its pulp removed and the remaining structure properly treated can last the lifetime of the patient. This fact is the basis for modern endodontic therapy.

The procedures to be discussed in this chapter all have a common principal goal. Regardless of what specific technique is used, the principal goal is to create an absolute seal in the root portion of the tooth. This is essential so that neither tissue fluids nor microorganisms can enter or leave the pulp canal of the nonvital tooth. The accomplishment of an adequate seal will prevent continued irritation of the periapical tissues and allow them to heal.

Pulpectomy

The most common endodontic procedure is the pulpectomy, which is the complete removal of the entire pulp. After the removal of the pulp, the empty canal is completely filled to create a seal that will eliminate further periapical irritation.

Armamentarium. In addition to rubber dam isolation materials that are required at each appointment, a standardized armamentarium can be established for the pulpectomy procedure. This standardized setup can be used during each phase of treatment. Additional items are added to the setup during the specific phase in which they are needed.

Instruments and materials that are a part of the standard pulpectomy armamentarium are shown in Fig. 22-11.

Phases of treatment. A typical scheme of accomplishing the pulpectomy procedure involves several phases of treatment, as follows:

1. Isolation
2. Endodontic preparation (openings)
3. Culturing
4. Canal cleaning
5. Canal medication
6. Canal filing
7. Root canal filling

The specific sequence of events is rather variable, since it is largely dependent on the condition of the individual patient. In other words, a patient with a periapical abscess may be treated in a slightly different sequence from one with a painless granuloma.

Isolation. Pulpectomy procedures involve not only removal of the pulp and sealing of the empty canal but also sterilization of the canal as part of the procedure. Canal sterilization further ensures against future infection by eliminating bacteria before the canal is sealed. To achieve sterilization of a root canal requires an absolutely dry field, free from bacteria-laden saliva. This dry field is accomplished best under rubber dam isolation. Application of the rubber dam, followed by painting it with a disinfectant such as nitromersol (Metaphen) or Mercresin, should be considered essential parts of the sterile technique. A new dam is applied at the beginning of each appointment.

Endodontic preparations. After the tooth has been isolated, an opening is made through the crown of the tooth to gain access to the pulp chamber and pulp canal. The openings are made through the occlusal surface on posterior teeth and through the lingual surface on anterior teeth (Fig. 22-12). The main objective of any endodontic preparation is to gain easy access to the pulp cavity, which permits smooth entry into the root canals during cleaning, filing, and filling procedures.

Culturing. This is a term used to designate the procedure of collecting a sample of the contents of the pulp cavity to test it for the presence of bacteria. A common method is to place a sterile paper point into the pulp cavity. The paper point will collect bacteria on its surface if they are present in the canal. The point is removed and immediately dropped into a test tube or vial of culture medium. The test tube containing the paper point is placed in an incubator at body temperature for 48 hours. This incubation process is called culturing; however, the common reference to culturing implies the whole process of sample collection and incubation.

After the 48-hour incubation period the test tube is checked for growth of bacteria. If the culture medium is clear with no growth around the point, the canal is probably free of bacteria. If the culture medium is cloudy or if a fuzzy growth appears around the point, it indicates that the canal contains bacteria that must be destroyed (Fig. 22-13).

The operating team must take extreme care in the culturing procedure so that the paper point remains untouched by contaminated surfaces such as fingers or counter tops. Bacteria would be picked up by the

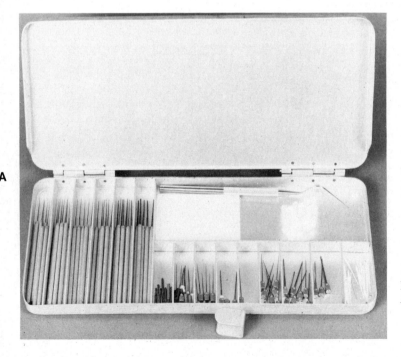

A

Complete size range of endodontic files
  (long and short handled)
Absorbent paper points, assorted sizes
Cotton pellets
Small glass mixing slab
Gutta-percha condenser
Burs: R.A. No. 4, No. 6, No. 8, and
  flame-shaped cross-cut
Barbed broach
Cement spatula

Fig. 22-11. Pulpectomy armamentarium. **A,** Sterile endodontic kit.

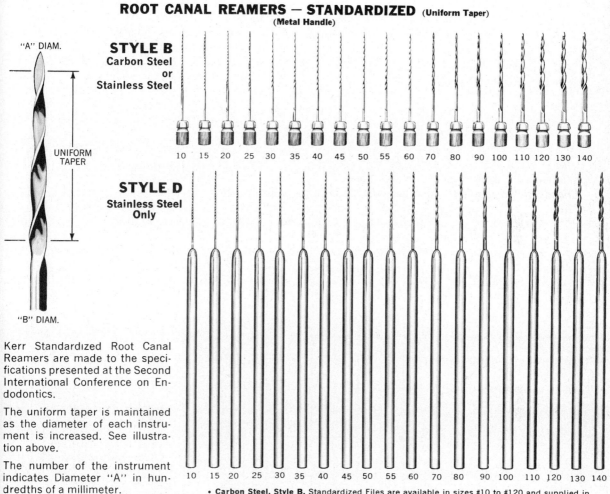

ROOT CANAL REAMERS — STANDARDIZED (Uniform Taper)
(Metal Handle)

"A" DIAM.

UNIFORM TAPER

"B" DIAM.

STYLE B
Carbon Steel
or
Stainless Steel

10 15 20 25 30 35 40 45 50 55 60 70 80 90 100 110 120 130 140

STYLE D
Stainless Steel
Only

10 15 20 25 30 35 40 45 50 55 60 70 80 90 100 110 120 130 140

Kerr Standardized Root Canal Reamers are made to the specifications presented at the Second International Conference on Endodontics.

The uniform taper is maintained as the diameter of each instrument is increased. See illustration above.

The number of the instrument indicates Diameter "A" in hundredths of a millimeter.

Diameter "B" is always .30 mm larger than Diameter "A", providing a constant uniform taper in all sizes of instruments.

- **Carbon Steel, Style B,** Standardized Files are available in sizes #10 to #120 and supplied in 21 MM, 25 MM, and 30 MM lengths.
- **Stainless Steel, Style B,** Standardized Files are available in sizes #10 to #140 and supplied in 25 MM length.
- **Stainless Steel, Style D,** Standardized Files are available in sizes #10 to #140 and supplied in 25 MM length.

Fig. 22-11, cont'd. B, Endodontic reamers. (Courtesy Kerr Dental Mgr. Co., Romulus, Mich.)

Continued.

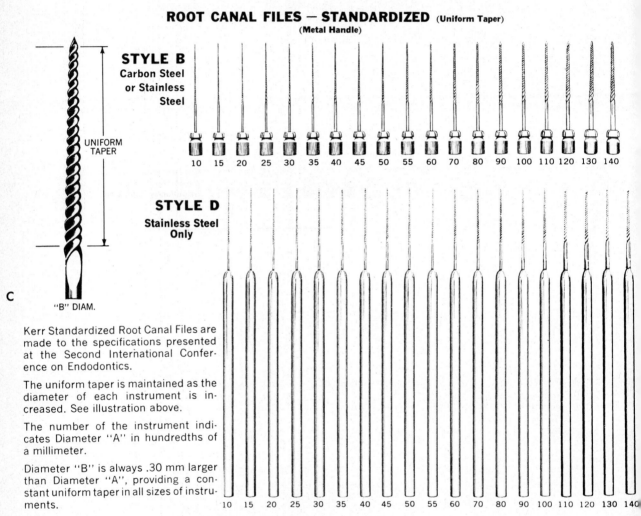

ROOT CANAL FILES — STANDARDIZED (Uniform Taper)
(Metal Handle)

STYLE B
Carbon Steel
or Stainless
Steel

UNIFORM TAPER

"B" DIAM.

10 15 20 25 30 35 40 45 50 55 60 70 80 90 100 110 120 130 140

STYLE D
Stainless Steel
Only

10 15 20 25 30 35 40 45 50 55 60 70 80 90 100 110 120 130 140

C

Kerr Standardized Root Canal Files are made to the specifications presented at the Second International Conference on Endodontics.

The uniform taper is maintained as the diameter of each instrument is increased. See illustration above.

The number of the instrument indicates Diameter "A" in hundredths of a millimeter.

Diameter "B" is always .30 mm larger than Diameter "A", providing a constant uniform taper in all sizes of instruments.

- **Carbon Steel, Style B,** Standardized Reamers are available in sizes #10 to #120 and supplied in 21 MM, 25 MM, and 30 MM lengths.
- **Stainless Steel, Style B,** Standardized Reamers are available in sizes #10 to #140 and supplied in 25 MM length.
- **Stainless Steel, Style D,** Standardized Reamers are available in sizes #10 to #140 and supplied in 25 MM length.

Fig. 22-11, cont'd. C, Endodontic files. (Courtesy Kerr Dental Mgr. Co., Romulus, Mich.)

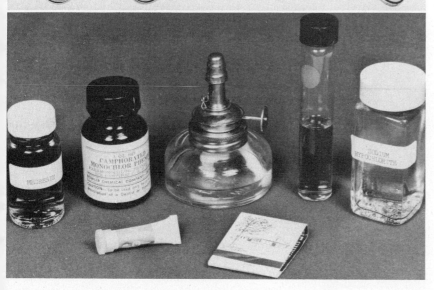

Preset endodontic tray

Burs, F.G. No. 4 and No. 35
Fingernail clipper
Hemostat, small
Scissors
Endodontic pliers, self-locking, two pair
Wesco plugger, No. 25
Plastic instrument, F.P. No. 1
Spoon excavator
Ball burnisher, hand type
Cowhorn explorer, No. 3
Mouth mirror, No. 4
Irrigation syringe, 2 ml

Add-on items

Culturing and medication appointments
  Rubber dam disinfectant (Mecresin or
    Metaphen)
  Root canal disinfectant (camphorated
    monochlorophenol)
  Temporary cement (Cavit)
  Alcohol lamp
  Matches
  Culture media tube
  Root canal cleaning agent
    (sodium hypochlorite)
Final filling appointment (not shown)
  Root canal cleaning agent
  Alcohol lamp and matches
  Root canal filling points (silver and
    gutta-percha)
  Root canal sealer
  Radiographic film
  Cement material (zinc phosphate)

Fig. 22-11, cont'd. D, Preset endodontic set-up. (Use sterile towel wrap.) **E,** Add-on items.

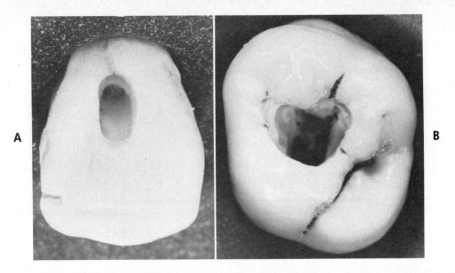

Fig. 22-12. Preparation of teeth for endodontic treatment. **A,** Lingual opening on anterior tooth. **B,** Occlusal opening on posterior tooth.

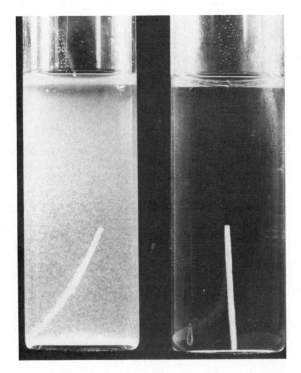

Fig. 22-13. *Left:* Culture of pulp sample is positive for presence of bacteria. *Right:* Culture is negative.

sterile paper point and be transferred into the culture medium. Then the result would be a false reading of the actual bacterial status of the pulp cavity.

If the dentist chooses to do a culture test during the endodontic procedure, it is done as the first step after the opening into the pulp cavity is made. This will give the most accurate indication of the true bacterial status of the pulp.

Culturing should be considered a diagnostic tool that assists the dentist in determining the presence of bacteria in the canal. In recent years the trend seems to be away from routine culturing of every case. This decision is left to the individual dentist.

Canal cleaning. After the pulp cavity is opened and cultured, the pulpal remnants must be removed, and the walls of the pulp canals thoroughly cleaned. A common method is to gently inject either a mild solution of sodium hypochlorite or hydrogen peroxide into the canal using an irrigating syringe. A small root-canal file, or reamer, is then placed into the canal and swirled like a cocktail "swizzle stick." The solutions are mild disinfectants that assist in destroying bacteria. The rubbing of the file against the pulp canal walls has a scrubbing effect that loosens debris and bacteria. This process is called biomechanical cleaning and is an essential part of the canal sterilization process. It is repeated at each subsequent appointment until the canal is filled.

After the canal is cleaned, it is flushed gently with

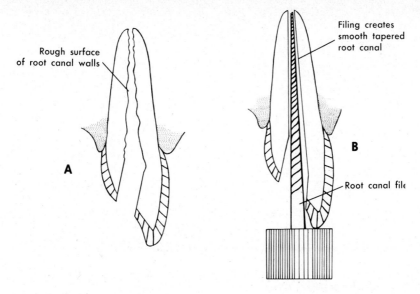

Fig. 22-14. Filing root canal. **A,** Root canal before filing (exaggerated). **B,** Canal being filed.

the irrigation syringe and dried thoroughly with the same type of paper points that were used to culture the canal. A completely dry canal is necessary to allow the subsequent cavity medication to work effectively.

Many endodontists believe that biomechanical cleaning is the most important part of the sterilization process.

Canal medication. After biomechanical cleaning and drying of the pulp canal, a strong disinfectant is placed in the canal to destroy any remaining bacteria. This disinfectant is sealed inside the canal between appointments.

A typical method of placing the medication is to cut a paper point to a length that will fit into the canal and not protrude out of the opening in the crown.

Then a cotton pellet is moistened with the disinfectant and brought to the canal opening and touched to the dry paper point. The medication will be drawn down the length of the absorbent paper point. This is a favorable method, since dipping the paper point into the disinfectant before introduction into the canal softens the point and makes it difficult to place into the canal. This method also helps to prevent excessive medication of the canal, which can cause patient discomfort.

Three of the most common disinfectants that are used are camphorated paramonochlorophenol, cresatin, and cresol and formaldehyde (Formocresol).

All these disinfectants lose their effectiveness after 2 to 3 days. Thus the patient should have appointments at frequent intervals for maximum sterilization effect from the medication.

After the medication is placed, the canal is closed by placing a dry cotton pellet in the crown opening, and a temporary cement is used to seal the opening. The rubber dam is removed, and the patient can be dismissed. The same procedure is repeated for two or three appointments until the canal is sterile. Most dentists prefer to have the canal sterile before doing extensive filing of the canal.

Canal filing. Root canal filing is a process of shaping the walls of the root canal so that they are smooth and so that the entire root canal obtains a specific shape and size (Fig. 22-14). This is accomplished by using endodontic files and reamers (Fig. 22-11, *B* and *C*). These instruments are available in a range of different diameters. The length of the cutting portion of each instrument is the same, regardless of its diameter.

The filing procedure begins by first establishing the approximate length of the root canal. This can be done from an accurate radiograph of the tooth to be treated. The file is held against the radiograph with the tip of the file at the apex. A rubber file marker is slid along the file so that it is even with a reference point on the crown portion of the tooth. Good refer-

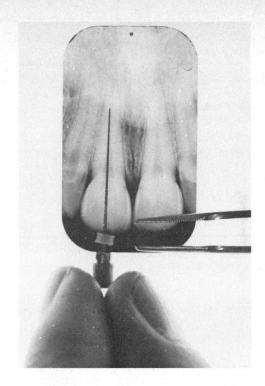

Fig. 22-15. Adjusting file marker to proper length of root canal, with incisal edge of tooth used as reference point.

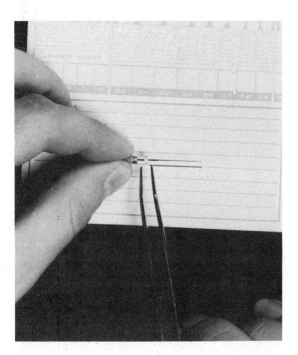

Fig. 22-16. Using reference line on patient's dental chart to record length of root canal. File markers for all files needed can be set to length of this reference line.

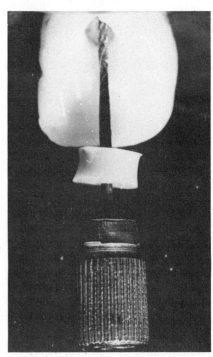

Fig. 22-17. Using incisal edge as reference point to determine proper length of root canal. When preset file marker touches incisal edge, tip of file is at apex of root.

ence points are the incisal edges of anterior teeth and a cusp on a posterior tooth (Fig. 22-15). This length can be transferred to the patient's record by drawing a straight line the same length as the measured canal. As filing progresses, file sizes are increased to enlarge the size of the canal. Every time a different file is used, the rubber file marker is adjusted so that the file length is the same length as the reference line marker on the patient's record (Fig. 22-16). When the file is inserted in the root canal, the rubber file marker will touch the reference point on the crown when the tip of the file is at the apex (Fig. 22-17).

The proper size of file to use first is any size that will slide easily to the apex of the root. The size to finish the filing procedure is determined by the dentist according to the resistance that is felt on inserting a larger file. Table 22-1 lists average sizes that are used for the various root canals in the adult dentition.

It should be noted that in teeth with more than one

canal, it is essential that each canal be filed to its predetermined length. Each canal may well be filed to diameters of different size, as can be seen in Table 22-1.

Filing is aided greatly by flooding the root canal with either sodium hypochlorite or hydrogen peroxide. These solutions keep the dentin shavings from clogging the cutting edges of the file as they are removed from the walls of the canal.

After filing is complete, the canal is flushed thoroughly with a biomechanical cleaning solution and dried. The canal is now ready to be filled.

Root canal filling. Three principal types of root canl fillings are in common use: (1) silver point, (2) gutta-percha point, and (3) combination gutta-percha and silver point. The selection of the appropriate filling materials is dependent on the personal preference of the dentist and the specific tooth being treated.

Silver point technique. After the canal has been

Table 22-1. File sizes and filling materials

Tooth	Canal	File size	Size and type of filling material
Maxillary			
Central incisor	Central	70	70 Silver point and gutta-percha
Lateral incisor	Central	40	40 Silver point and gutta-percha
Canine	Central	50	50 Silver point and gutta-percha
First premolar*	Buccal	30	30 Silver point
	Lingual	30	30 Silver point
Second premolar*	Buccal	30	30 Silver point
	Lingual	30	30 Silver point
First molar	Mesiobuccal	25	25 Silver point
	Distobuccal	25	25 Silver point
	Lingual	40	40 Silver point
Second molar	Mesiobuccal	25	25 Silver point
	Distobuccal	25	25 Silver point
	Lingual	40	40 Silver point
Mandibular			
Central incisor	Central	40	40 Silver point and gutta-percha
Lateral incisor	Central	30	30 Silver point and gutta-percha
Canine	Central	50	50 Silver point and gutta-percha
First premolar*	Central	50	50 Silver point and gutta-percha
Second premolar*	Central	50	50 Silver point and gutta-percha
First molar	Mesiobuccal	25	25 Silver point
	Mesiolingual	25	25 Silver point
	Distal	50	50 Silver point and gutta-percha
Second molar	Mesiobuccal	25	25 Silver point
	Mesiolingual	25	25 Silver point
	Distal	50	50 Silver point and gutta-percha

*Note: No. 25 size files and silver points can be used in the canals of these teeth if they are bifurcated.

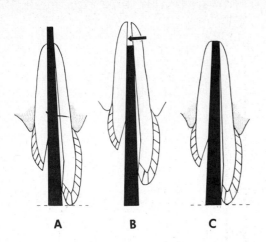

Fig. 22-18. Trial point radiographs would reveal accuracy of silver point fitting. **A,** Too long. **B,** Too short; arrow indicates space left unfilled. **C,** Accurately fitted.

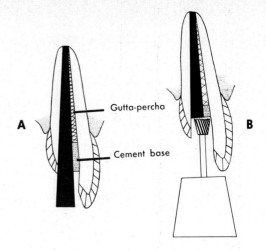

Fig. 22-19. A, Combination silver point and gutta-percha root canal filling. **B,** Removing excess length of silver point with inverted cone bur in ultraspeed handpiece.

filed to the desirable size, cleaned, and dried, the silver point is selected and cut to the predetermined length. The selection of the proper size silver point is rather simple. Manufacturers of endodontic files and silver points have coordinated the size and taper of the files with their silver points. For example, if a canal was filed to completion with a No. 50 size file, a No. 50 size point would be used to fill the canal.

The silver point can be cut to length very easily by using the same reference length that was established during the filing procedure. A handy suggestion for cutting silver points is to use an ordinary fingernail clipper to cut the silver point.

The silver point can now be placed in the canal and checked for length. If the point does not seat far enough in the canal, additional filing may be required to allow the point to slide further into the canal to seal the apical foramen. If the point extends beyond the apex, the excess can be cut off the apical end of the silver point.

The proper length of the point is verified by taking a periapical radiography of the tooth with the silver point in the canal. The tip of the silver point should be within 1 mm of the apex of the root. This relationship will adequately seal the apical foramen. This periapical radiograph is commonly referred to as a trial point radiograph. If any adjustment is needed to achieve the proper length of the silver point, additional trial point radiographs may be taken to confirm the proper point length (Fig. 22-18).

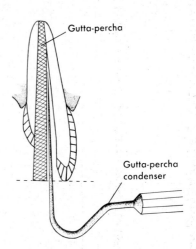

Fig. 22-20. Lateral condensation of gutta-percha. Additional fine gutta-percha points are inserted and condensed to completely fill canal.

With the silver point properly prepared, it is now ready to be seated in the canal. A thin mix of zinc oxide–eugenol cement called root canal sealer is prepared. The apical end of the silver point is coated with the sealer, and the point is seated firmly into the canal. The sealer is further assurance of a perfect seal at the apical foramen.

If any space exists between the silver point and the walls of either root canal or the pulp chamber, this

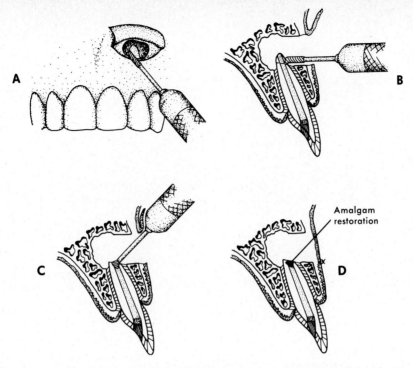

Fig. 22-21. Apicoectomy procedure. **A** and **B,** Reflection of mucoperiosteal flap and removal of end of root with a bur. **C,** Forming a small cavity preparation on cut end of root. **D,** Preparation is filled with amalgam to create seal in end of root. Incision is closed with silk sutures.

space can be filled with gutta-percha. Gutta-percha is a soft rubber material that can be condensed into small spaces. If this is done, the filling is referred to as a combination endodontic filling (Fig. 22-19, *A*).

The remainder of the endodontic opening can now be filled with zinc phosphate cement base. After the cement has hardened, any excess in length of the silver point can be removed with a high-speed handpiece (Fig. 22-19, *B*). The tooth is now ready to be restored with the appropriate restoration.

Gutta-percha technique. If the dentist chooses to fill the canal with gutta-percha points, the same basic steps are used as in the silver point technique with a few exceptions.

The size and length of the gutta-percha points are established in the same way as those of the silver point. After the gutta-percha point is coated with root canal sealer, it is sealed in the canal. Since gutta-percha is soft, it can be condensed against the walls of the root canal with a gutta-percha condenser (Fig. 22-20). Additional smaller gutta-percha points can be

added to fill any voids between the filling material and the walls of the pulp cavity.

Any excess in length of gutta-percha can be easily removed with a hot spoon excavator. Zinc phosphate cement base can be placed over the gutta-percha before the tooth is restored.

It should be noted that if the tooth has more than one root canal, each canal will be filed individually and each will require a properly fitted silver or gutta-percha point to be sealed in it. A perfect sealing of the apical foramen in the roots of teeth is essential to eliminate irritation of periapical tissue.

Apicoectomy

An apicoectomy is the surgical removal of the apical portion of the root of a tooth. To gain access to the apex of the root, an incision must be made on the facial aspect of the alveolar ridge in the area of the tooth to be treated. After the incision is made, the soft tissue is retracted, and the bony covering of the apical portion of the tooth is removed. After the apex of the

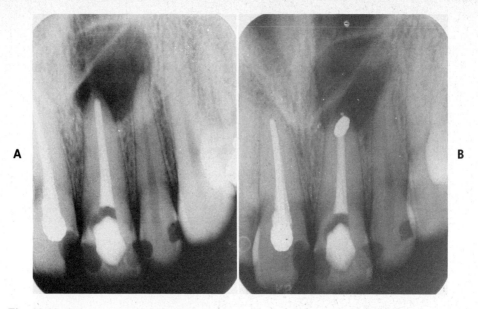

Fig. 22-22. Apicoectomy. **A,** Preoperative radiograph. **B,** Postoperative radiograph. (Courtesy Dr. J.F. Corcoran, Jr., Ann Arbor, Mich.)

root is uncovered, it can be removed with a sterile dental bur (Fig. 22-21, *A* and *B*).

When the root tip is removed, the opening into the root canal can be sealed with dental amalgam, using a procedure called a reverse filling technique. This simply means that the root canal is filled from the opposite end of the tooth instead of the approach through the crown that was described before. A small cavity preparation is made in the end of the root, and it is filled with amalgam. This ensures that a perfect seal exists at the root end (Fig. 22-21, *C* and *D*).

Before the incision is closed, the periapical area is curetted (scraped) clean of any abnormal tissue that may have formed in response to the offending tooth. Such tissue may be a granuloma or a periapical cyst.

An apicoectomy is usually done when a standard approach through the crown cannot be done. The reason a standard approach cannot be done may be any of the following conditions:

1. The root canal may be hypercalcified, so that the canal is obstructed.
2. An extreme curvature may prevent a file from reaching the apex of the root.
3. A previous endodontic filling may have been placed in the canal but may have not achieved an adequate apical seal.

4. A coronal approach may not be possible because of the presence of a coronal restoration that would have to be sacrificed if an opening were made through it.

The apex is removed to facilitate the reverse filling procedure and to eliminate any additional foramen that might exist. Often a tooth has more than one apical foramen for each canal. These will be eliminated by the apicoectomy.

The apicoectomy procedure is usually limited to anterior teeth and some premolars because of anatomic limitations that prevent access to most posterior teeth (Fig. 22-22).

Root amputations

On occasion, a multirooted tooth requiring a pulpectomy may have a root that is impossible to file completely to obtain an adequate apical seal. Yet the other roots of the teeth may be treatable. Instead of extracting the entire tooth, the untreatable root can be amputated from the rest of the tooth and removed from the alveolus. The remainder of the tooth can be treated by standard pulpectomy procedures. The opening to which the amputated root was attached can be sealed with amalgam in a similar fashion to that for the apicoectomy procedure.

DENTAL ASSISTANT'S ROLE

The specific role of the dental assistant in pulpectomy procedures will depend greatly on the dental law within each state. Presently, states permit the assistant to set up the armamentarium, assist the dentist in rubber dam application, deliver instruments and materials to the dentist during treatment, and take and process trial point radiographs.

States that permit dental assistants to perform "expanded duties" might include other tasks in the dental assistant role. Placement and removal of the rubber dam and the culturing procedure are the most likely expanded duties for the dental assistant in endodontics.

BIBLIOGRAPHY

Boucher, C.O.: Current clinical dental terminology, ed. 2, St. Louis, 1974, The C.V. Mosby Co.

Sommer, R.F., Ostrander, F.D., and Crowley, M.C.: Clinical endodontics, ed. 2, Philadelphia, 1965, W.B. Saunders Co.

Weine, F.S.: Endodontic therapy, ed. 3, St. Louis, 1982, The C.V. Mosby Co.

CHAPTER 23

PEDODONTICS

Dentistry for children differs from dentistry for adults in three major areas: patient management, problems relating to growth and development, and restorative procedures concerned with the developing dentitions. The problems relating to the emotionally and physically developing child are so unique that children's dentistry has stimulated the growth of the two dental specialty areas of pedodontics and orthodontics. Pedodontics predominantly deals with problems related to patient management and education, restorative procedures, and interceptive orthodontics. Orthodontics deals principally with problems relating to growth of the face and the development of the dentitions. However, orthodontic treatment is not limited to children.

Obviously, the vast subject of dentistry for children cannot be totally discussed in the limited confines of one chapter or even an entire textbook. The intention of this chapter is to introduce the dental assistant to some of the most common challenges faced in this area of dentistry.

PATIENT MANAGEMENT

Virtually all successful treatment of any patient centers around how well the patient is managed. This is particularly true of children. Children live in a world of their own. It is a world of limited life experiences and one that is greatly influenced by the child's environment and the people in it.

The success of the dental team in providing dental services for a child will depend on how well the team relates to the world of the child. Both the dentist and the auxiliaries must continually nurture a positive relationship with child patients. A basic understanding and fondness for children must exist within the minds of the operating team for positive relationships to develop. Children are experts in detecting the feelings of others around them. They form rapid opinions of others from facial expressions, tone of voice, conver-

sational topics, and physical actions. If one is truly sincere and honest with a child, he will sense it almost immediately and react in a positive manner. Conversely, if one betrays the child and is dishonest and insincere, it is safe to assume that the child will react in a negative manner. Dental assistants should analyze their own feelings toward children to determine if they possess the fundamental personality that is so necessary in relating to children. Many experts agree that the dentists and their auxiliaries who are not successful in patient management fail because they do not enjoy working with children.

Treating a child patient is much like being a parent. The operating team tries to guide and modify the child's behavior during the dental appointment. The same parental techniques that are used to modify behavior at home can be used in the dental office. Displays of fondness, firmness, fairness, honesty, sincerity, authority, and consistency are integral parts of behavior modification. However, like parents themselves, the dental team does not always succeed, and other measures utilizing premedication may have to be employed, at least on a temporary basis.

With the recognition that there will be some successes and failures in managing children, it is important that the operating team establish basic guidelines for their behavior to avoid unnecessary management problems. The dentist and the staff should have a clear understanding of each person's role in patient management. Constant communication between the dentist and staff is essential so that the operating team is compatible in the eyes of the child who enters the dental office.

General behavior characteristics of children

Children constantly undergo both physical and psychological growth. Psychological growth occurs at different rates within each individual just as physical growth varies. Psychological growth is influenced by age, the child's environment, and the influence of other people around him.

Following is a general characterizaton of children in various age groups, which may be of assistance to the dental assistant in anticipating a child's behavior.

At 3 years of age

1. Still desires the comfort of mother.
2. Apprehensive of strangers until accustomed to new surroundings and new people.
3. May use dental assistant as a substitute mother.
4. Desires to talk to people, especially after becoming familiar with them.
5. May resort to infantile behavior.
6. Can communicate and understand simple explanations.
7. Responsive to positive, concise directions.

At 4 years of age

1. Generally more sociable.
2. Fear of strangers gradually decreases.
3. Is in peak period for fear of the unknown, the unexpected, falling, and noise.
4. Often the most difficult management age.
5. Fantasizes to combat fear; may play "going to the dentist" at home to develop courage.
6. Tends to exaggerate stories.
7. Can become defiant and even start "name-calling."
8. Very talkative age.
9. Responsiveness to specific, positive directions.

At 5 to 6 years of age

1. Usually has no fear of leaving parents for social activities (including dental appointments).
2. Personal and social relationships are better developed.
3. Pinnacle of ego development; proud of self and possessions.
4. Responsive to admiration and compliments, especially of appearance and behavior.
5. Willing to transfer confidence from only parents to people the child admires.
6. Has a burning desire to try out new things (dental instruments, air-water syringes, etc.).
7. Increased fear of bodily injury; often reacts out of proportion to a pain stimulus.
8. Tends to associate pain with punishment (spankings). Therefore since a dentist can cause discomfort, the child may interpret the dental visit as a punishment.

At 7 years of age

1. More confident.
2. Willing to experience things without parent.
3. Alternates cowardice with courage.
4. Increased emotional control.
5. Dislikes the belittlement by others.
6. Often becomes attached to the dental assistant.

7. Girls tend to regress to earlier fears at times.
8. Boys may tend to conflict more with a male dentist and favor the female assistant.

At 8 to 13 years of age

1. Usually does not differentiate strongly between pleasant and unpleasant experiences.
2. Generally obedient.
3. Retains emotional control.
4. Resents belittlement.
5. Usually very manageable.

Teenage

1. Great social awareness.
2. Sensitive to peer group.
3. Great concern regarding appearance and mouth odors.
4. Very manageable.
5. Enjoys adult level conversation.
6. Needs constant oral hygiene motivation.

These characteristics are by no means absolute; neither are they limited only to the age groups stated. They may extend either way from the ages stated because of individual variability. An analysis of these characteristics may aid the dental assistant in establishing rapport with a child and developing a more relaxed conversation geared to the patient. It is hoped that a better understanding of children's behavior will contribute to more successful patient management.

Office environment

Children are sensitive to their environment. They like bright colors and a cheery decor. Every dental office that treats children should have at least a portion of the reception room designed for the young patient. Small tables and chairs geared to children's physical size give them a sense of belonging. A variety of toys, books, and activities should be available for different age groups to enhance this sense of belonging and to occupy the child waiting to be treated. It is good to include some pictures or posters of current cartoon characters on the walls of the children's area to add familiarity to the room.

Children show a marked dislike for gloomy surroundings, unpleasant room odors (medical and otherwise), and white uniforms. The white uniform is often associated with unpleasant experiences the child may have endured earlier in life, such as previous medical or dental treatment. Colored uniforms have helped in this regard. Some dentists who treat a lot of children prefer to wear no uniform of any kind.

Pleasant music is as acceptable to children as it is to adult patients. Music can create a favorable mood, occupy one's mind, and mask other noises in the offices.

Sound control is a factor in the office. Patients in the reception room can be readily upset by a crying child in the treatment area. Office designers should take this into account when the office is built.

Parental management

Children have no natural fear of going to the dentist. Their fears are acquired either through the negative influence of others or by their own unfavorable dental experiences. Unfortunately, many parents contribute significantly to the development of fear of dental treatment. Parents often prejudice the child against dentistry by relating their unfavorable experiences or their fears to the child at home. It is essential that parents be cautioned to let children experience dental treatment on their own without any preconceived fears passed on through the family.

It is quite common for parents to "overprepare" children for their first dental visit. Although the intent may be favorable, the results are often negative. When a parent dwells on the ease of going to the dentist, the child often senses that the parent is trying to be deceptive. Parents are better advised to minimize the significance of the visit to the dentist. Children should be informed that the dentist will look at their teeth and probably take pictures. They should be encouraged to *ask the dentist* what other things might be done at any appointment. The first dental appointment should be standardized, so that the parent knows what will be done. It is a real sign of deceit in the mind of children if they are told that the dentist will only look at their teeth and take pictures and then the dentist gives an injection and restores a tooth. More often than not, children will believe that the dentist deceived them rather than the parent. Honesty is the best policy with children. If a parent is unsure of what the dentist is going to do, children should be instructed to ask. Then the dentist can deal with the answer.

Parents, particularly mothers, are tempted to enter the operatory with children, especially at the first appointment. There is some disagreement among dentists as to whether they want the parent in the operatory during the appointment. Generally the operating team can handle a child more favorably if the parent remains in the reception area. This practice allows children to experience dentistry on their own. It also allows the dentist and auxiliaries the opportunity to establish rapport with the patient without interference from the parent. Typically, the dental team makes the child the center of attention. Conversation should be directed toward the youngster, and the patient will accept directions from the dentist. If the parent is present, the child's attention is often diverted from the dentist to the parent. In addition, the child may not easily accept the dentist as an authority figure. A female dental assistant should be aware of the possibility of the child placing her in the role of a mother figure. An effective pedodontic assistant will graciously accept this affection while redirecting the child's attention to the wishes of the dentist.

There are exceptions to the rule of child-parent separation. This is particularly true in children under 3 years old and handicapped children. Children who speak a different language (verbal or sign language) are also possible exceptions. This decision is made entirely by the dentist on the basis of personal experience and ability.

Dental assistants must be aware of the dentist's policies regarding managing both the parent and the child so that the parents can be informed of their role in cooperation with the dentist. Most parents are extremely willing to cooperate if they are aware of the office policy.

Timing of an appointment is sometimes a key factor in patient management. Some children can accept treatment more favorably at a certain time of day or even on certains days of the week. Parents can be more helpful in setting up appointments for the child at favorable times. This may mean some inconvenience to the parents and school officials, yet timing may be of great significance in achieving success. It is often wise to schedule shorter, more frequent appointments for very young children until they become accustomed to dental treatment.

Suggestions for patient management

Verbal communication

1. *Dental staff communication*. The dentist and staff must be in constant communication at staff meetings and throughout the day so that there is good coordination between staff members. There should be no question as to the role each member plays in patient management.

2. *Give specific positive directions*. Avoid confusing the child with inadequate directions. The directions should be positive and specific. Avoid saying "Would you like to come in now, Johnny?" or "Don't you want to sit in our big chair?" (Fig. 23-1). The child is given a choice with this type of direction

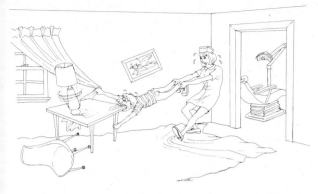

Fig. 23-1. ''Would you like to come in now, Johnny?''

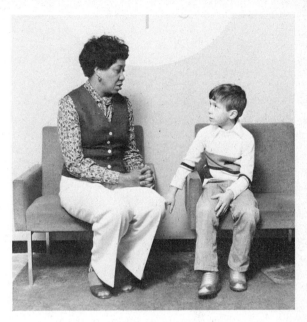

Fig. 23-2. Response to positive directions.

and has to decide what to do—stay with mother or please the dentist. The same directions given in a specific and positive manner will avoid this dilemma. ''Hi, Johnny, it's time to come in now'' and ''Now climb into the big chair'' tell the child exactly what you want and give him no choice in the matter. Most children will respond more favorably to positive directions (Fig. 23-2).

3. *Keep the child the center of attention.* On arriving, the patient must become the center of attention. All conversation should be directed toward the child. Select topics of conversation that pertain directly to the child and not someone else. A child enjoys being the center of attention. Suggested topics of conversation are clothes the child is wearing, television shows, pets, favorite toys, sports, and favorite stories. An alert assistant will take the time to watch some children's programs and review some popular children's stories so that conversation is easier to initiate, especially with shy children. Some dentists are not particularly good at initiating conversation, and the assistant may be depended on to ''break the ice.'' These conversations can be the real joy of the working day—in fact, some of the things children say will be remembered for many years to come. Raise the chair to eye level during conversation so that the child does not feel dwarfed by people towering over him.

4. *Adjust language level to the child.* Avoid ''baby talk'' to all children. It is better to adjust the vocabulary from a higher level to a lower one as needed than to assume children know nothing and talk down to them. This level is achieved as the operating team becomes more familiar with the youngster.

5. *Voice tone to be used.* During conversation, use normal voice tones. The high-pitched, ''singsong'' voice level should be avoided because a change to normal voice tone during the procedure may be interpreted by the child as a change in the relationship from friendliness to seriousness. Voice tone during the procedure is an important communication device. A singsong-like ''Open wide, Johnny'' may not get the same result as a firm-toned ''Open wide, Johnny.'' The tone need not be harsh or unfriendly, just firm and definite.

6. *Inform the child.* An informed child is usually less fearful. Procedures should be explained in a concise manner using nonthreatening terminology. Children experiencing the first dental appointment should be shown various nonthreatening instruments such as a mouth mirror, ''tooth polisher'' (polishing cup), ''whistle'' (the high-speed handpiece without a bur), and ''Mr. Thirsty'' (saliva ejector) (Fig. 23-3). Before an injection tell the child that a mosquito bite will be felt. This should be done just an instant before the sensation is felt so that the child does not have an opportunity to react to the thought. Timing of this kind of information can be as influential on the child as the information itself. Avoid words that promote fear such as *hurt, shot, drill, pick,* and *bleeding.* Substitute descriptive terms that have less unpleasant-

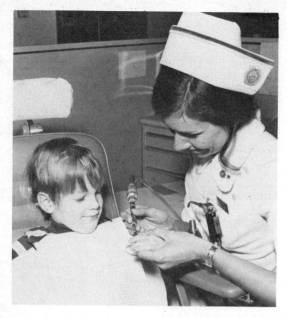

Fig. 23-3. Introduction of child to dental operatory on his first visit.

ness associated with them, or none at all, such as *slightly uncomfortable, mosquito bite, polisher,* and *cavity finder.* Care should be taken in using words that limit the procedure, such as *just* or *only.* If the assistant says, "Dr. Jones is only going to look at your teeth," the assistant had better be sure that only that is planned. It is preferable to say, "Dr. Jones will look at your teeth, and then we'll see if anything else has to be done."

7. *Talkative patients.* A talkative youngster may be using this as a device to vent anxiety or as a defense mechanism to delay treatment. A patient who asks a lot of questions should be suspected of this delaying tactic. It can be halted by simply stating that it is time to go to work now and any other questions the child wants to ask will be answered after the work has been completed. It is not surprising to find that after treatment previously talkative youngsters have no further questions, but they should be given the opportunity to ask them as they were promised.

Nonverbal communication

1. *Facial expression.* Children are not unlike adults in that they read facial expressions and form opinions. A friendly facial expression is worth a thousand kind words. On the other hand, a firm look at the right time often achieves effective results.

2. *Touch.* By and large, young children like to be fondled as a means of expressing affection for them. A gentle pat, holding hands, and putting an arm around them occasionally are often well received by the youngster. A squirming child will know exactly what you mean when a firm grip is applied to an arm or leg.

3. *Eye contact.* Maintenance of eye contact during conversation enhances the sincerity of what is being said and enforces the attention being given to him.

Appearance

1. *Uniforms.* Many children fear white uniforms because of the association with previous medical or dental experiences that were not particularly favorable. Colored uniforms have helped to eliminate this association. Some dentists prefer to remove clinic jackets when seeing a child patient to further dissolve the unpleasant association.

2. *Personal hygiene.* Children, like adults, prefer neat, attractive people. They dislike people with body and breath odors, and often say so! Attention to personal hygiene cannot be relaxed because one is treating "just kids."

3. *Face masks.* The face covered by a surgical face mask is often a fearsome sight to the child. If it is necessary to wear one, the child should be told that you do not want to "give him or her your germs." Drawing a friendly smile on the mask can be amusing to the child and may relieve the fear associated with the mask.

Controlling emotions. The operating team must control their negative emotions toward a child. If both the dentist and the patient are angry, the procedure is doomed to failure. It is better for the dentist to leave the room to "cool off" when this happens. Another appointment for the child may be necessary—with premedication if all else fails.

Praise. Youngsters thrive on praise. Reinforcement of positive behavior during the appointment should be done by offering various forms of praise. "Boy! Johnny can sure open wide, can't he, Dr. Jones?" This is an example of indirect praise that the assistant can offer during a procedure.

Every appointment should end on a good note. There should be at least one thing that even the most misbehaved youngster has done during the appointment that merits praise. A few moments should be taken at the end of each appointment for some form of praise from the dentist and the assistant. A trip to the "treasure box" for a toy reward is in order for all kids of the appropriate age.

Consistency. The operating team should establish consistency in office policy, operating technique, terminology, and patient management techniques. Children respond much better to consistency. They know what to expect from you and will react with greater predictability.

Role of the dental assistant

The specific role of the assistant in patient management will vary from one dental office to another. The important thing is to have the role clarified by the dentist to avoid misunderstandings. Some dentists rely heavily on the assistant's involvement in handling children, whereas others prefer to minimize the assistant's role.

A typical format is to have an assistant play the predominant role in introducing the child to the office and its equipment. Establishing conversation with the youngster is an important part of this task. As the dentist enters the operatory, the assistant introduces the child to the dentist, and as the dentist establishes rapport with the child, the assistant's involvement in the conversation is gradually reduced. As the procedure progresses, the assistant should slowly aid the dentist in the establishing of an authority image. This is especially important if the child attempts to cling too heavily to the newly adopted mother—the assistant. The amount of verbal input the assistant should offer during a procedure is a matter of opinion. However, most dentists agree that directions to the child should be given by the dentist. Directions from two sources tend to confuse the patient and may generate problems. The assistant again plays a prominent role in directing the youngster after the procedure is finished. The dental assistant often gives postoperative instructions and dismisses the child.

This format changes somewhat for expanded duty assistants and dental hygienists, since they assume the role of the operator. They must therefore assume a greater authority figure role.

COMMON OPERATIVE AND RESTORATIVE PROCEDURES

Dental care for the young patient involves treatment of the primary and permanent dentitions, or a combination of both (the mixed dentition), depending on the age of the patient. Generally parents do not question the validity of restoring carious or fractured permanent teeth. However, parents often question the restoration of primary teeth, since "the child will shed them anyway!"

Restoration of the primary teeth is important for the following reasons:

1. A restoration maintains the function of the teeth in chewing, speech, and appearance.
2. A restoration helps to ensure symmetrical growth of the developing jaws.
3. The primary teeth maintain space on the jaws for the permanent teeth that replace them. Primary teeth also guide the path of eruption of the permanent teeth into proper position.
4. The child should be free of discomfort and mouth odors, as is the adult patient.

The preservation of the primary teeth until they are lost by natural exfoliation (shedding) is a principal goal of operative and restorative dentistry.

Operative dentistry

Operative dentistry techniques for children differ very little from those used for adults as far as the assistant's duties are concerned. The same basic steps are used in the fabrication of composite and amalgam restorations as described in Chapters 16 and 17. Gold inlays and cohesive gold restorations are not usually done on primary teeth.

Additional features of rubber dam isolation that are beneficial in children's dentistry are that it assists the patient in keeping the mouth open, has a quieting effect on the child, and protects the tongue and cheek.

Pulpotomy. Pulpotomy is a procedure that involves partial removal of the dental pulp after it has been extensively exposed. This is in contrast to the pulpectomy, which involves the complete removal of the pulp. Pulpectomy procedures are discussed in Chapter 22.

Pulpotomy procedures are usually done on primary and young permanent teeth. Success rates drop markedly when attempts are made to treat permanent teeth of individuals past their teens. Extensive pulp exposures in older adult teeth are usually treated with a pulpectomy procedure. Pulpal circulation is reduced significantly in adult patients as a result of the constriction of the apical foramen that is a part of normal tooth development. Ample blood supply to the remaining portion of the pulp is essential to the success of a pulpotomy. Another factor in the success of a pulpotomy is the condition of the pulp at the time of treatment. Infected pulp tissue is a poorer candidate than healthier pulp tissue.

The pulpotomy is a surgical procedure, so that care must be exercised to maintain a sterile operating field as much as possible. Rubber dam isolation is indicated to prevent salivary contamination. The standard amalgam armamentarium can be used for this procedure with the following additional items:

Formocresol

No. 6 sterile round bur

Zinc oxide–eugenol cement (IRM)

After the administration of anesthesia and the placement of the rubber dam, a large opening is made into the pulp chamber to expose the entire coronal portion of the pulp. A No. 6 round bur in a conventional-speed handpiece is used to remove this portion of the pulp to the level of the openings of the root canals (Fig. 23-4, *A* and *B*).

A small cotton pellet wetted with Formocresol solution is placed over the remainder of the pulp and allowed to remain for 5 minutes. This solution fixes, or mummifies, a thin layer of the remaining pulp, which stops the bleeding from the amputated pulp tissue. The cotton pellet is then removed, and a thick layer of rapid-setting zinc oxide–eugenol base material is placed over the pulp (Fig. 23-4, *C* and *D*).

After completion of the pulpotomy, the final restoration, such as amalgam or a stainless steel crown, can be placed. Dentists sometimes prefer to delay placement of the final restoration until the injured pulp has an opportunity to recover from the surgical procedure. In these cases, the zinc oxide–eugenol

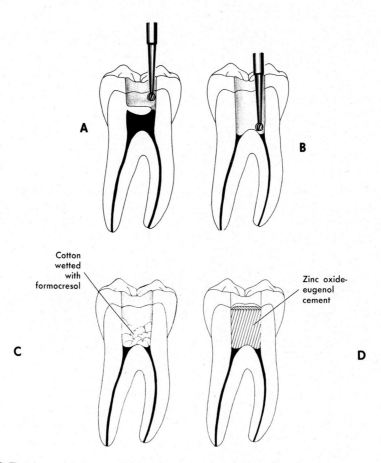

Fig. 23-4. Formocresol pulpotomy. **A,** Caries removal. **B,** Removal of coronal portion of pulp. **C,** Application of formocresol. **D,** Placement of cement.

cement is used to completely fill the cavity preparation and thus act as a temporary restoration.

Spot-welded matrix band. One variation that is common in the fabrication of an amalgam restoration for primary teeth is the use of a spot-welded matrix band for Class II and VI restorations (Table 15-1). Some dentists prefer these to the conventional matrix bands that are held in place by a matrix retainer.

The spot-welded matrix band can be quickly made as follows:

1. The matrix band material is placed around the tooth and pinched tightly with a Howe pliers or a hemostat (Fig. 23-5, *A*). The excess length of the band (½ inch) is bent to one side to mark the proper size of the tooth.
2. The band is carried to the spot welder and welded at the bend in the band made by the pliers (Fig. 23-5, *B*).

3. The excess band material can be cut away, and the band contoured to fit the tooth (Fig. 23-5, *C*).
4. After the band is placed around the tooth, interproximal wedges are placed as when conventional bands are used. After the insertion of the amalgam, the band is removed by cutting the band on the lingual aspect and pulling it in a buccal direction with cotton pliers.

Restorative dentistry

Elaborate cast gold restorations are usually only done on primary teeth under very special circumstances. Typically, primary teeth that are extensively destroyed because of caries or fracture are restored with "temporary" crowns that are cemented to the involved teeth with a permanent cementing agent. Stainless steel crowns are used on posterior teeth, and

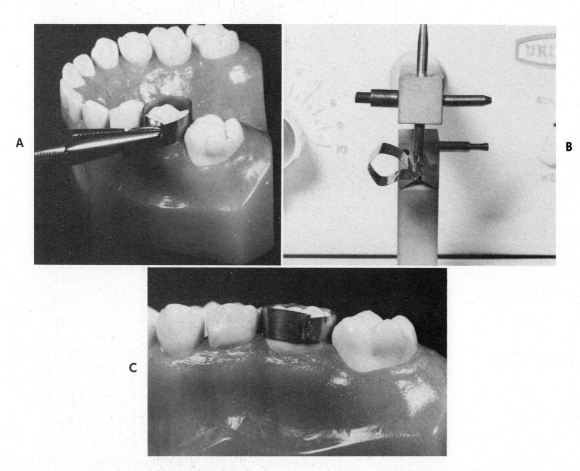

Fig. 23-5. Fabrication of a spot-welded matrix band. **A,** Pinching band with hemostat. **B,** Welding band. **C,** Finished band in place.

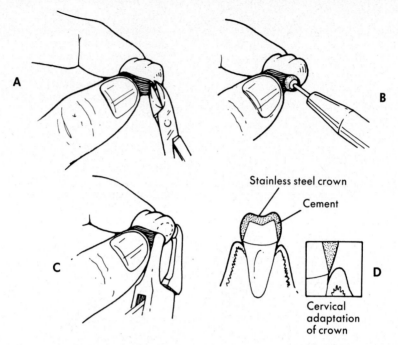

Fig. 23-6. Fabrication of stainless steel crown. **A,** Trimming crown to proper length with crown and collar scissors. **B,** Smoothing rough edges with a green stone followed by abrasive rubber wheel (Craytex). **C,** Contouring crown with contouring pliers. **D,** Longitudinal section of completed crown.

polycarbonate preformed crowns are used on anterior teeth.

Stainless steel crowns. These can be used as interim restorations on primary teeth until they are exfoliated or on permanent teeth until a more accurately contoured cast gold crown can be fabricated. These crowns are available in kits that contain a range of sizes for the various primary and permanent posterior teeth. The technique used in their fabrication follows:

Procedure

1. The tooth is prepared in a fashion similar to that for a cast gold crown, with the tapered diamond in the high-speed handpiece. The entire circumference of the tooth is reduced, as well as the height of the tooth. Caries is removed with conventional methods, and cavity medications are placed.
2. The proper-size crown is selected from the kit. It must both fit the circumference of the prepared tooth and duplicate the mesiodistal dimension of the original crown of the tooth.
3. The occlusocervical height of the crown is adjusted so that it extends approximately 1 mm below the free gin-

gival margin. The crown is trimmed along the cervical margin with the crown and collar scissors. The rough-cut edges are then smoothed with the green stone, followed by polishing with the rubber abrasive wheel (Fig. 23-6, *A* and *B*).
4. The occlusion is checked and adjusted as needed.
5. The contouring pliers are used to bend the cervical margins of the crown in toward the tooth to assure a snug fit and a proper cervical contour (Fig. 23-6, *C*).
6. The prepared tooth is dried thoroughly, and the crown is filled with permanent cement and seated in place (Fig. 23-6, *D*).
7. Excess cement is removed from around the tooth, and the patient can be dismissed.

Polycarbonate crowns. These are fabricated for primary and permanent teeth in the same manner as described in Chapter 20.

• • •

It is uncommon that a fixed bridge is used to replace a missing primary tooth. Usually a space-maintaining device, as described on p. 337, is used. If

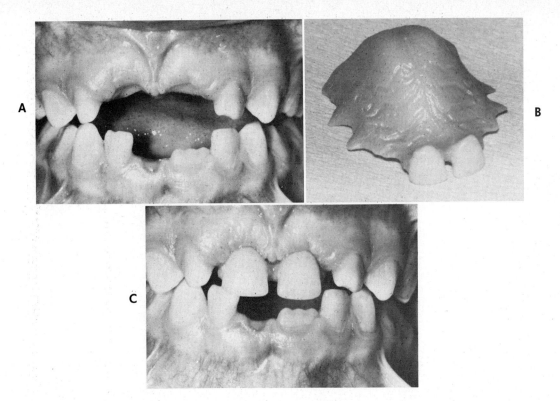

Fig. 23-7. A, Missing primary incisors. **B,** Replaced with removable partial denture. **C,** Denture in place. (From Law, D., and others: An atlas of pedodontics, Philadelphia, 1969, W.B. Saunders Co.)

several teeth are missing so that there is difficulty in speech or mastication (chewing) and significant impairment to the child's appearance, a removable partial denture can be made (Fig. 23-7). Crown and bridge procedures are sometimes required for the restoration and replacement of permanent teeth in both the mixed and permanent dentitions.

EMERGENCY TREATMENT FOR TRAUMATIZED TEETH
Fractured anterior teeth

Fractured anterior teeth are common emergencies among children. The active nature of children predisposes them to this type of emergency. Table 23-1 outlines the Ellis classification of crown fractures and a recommended treatment for each class.

Since it is difficult for parents to accurately assess the extent of damage done to a tooth and the surrounding tissue, it is advisable for the dentist to see the patient as soon as possible. Clinical examination,

documentation of the history of the accident, and radiographs are essential elements of the initial visit. Pulpal treatment and temporization is carried out as described in Table 23-1. Generally speaking, dentists prefer to delay treatment that involves further trauma to the pulp of an injured tooth for 3 to 6 months. This gives the delicate pulp tissue a greater opportunity to recover without added insult. Radiographic documentation at subsequent appointments is mandatory to determine the status of the injured teeth. Vitality tests are carried out initially to establish a basis of comparison for tests done in the future.

After a 6-month interval more definitive restorative procedures can be done on injured teeth with still vital pulps. Less severe fractures (Classes I and II) can be restored with composite restorations utilizing a retention pin, acid-etch techniques, or both. More extensive fractures (Classes II and III) that will require a permanent crown to be placed on a still vital tooth may have to be delayed until the tooth erupts suffi-

Table 23-1. Classification of crown fractures and treatment method for permanent anterior teeth*

Class	Definition	Treatment
I	Fractures of enamel layer only, or very little dentin involvement	1. Smooth rough edges. 2. Check radiographically and perform vitality tests at 3- or 6-month intervals. 3. Reshape after 6 months; check to improve esthetics.
II	Extensive fracture of dentin layer but no pulp exposure occurring	1. Coat exposed dentin with zinc oxide–eugenol paste (Cavitec). 2. Cement a temporary crown on tooth for 3 to 6 months. 3. Radiograph and perform vitality test at 3 to 6 months. 4. Place permanent crown when tooth has erupted fully and pulp receded enough.
III	Extensive fracture where pulp is exposed	1. Pulpotomy or pulpectomy depending on status of patient. 2. Place temporary crown until teeth erupt and pulp recedes enough for a permanent crown to be placed.
IV	Fractures that involve loss of crown of tooth	1. Pulpectomy procedure must be done. 2. Post crown has to be done after endodontic treatment is completed

*Primary teeth are treated similarly except that teeth that undergo pulp death at a later date may require endodontic treatment like the permanent incisor or extraction. If endodontic therapy is done on severely fractured teeth, then temporary crowns are placed until they are exfoliated.

ciently and the apex of the root has completely developed. If the pulp has not been altered (Class II cases), the fabrication of a permanent crown may have to be delayed until the large young pulp recedes with age. (A smaller pulp allows the dentist to prepare the tooth for the permanent crown without exposing the pulp during the preparation.) Long-term temporary crowns are used in these cases.

Traumatic intrusion

Traumatic intrusion of primary and permanent teeth is another common injury to maxillary anterior teeth. The tooth is forcibly driven into the alveolus so that only a portion of the crown is clinically visible (Fig. 23-8). Primary and permanent teeth that are intruded should be allowed to reerupt on their own. Since intruded teeth may undergo devitalization, endodontic treatment may be required later.

Intrusion of a primary tooth can present a threat to the underlying developing permanent tooth. The permanent tooth can be damaged either from the physical injury caused by the intruded primary tooth or by a developing infection in a devital primary tooth after the injury. There is no way in which damage to the permanent tooth can be determined for certain until it erupts. However, previously injured primary teeth should be observed so that if they should become infected, endodontic treatment can be done or the offending tooth can be extracted.

Displaced teeth

Displaced primary teeth other than those displaced by intrusion should be repositioned by the dentist and splinted as soon as possible. Primary teeth tend to undergo root resorption more quickly after these injuries and become very mobile. They should be observed for possible development of infection and removed if indicated. Permanent teeth should be repositioned as soon as possible and stabilized with a temporary splint using self-curing acrylic or wire ligatures (Fig. 23-9, *C*) or orthodontic bands and arch wires. Endodontic treatment is often required in the future for these teeth.

Avulsed teeth

A permanent tooth that has been completely dislodged (avulsed) from the alveolus can be replanted with varying degrees of success. A big factor in the

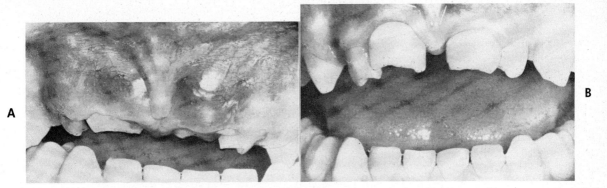

Fig. 23-8. Traumatic intrusion. **A,** Intruded incisor. **B,** Reeruption. (From Law, D., and others: An atlas of pedodontics, Philadelphia, 1969, W.B. Saunders Co.)

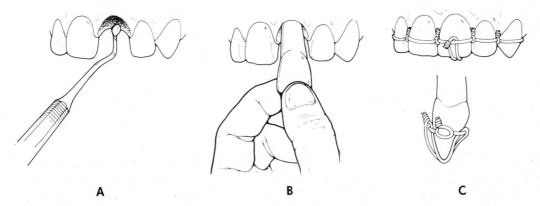

Fig. 23-9. Treatment of avulsed tooth. **A,** Clotted blood is removed from alveolus with surgical curette. **B,** Avulsed tooth is inserted and positioned in alveolus. **C,** Tooth is splinted in place with wire, acrylic, or orthodontic splints.

success or failure in a replantation procedure is the amount of time that elapses between avulsion and replantation. One study* demonstrated that a 90% success rate was achieved when an avulsed tooth was replanted within 20 minutes after the accident. The success rate dropped to 43% when replantation was attempted after 90 minutes. The essence of this study is to point out the need for parents and school officials to notify the dentist immediately when a youngster has a tooth dislodged from the alveolus. The more

*Andreason, J.O., and Hjorting-Hansen, E.: Replantation of teeth. I. Radiographic and clinical study of 110 human teeth replanted after accidental loss, Acta Odontol. Scand. **24:**263-286, 1966.

quickly the tooth can be replanted, the greater the chances for success.

If such an injury should occur, parents should be instructed to recover the tooth immediately, wrap it in a moistened gauze, and come straight to the office. The child should be given a small gauze or tissue pad to bite on over the alveolus to control bleeding while en route to the office.

The replantation procedure is as follows:

1. Anesthesia is administered.
2. The alveolus is cleared of clotted blood with a surgical curette (Fig. 23-9, *A*).
3. The avulsed tooth is washed in saline solution and inserted into the alveolus (Fig. 23-9, *B*).

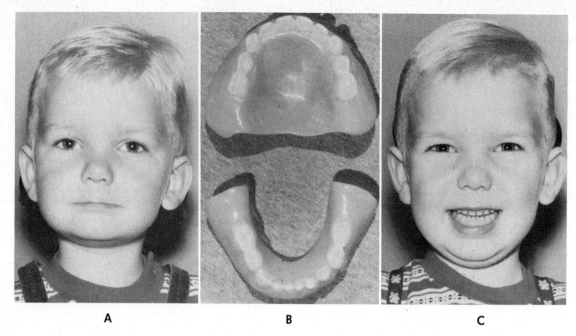

Fig. 23-10. Replacement of all primary teeth with a complete denture. **A,** Patient without denture. **B,** Complete dentures. **C,** Dentures in place. (From Law, D., and others: An atlas of pedodontics, Philadelphia, 1969, W.B. Saunders Co.)

4. The tooth is splinted in place with wire, acrylic, or orthodontic splints (Fig. 23-9, *C*).
5. Both preoperative and postoperative radiographs are taken.
6. Endodontic treatment* is carried out 6 to 8 weeks after replantation.

Avulsed primary teeth are usually not replanted.

PROSTHODONTICS FOR CHILDREN

Removable partial dentures and even complete dentures are sometimes necessary to replace missing teeth in the child. The use of the removable partial denture appliance is most often limited to the replacement of more than one tooth, unless the missing tooth is in the maxillary anterior and esthetics would be greatly improved (Fig. 23-7).

Children's primary teeth may be missing because of (1) lack of development of the teeth (congenitally

missing), (2) developmental diseases of the teeth, resulting in extraction, or (3) premature loss of teeth caused by caries or trauma. The number of missing teeth may range from one to all of the teeth. The treatment for missing teeth varies from no treatment at all to space-maintaining appliances, to partial dentures, and to complete dentures if all the primary teeth are missing (Fig. 23-10). The dentist has to judge each case individually to determine the appropriate treatment plan.

PREVENTIVE DENTISTRY FOR CHILDREN

The presence of dental caries in patients under 20 years old is of staggering proportions. The only rational approach to conquering the problem is to emphasize the benefits of a preventive program to all patients including children.

Diet control, oral hygiene procedures, and the use of fluorides and pit and fissure sealants all play an important role in preventive dentistry for the young (Chapters 1 and 2).

Youngsters who engage in athletic activities should

---

*Some dentists prefer to do the endodontic procedure on the tooth before replantation. Although this is convenient, it does involve more handling of the avulsed tooth and a delay of time before replantation is done.

be encouraged to wear protective mouth guards to help prevent traumatic injuries to oral structures.

INTERCEPTIVE ORTHODONTICS

For a discussion of interceptive orthodontics, see Chapter 24, p. 334.

BIBLIOGRAPHY

Andreason, J.O., and Hjorting-Hansen, E.: Replantation of teeth. I. Radiographic and clinical study of 110 human teeth replanted after accidental loss, Acta Odontol. Scand. **24:**263-286, 1966.

Finn, S.: Clinical pedodontics, Philadelphia, 1957, W.B. Saunders Co.

Law, D.B., et al.: An atlas of pedodontics, Philadelphia, 1969, W.B. Saunders Co.

McDonald, R.E., and Avery, D.R.: Dentistry for the child and adolescent, St. Louis, ed. 4, 1983, The C.V. Mosby Co.

Pike, J.S.: Patient and parent management in dentistry for children, J. Ala. Dent. Assoc. **56:**20-23, Oct., 1972.

Till, M.J., and Brearley, L.J.: Communicating with children, North West Dent. **50:**392-397, 1971.

CHAPTER 24

ORTHODONTICS

Orthodontics is a specialty area of dentistry that deals with problems related to the undesirable development of the jaws, the positions of the teeth, and the oral and facial muscles that influence speech, mastication, and swallowing. Patients often seek orthodontic treatment simply to improve their own appearance by having their teeth repositioned, whereas orthodontists (specialists in orthodontics) concern themselves not only with a patient's appearance, but also with the functional aspects of chewing, swallowing, and speech mechanisms. Although orthodontists provide treatment for complex cases, it is common practice for pedodontists and general practitioners to provide preventive and interceptive orthodontic services for their patients.

ETIOLOGY OF ORTHODONTIC PROBLEMS

The etiology, or causes, of orthodontic problems can be grouped into three basic categories. These categories are (1) hereditary influences, (2) systemic influences, and (3) local influences.

Hereditary influences

Since a child is a biological product of two different adults, the child often displays characteristics unique to one or both of the parents. This is true of oral facial characteristics. Therefore a variety of discrepancies can occur that are genetic in origin. Some of these discrepancies are as follows:

1. *Poor tooth-jaw ratio*. A child can have teeth that are not the proper size to match the size of his jaws. Simply stated, the teeth may be either too large or too small for the jaws of the child.

2. *Poor skeletal relationships*. The maxilla and the mandible may not grow in harmony with each other. A child can have one jaw grow so that it is larger than the other, which causes both functional and esthetic problems. The disharmony in growth may result in a mismatch of the jaws in an anteroposterior or lateral direction, in the vertical distance between upper and lower jaws, or in combinations of these disharmonies. In other words, the jaws may not be in proper alignment with each other, or both jaws are not aligned properly in relation to the rest of the skeletal portion of the head.

3. *Miscellaneous discrepancies*. There are a variety of other hereditary problems that can influence the orthodontic status of an individual. Some of these are as follows:

   a. Deformed teeth
   b. Congenitally missing teeth
   c. Supernumerary teeth
   d. Cleft palate
   e. Abnormal jaw shape
   f. Abnormal eruption of teeth
   g. Abnormal exfoliation of teeth
   h. Excessive tongue size
   i. Inadequate lip size
   j. Improper frenum development

Any combination of these discrepancies can occur because a child is a product of two individuals who each contribute genetically to the characteristics of the child.

Systemic influences

A variety of systemic conditions can influence the development of the teeth, jaws, and muscles. Among these are nutritional deficiencies, infectious diseases, and endocrine (hormonal) disturbances. These systemic influences can affect the development of tissues, affect the eruption pattern of the teeth, and influence the susceptibility of the child to dental caries. Any of these influences can contribute to an orthodontic problem.

Local influences

After birth, an individual is subject to a variety of conditions that can contribute to the development of orthodontic problems in varying degrees of severity. Some of the more common conditions are as follows:

1. Premature loss of primary teeth
2. Overretained primary teeth
3. Loss of permanent teeth
4. Injuries
5. Habits
6. Abnormal growths and cysts that occur in the jaws, putting pressure on teeth and displacing them from their normal positions

The etiology of orthodontic problems is varied and complex. The purpose of this brief summary is to introduce dental assistants to some of the possible factors involved in the cause of orthodontic problems so that assistants may be better able to understand and assist the dentist during treatment.

DIAGNOSIS

The object of diagnostic procedures is to identify what is wrong with a patient so that appropriate treatment can be carried out. In the field of orthodontics, diagnostic procedures are geared toward the evaluation of the teeth and the skeletal relationships of the head, as well as the surrounding oral and facial soft tissues. Some of these procedures will be discussed here.

Of primary concern to the dentist making an orthodonic diagnosis is the patient's occlusion. Occlusion is the relationship of the maxillary and mandibular teeth when they are in contact. To diagnose an orthodontic problem, the orthodontist uses the characteristics of a normal occlusion as a reference. A general description of a normal occlusion is as follows:

1. The term *normal* implies that the occlusion does not deviate from the average patient on a statistical basis.

2. Mandibular teeth are in maximum contact with the maxillary teeth throughout the entire dentition.

3. The maxillary anterior teeth should overlap the mandibular anterior teeth by approximately 1 to 2 mm (overbite). The labial surfaces of these maxillary teeth should not be more than 1 to 2 mm anterior to the mandibular anterior teeth (overjet) (Fig. 24-1, *A*). There should be contact between the upper and lower anterior teeth.

4. The maxillary posterior teeth are located one cusp buccal to the mandibular posterior teeth (Fig. 24-1, *B*).

5. The mesiobuccal cusp of the maxillary first permanent molar should rest in the mesiobuccal groove of the mandibular first permanent molar (Fig. 24-1, *C*).

6. The cusp tip of the maxillary cuspids should rest between the mandibular cuspid and the first premolar when the teeth are brought together (Fig. 24-1, *C*).

7. There should be no rotated teeth or abnormal spaces between the teeth (diastemas).

Malocclusion is any deviation from normal occlusion. Malocclusion may result from the improper jaw relationships described previously, from malposed teeth, or from a combination of both, which is generally the case.

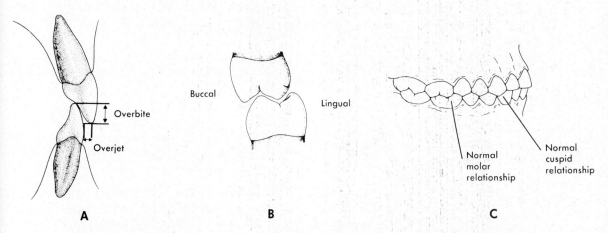

Fig. 24-1. Characteristics of "normal" occlusion. **A,** Normal overbite and overjet. **B,** Buccolingual relationship of posterior teeth. **C,** Anteroposterior relationship of upper and lower permanent first molars and cuspids.

It is rare that a patient has an absolutely ideal occlusion. However, dentists generally classify a patient's occlusion as normal if the relationships just described exist to the extent that the patient has a favorable chewing mechanism, has an acceptable appearance from a dental standpoint, and has no potential for injury to other tissues present. Since "normal" occlusion is unique to the individual and is rarely an ideal occlusion, some dentists prefer to substitute the term *satisfactory* for "normal" occlusion.

Angle's classification of malocclusion

To establish a common terminology that can be used to describe common forms of malocclusion, Edward Angle established a classification system in 1899 that is still in common use today. Angle established three broad classes of malocclusion, using as a reference the relationship of the maxillary and mandibular first permanent molars when the jaws are closed. The classification system is as follows:

Class I malocclusion (Figs. 24-2, *A* and 24-3, *A*)

1. The mesiobuccal cusp of the maxillary first permanent molar rests in the mesiobuccal groove of the mandibular first permanent molar.
2. The cusp tip of the maxillary cuspid rests between the mandibular cuspid and the first premolar.
3. The jaws are in a normal relationship.
4. There is some dental discrepancy, such as malposed teeth, excessive spacing, missing teeth, open bite, overbite, crossbite, or unerupted teeth. The presence of one or more of these discrepancies differentiates between a normal occlusion and a Class I malocclusion.

Class II malocclusion (Figs. 24-2, *B* and 24-3, *B*)

1. The molar relationship differs from normal in that the distobuccal cusp of the maxillary first permanent molar rests in the mesiobuccal groove of the mandibular first permanent molar.
2. The maxillary cuspid is located mesial to the mandibular cuspid.
3. The lower jaw is retruded relative to the upper jaw.
4. Dental discrepancies frequently exist. Crowding of teeth, deep overbites, tipped incisors, and overlapped maxillary lateral incisors are commonly found in this class of malocclusion.

The Class II malocclusion is divided into two divisions based on the relationship of the maxillary incisor teeth:

Class II–Division 1 malocclusion

1. Jaw, molar, and cuspid relationships are as just described for the Class II malocclusion.

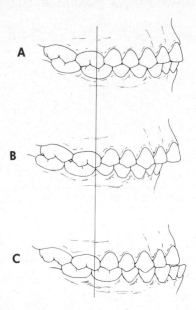

Fig. 24-2. Angle's classes of malocclusion. **A,** Class I. **B,** Class II. **C,** Class III.

2. The maxillary incisors are tipped in extreme labioversion (toward the lip) (Fig. 24-3, *B*).

Class II–Division 2 malocclusion

1. Jaw, molar, and cuspid relationships are as just described for the Class II malocclusion.
2. The maxillary central incisors are in a near normal position or tipped slightly in linguoversion (toward the tongue). The maxillary lateral incisors are tipped labially and mesially. They often overlap the adjacent central incisors (Fig. 24-3, *C*).

Class III malocclusion (Figs. 24-2, *C* and 24-3, *D*).

1. The mesiobuccal cusp of the maxillary first permanent molar rests distal to the mandibular first permanent molar.
2. The maxillary cuspid is in an exaggerated distal relationship to the mandibular cuspid.
3. The lower jaw is protruded relative to the upper jaw.
4. Dental discrepancies can exist. Crossbites are frequently found in Class III malocclusions.

Common dental discrepancies

There are a variety of dental discrepancies that can be found in any of the classes of malocclusion just described. Dental discrepancies are irregularities that are associated with the teeth. These discrepancies are variations in the positions of the teeth in the jaws, the

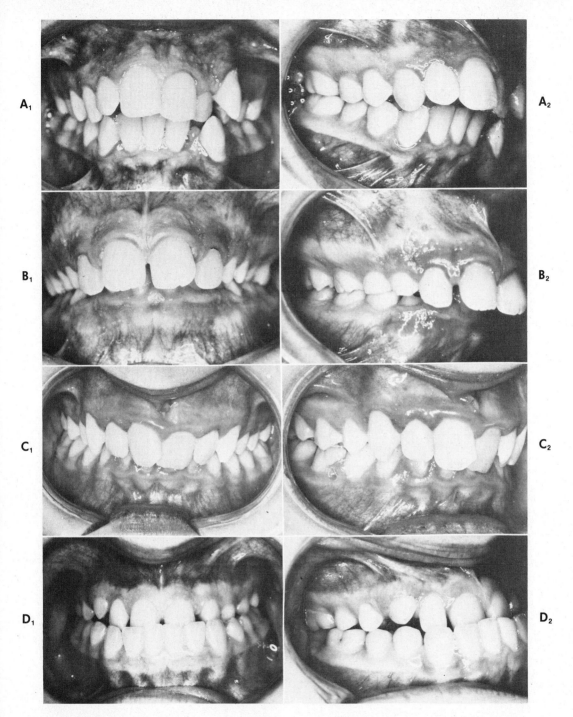

Fig. 24-3. Clinical examples of Angle's classes of malocclusion (anterior and lateral views). **A,** Class I. **B,** Class II, Division 1. **C,** Class II, Division 2. **D,** Class III.

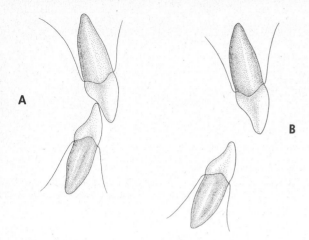

Fig. 24-4. Anterior open bite. **A,** Normal incisor relationship. **B,** Open bite when posterior teeth are occluded.

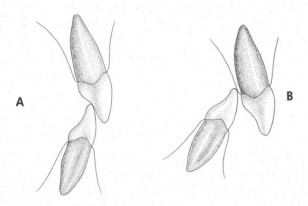

Fig. 24-5. Impinging overbite. **A,** Normal. **B,** Deep and impinging overbite.

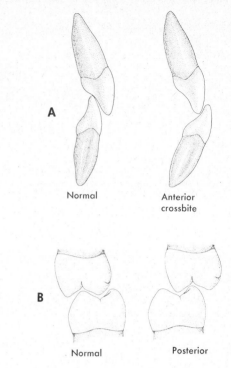

Fig. 24-6. Crossbite. **A,** Anterior teeth; normal and crossbite. **B,** Posterior teeth; normal and crossbite.

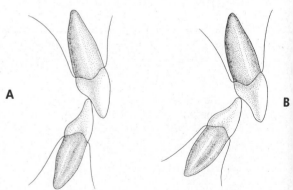

Fig. 24-7. Overjet. **A,** Normal. **B,** Excessive.

number of teeth present, or the size or shape of the teeth.

Aside from the more obvious discrepancies such as supernumerary, missing, malformed, and rotated teeth, there are some that require further description.

open bite When the jaws are closed the mandibular anterior teeth should contact the lingual surfaces of the maxillary anterior teeth. If they do not, an open bite exists (Fig. 24-4). Open bites can also exist in posterior areas but are more frequently found in anterior areas (Fig. 24-21).

overbite The amount of overlap of the upper anterior teeth over the lower anterior teeth is called overbite. If the over-

lapping is excessive, it is referred to as a deep overbite. If the incisal edges of the lower anterior teeth contact the soft tissue of the palate, the patient is said to have an impinging overbite (Fig. 24-5).

crossbite In normal occlusion the upper teeth overlap the lower teeth buccally or labially. If the opposite exists, that is, if the lower teeth overlap the upper teeth, the teeth are in crossbite (Fig. 24-6). Crossbite can be limited to one or more teeth in either the anterior or posterior regions of the dental arches.

overjet The distance between the labial surface of a maxillary incisor and the mandibular incisor in an anterior-posterior dimension is called overjet (Fig. 24-7). If this distance is increased as a result of malposition of the incisors, the patient is described as having an excessive overjet. The common and somewhat unkind term "buckteeth" refers to an excessive overjet condition.

Tooth positions

There are common terms that are used in orthodontics to describe abnormal tooth positions. This terminology adds the suffix *-version* to a root word to indicate in what direction from normal a tooth (or teeth) is positioned. The following are some common terms used to describe abnormal tooth positions.

mesioversion Mesial to normal position
distoversion Distal to normal position
linguoversion Lingual to normal position
labioversion Labial to normal position
buccoversion Buccal to normal position

The dental assistant's understanding of the classification system and of terminology associated with the diagnosis of orthodontic conditions facilitates communication with the dentist and the patient and aids in recording information on dental records and in referral letters.

Radiography

Both intraoral and extraoral radiographs are used in the diagnosis of orthodontic conditions. The following are some of the most common radiographs that are used to document the patient's condition:

1. Panoramic radiograph (Fig. 3-4, *C*)
2. Cephalometric radiographs: (a) lateral view (Fig. 24-8); (b) anterior-posterior view (not shown)
3. Posterior bite-wing radiographs (Fig. 3-4, *B*)

Some orthodontists use radiographs of young patients' wrists to analyze individual growth status.

A cephalometric radiograph is taken using a cephalostat. The cephalostat is a unit that holds the patient's head in a stationary position relative to the x-ray source (Fig. 24-9). This device allows the dentist to take a series of cephalometric radiographs from a standard position so that the developmental pattern in the skull can be compared as the patient grows or as treatment is rendered. These radiographs can be com-

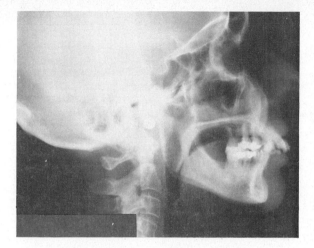

Fig. 24-8. Cephalometric radiograph (lateral view).

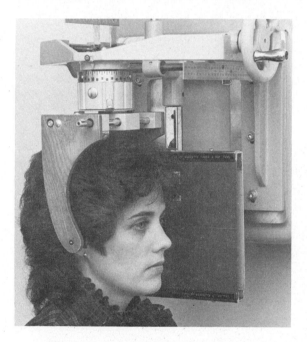

Fig. 24-9. Patient positioned in cephalostat.

pared over a period of time to assess not only the growth pattern of the patient, but also the effect orthodontic therapy is having on skeletal development.

Photography

Photographs are generally considered a mandatory part of the orthodontic patient record. Both intraoral

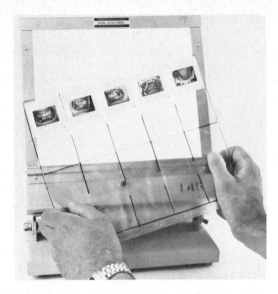

Fig. 24-10. Slide holder for storage of slide photographs.

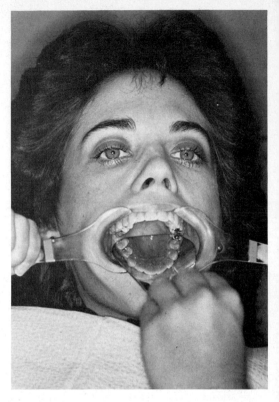

Fig. 24-11. Cheek retractors and intraoral photographic mirror in use.

and extraoral views of the patient's head are taken at the diagnostic appointment and at various intervals as treatment progresses. These photographs document the starting point in treatment and visually record the progress of treatment for both the dentist and the patient.

Slide photography is the most common form in use today. Slides are small and easy to store in a patient record. Dates that the photographs were taken can be recorded on the slide mounts for future reference (Fig. 24-10). A standard photographic series that is taken includes the following:

Extraoral
  Right lateral view
  Front view (not smiling)
  Front view (smiling)
Intraoral
  Right lateral view (teeth occluded)
  Front view (teeth occluded)
  Left lateral view (teeth occluded)
  Maxillary occlusal view (mouth open)
  Mandibular occlusal view (mouth open)

Soft tissue retractors and large intraoral mirrors are used to gain access to the intraoral view that is required (Fig. 24-11). The air-water syringe is used to dry the teeth just before the photograph is taken, to improve the detail in the picture. A dental assistant can hold these devices with the help of the patient while the orthodontist or another assistant operates the camera. The orthodontist can view patient photographs to analyze tooth relationships, skeletal contours, and the soft tissue configuration of a patient.

Study models (Fig. 24-12)

A discussion of study models is presented on p. 40. It should be emphasized that study models provide the dentist with a unique three-dimensional record of the patient's dentition and contour of the alveolar processes. Study models are the only diagnostic tool that a dentist has that will permit a view of the lingual aspect of the patient's occlusion. Like photographs, study models can be used to document the starting point of treatment and record the progress of treatment as subsequent sets of models are taken.

Making study models. Since many states permit dental assistants to take impressions for study models, a description of a technique will be presented here:

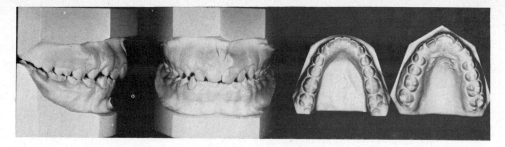

Fig. 24-12. Study models.

Materials required (Fig. 24-13)
1. Alginate material is generally used for this technique.
2. Impression trays are selected to fit the size and shape of the patient's dental arches (various types are available).
3. Rope-style utility wax is used to extend the vertical height of the trays to record the shape of the alveolar processes.
4. The material is mixed in a flexible rubber bowl with a still wide-bladed spatula.

Impression technique
1. Try each of the impression trays in the patient's mouth to determine the appropriate size and shape of the impression tray. There should be 3 to 4 mm of space between the inside of the tray and the teeth and soft tissue when the tray is in place.
2. Press soft rope-shaped utility wax onto the edges of the trays to extend their vertical height (Fig. 24-14, *A*). Try the trays again to confirm the fit.
3. Mix the alginate material with water for one impression at a time in the flexible rubber bowl according to the manufacturer's instructions. The wide-bladed spatula is used to press the material against the side of the bowl to create a smooth, creamy mix that is free of air bubbles. Mixing time is approximately 1 minutes (Fig. 24-14, *B*).
4. Instruct the patient to rinse vigorously with mouthwash to remove thick saliva and food particles that can cause voids on the surface of the impression.
5. Load the maxillary tray with the mixed material as the patient rinses with mouthwash. The tray should be loaded in one large increment with a wiping motion of the spatula to avoid trapping air in the material.
6. Wipe off excess material to the level of the waxed edges of the tray, using a wet finger to smooth the surface of the material (Fig. 24-14, *C*).
7. With the patient seated in an upright position use the left index finger to retract the patient's right cheek. Insert the loaded tray into the patient's mouth and use it to push the patient's left cheek out of the way (Fig. 24-14, *D*).

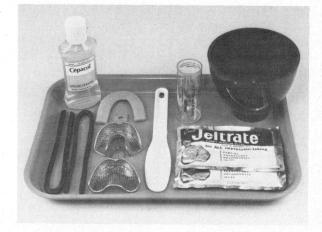

Fig. 24-13. Armamentarium for alginate impression taking.

8. Once the tray is in the patient's mouth, center it over the teeth. Press the posterior border of the tray up against the posterior border of the hard palate to form a seal (Fig. 24-14, *E*).
9. While maintaining this palatal seal, rotate the anterior portion of the tray upward slowly over the teeth. Use your left hand to lift the patient's lips and cheeks out of the way as the tray is seated completely. This retraction process allows the alginate material to flow upward into the vestibular fold areas (Fig. 24-14, *F*).
10. Pull the upper lip over the anterior portion of the tray to shape the anterior border of the impression once the tray is seated (Fig. 24-14, *G*). Average working time to accomplish this task is 1½ minutes. After this the material begins to set.
11. Check the posterior border of the tray to be sure that excess material has not escaped from the tray into the patient's throat area. If necessary, excess material can be quickly wiped away with a mouth mirror. Have the

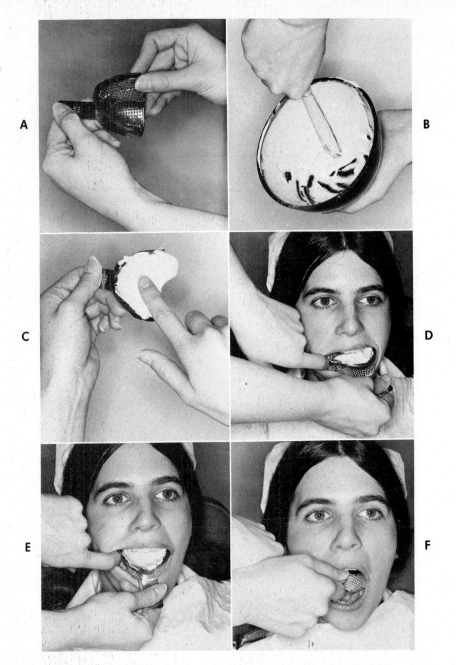

Fig. 24-14. Alginate impression taking. **A,** Trimming tray with utility wax. **B,** Mixing alginate. **C,** Smoothing surface of alginate. **D,** Tray insertion. **E,** Seating posterior border of tray. **F,** Lifting tray upward into place.

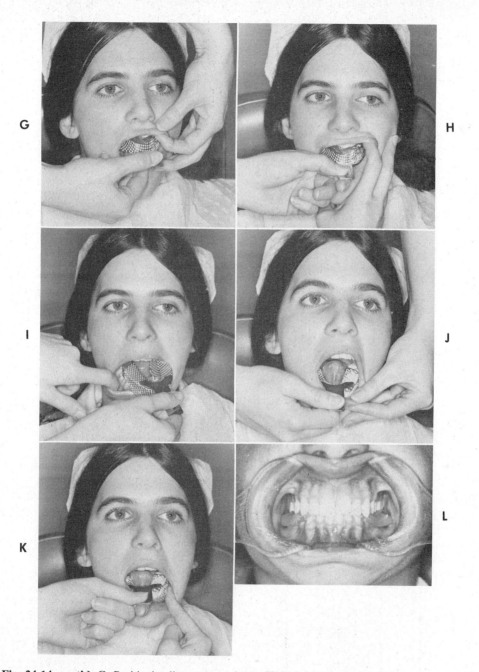

Fig. 24-14, cont'd. G, Positioning lip over seated tray. **H,** Releasing seal when alginate has set. **I,** Inserting lower tray. **J,** Positioning lip over seated tray. **K,** Releasing seal when alginate has set. **L,** Taking wax bite.

patient tip the head downward and breathe through the nose as the material sets. Hold the tray in place until the material has completely set.

12. Once the material has set, remove the tray by placing a finger along a lateral border of the tray and pushing downward to break the seal formed by the set material (Fig. 24-14, *H*). Remove the tray from the patient's mouth, rinse it with room temperature water and wrap it in a moist paper towel. Rinse the patient's mouth to remove residual impression material.

13. The mandibular impression is taken in a similar manner. In addition to retracting the lips and cheeks when the tray is inserted in the mouth, instruct the patient to life the tongue to permit the material to register an impression of the lingual aspect of the alveolar process (Fig. 24-14, *I*).

14. Once the tray is centered, press down the posterior border behind the last molars to form a seal. The anterior portion of the tray is rotated downward as the lips and cheeks are retracted.

15. After the tray is seated, pull the lower lip upward over the anterior portion of the impression tray (Fig. 24-14, *J*).

16. Once the material has set, the impression can be removed by lifting a posterior border of the tray upward to break the seal (Fig. 24-14, *K*).

17. Rinse the patient's mouth. Impressions should be poured as soon as possible.

18. A wax bite is recommended to aid in the trimming phase of study model fabrication. Instruct the patient to bite into a softened horseshoe-shaped piece of wax until the teeth are in maximum occlusion. Allow the wax to cool and then remove it from the patient's mouth. It is stored with the study models until it is needed during model trimming (Fig. 24-14, *L*).

Clinical evaluation

The clinical examination of a patient provides the dentist with an opportunity to analyze the patient's skeletal and facial profile, speech, swallowing pattern, and jaw movements as well as an examination of the patient's dentition. The occlusion is classified at the examination appointment and recorded along with other clinical data.

INTERCEPTIVE ORTHODONTICS

Interceptive orthodontics is a term used to describe various treatment procedures designed to intercept certain orthodontic problems that may develop if left untreated. Not all orthodontic problems can be prevented. However, many can be prevented entirely, or at the very least minimized in terms of severity through interceptive measures.

Interceptive orthodontic procedures have limitations. They do not, for example, alter skeletal disharmonies resulting from an undesirable growth pattern of the child. These procedures can be viewed as treatment techniques that assist in the development of a normal occlusion or at least in minimizing the severity of a developing malocclusion.

Following are some common interceptive orthodontic techniques:

Space maintenance
Space regaining
Crossbite correction
Habit control

The dentition stages

Before discussing interceptive orthodontics, it is necessary to review the basic principles of the development of the dentitions. Table 24-1 outlines the development and eruption sequence of the dentitions according to age.

Primary dentition stage. The function of the primary dentition is to aid in mastication and speech, provide favorable esthetics, and aid in guiding the eruption of the permanent teeth into proper position.

The primary dentition stage usually begins at 6 months of age, with the eruption of the mandibular central incisors, and ends at approximately 6 years when the first permanent tooth erupts. The primary dentition has usually completed eruption by 24 months of age. The typical sequence* of eruption of primary teeth is (1) central incisors, (2) lateral incisors, (3) first molars, (4) canines, and (5) second molars.

While the child remains in the primary dentition stage, the permanent teeth are developing in the jaws. At approximately 6 years of age the onset of the mixed dentition stage is marked by the loss of a primary tooth, eruption of the first permanent molars, or the eruption of permanent incisors. The permanent first molars erupt just distal to the primary second molars. An important function of the primary second molars is to help guide these permanent first molars into proper position during their eruption. If a second primary molar is lost prematurely because of dental caries, it cannot serve this important function. Then the permanent first molar can erupt out of position, and a discrepancy in the occlusion results (Fig. 24-15,

---

*The mandibular member of each type of tooth usually erupts before its maxillary counterpart; for example, the mandibular central incisors erupt before the maxillary central incisors. Next, the mandibular lateral incisors erupt, and so on.

Table 24-1. Chronology of the human dentition

Tooth	Hard tissue formation begins	Amount of enamel formed at birth	Enamel completed	Eruption	Root completed
Deciduous dentition					
Maxillary					
Central incisor	4 mo, in utero	Five-sixths	1½ mo	7½ mo	1½ yr
Lateral incisor	4½ mo, in utero	Two-thirds	2½ mo	9 mo	2 yr
Cupsid	5 mo, in utero	One-third	9 mo	18 mo	3¼ yr
First molar	5 mo, in utero	Cusps united	6 mo	14 mo	2½ yr
Second molar	6 mo, in utero	Cusp tips still isolated	11 mo	24 mo	3 yr
Mandibular					
Central incisor	4½ mo, in utero	Three-fifths	2½ mo	6 mo	1½ yr
Lateral incisor	4½ mo, in utero	Three-fifths	3 mo	7 mo	1½ yr
Cuspid	5 mo, in utero	One-third	9 mo	16 mo	3¼ yr
First molar	5 mo, in utero	Cusps united	5½ mo	12 mo	2¼ yr
Second molar	6 mo, in utero	Cusp tips still isolated	10 mo	20 mo	3 yr
Permanent dentition					
Maxillary					
Central incisor	3-4 mo	—	4-5 yr	7-8 yr	10 yr
Lateral incisor	10-12 mo	—	4-5 yr	8-9 yr	11 yr
Cuspid	4-5 mo	—	6-7 yr	11-12 yr	13-15 yr
First bicuspid	1½-1¾ yr	—	5-6 yr	10-11 yr	12-13 yr
Second bicuspid	2-2¼ yr	—	6-7 yr	10-12 yr	12-14 yr
First molar	At birth	Sometimes a trace	2½-3 yr	6-7 yr	9-10 yr
Second molar	2½-3 yr	—	7-8 yr	12-13 yr	14-16 yr
Third molar	7-9 yr	—	12-16 yr	17-21 yr	18-25 yr
Mandibular					
Central incisor	3-4 mo	—	4-5 yr	6-7 yr	9 yr
Lateral incisor	3-4 mo	—	4-5 yr	7-8 yr	10 yr
Cuspid	4-5 mo	—	6-7 yr	9-10 yr	12-14 yr
First bicuspid	1¾-2 yr	—	5-6 yr	10-12 yr	12-13 yr
Second bicuspid	2¼-2½ yr	—	6-7 yr	11-12 yr	13-14 yr
First molar	At birth	Sometimes a trace	2½-3 yr	6-7 yr	9-10 yr
Second molar	2½-3 yr	—	7-8 yr	11-13 yr	14-15 yr
Third molar	8-10 yr	—	12-16 yr	17-21 yr	18-25 yr

From Logan, W.H.G., and Kronfeld, R.: Development of the human jaws and surrounding structures from birth to the age of fifteen years, J. Am. Dent. Assoc. **20:**379-427, 1933. Copyright by the American Dental Association. Reprinted by permission.

A and *B*). Such discrepancies might include shifting of the first permanent molar in a mesial direction, which can cause occlusal interferences with opposing teeth, impaction of the developing second premolar, or the eruption of the second premolar in an abnormal position (ectopic eruption). This situation emphasizes the need to preserve the primary teeth whenever possible.

Mixed dentition stage. Once the first permanent tooth erupts, the child continues to have a dentition that is a combination of permanent and primary teeth. Hence the name mixed dentition stage.

As the child ages and jaw growth occurs, the primary teeth are exfoliated (shed) and replaced by newly erupted permanent teeth. The exfoliation of the primary teeth occurs in the same sequence as the eruption of their permanent replacements. The eruption sequence of the permanent teeth usually follows the order shown in Table 24-2.

The mixed dentition is probably the most critical stage of development for the permanent occlusion. The timing of the exfoliation of a primary tooth is rather critical, especially in the posterior areas. A posterior primary tooth must be kept in place until the

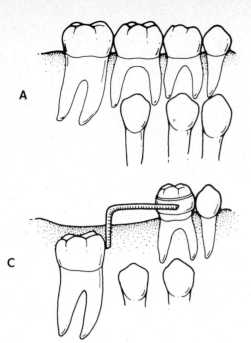

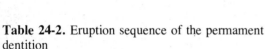

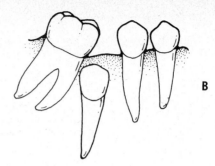

Fig. 24-15. Effects of premature loss of primary second molar. **A,** Normal eruption. **B,** Loss of primary second molar results in mesial shifting of permanent first molar. This can prevent normal eruption of permanent second premolar. **C,** Distal shoe appliance inserted after loss of primary second molar to guide eruption of permanent first molar into proper position.

Table 24-2. Eruption sequence of the permament dentition

Permanent teeth	Primary teeth replaced
Mandibular first molars	None; erupt distal to primary teeth
Maxillary first molars	
Mandibular central and lateral incisors	Mandibular central and lateral incisors
Maxillary central incisors	Maxillary central incisors
Maxillary lateral incisors	Maxillary lateral incisors
Mandibular canines	Mandibular canines
Mandibular first premolars	Mandibular first molars
Maxillary first premolars	Maxillary first molars
Mandibular second premolars	Mandibular second molars
Maxillary second premolars	Maxillary second molars
Maxillary canines	Maxillary canines
Mandibular second molars	None; erupt distal to primary teeth as jaws grow
Maxillary second molars	
Mandibular third molars	
Maxillary third molars	

permanent tooth that replaces it is ready to erupt. If a posterior primary tooth is lost too soon, the teeth adjacent to the tooth can drift into the empty space (Fig. 24-16). If this occurs, there is insufficient space left in the dental arch for the proper eruption of the under-lying permanent tooth when it is time for it to erupt. The result is that the permanent tooth may erupt in an undesirable position (be malposed) or it may not erupt at all (be impacted) because of insufficient space in the arch. Thus a discrepancy in the occlusion results.

A similar situation can result if a primary tooth is not exfoliated just before the eruption of its permanent replacement. These "overretained" primary teeth may prevent the eruption of the underlying permanent tooth or cause it to erupt in an undesirable (ectopic) position.

The dentist plays an important role in supervising the development of the occlusion of the child by seeing to it that the timing of the exfoliation of primary teeth corresponds with the eruption of their permanent counterparts. Caries prevention and restoration of decayed primary teeth become an integral part of preservation of the primary teeth so that the transition from the primary to the permanent dentition proceeds smoothly.

Permanent dentition stage. The permanent dentition should be completed by age 25, with the eruption of the third molars. However, in a great number of patients these teeth never erupt, since sufficient jaw space is lacking. The principal goal in dentistry is to preserve permanent teeth for a lifetime.

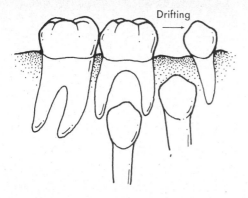

Fig. 24-16. Effect of premature loss of primary first molar.

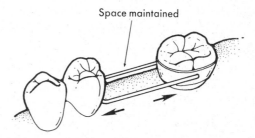

Fig. 24-17. Band and loop–style space maintainer.

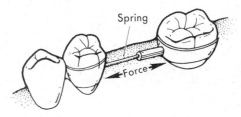

Fig. 24-19. Spring-activated space-regaining appliance.

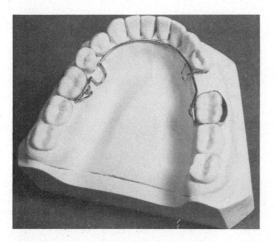

Fig. 24-18. Bilateral space maintainer, the "loop lingual appliance."

Common interceptive techniques

Space maintenance. If the child should lose primary teeth prematurely, the dentist has to prevent adjacent teeth from drifting into the empty (edentulous) space. This is accomplished through the use of devices called space maintainers. These are either removable or fixed appliances that provide a brace between the teeth adjacent to the edentulous space (Fig. 24-17). Space maintainers are kept in place until the eruption of the underlying permanent tooth begins. Thus they perform a function of the primary tooth had it not been lost prematurely.

If a primary second molar is lost before 6 years of age (before the eruption of the permanent first molar), a "distal shoe" space maintainer may be placed to guide the eruption of the permanent first molar into place (Fig. 24-15, *C*). The "shoe" portion of the maintainer is inserted into an incision just mesial to the unerupted first permanent molar and will guide the permanent tooth into proper position as it erupts. This space maintainer is often placed at the time of the extraction of the primary tooth, so that an incision into the soft tissue is unnecessary. The soft tissue will heal around the shoe.

When primary molars are lost on both sides of the arch, a bilateral space maintainer can be used (Fig. 24-18).

Sometimes the dentist may not see a child until long after a primary tooth is lost and the adjacent teeth have drifted into the edentulous space. Space maintainers could have prevented this. After drifting has occurred, the dentist is faced with the challenge of regaining the space.

Space regaining. Space-regaining appliances apply forces to teeth that have drifted out of place (Fig. 24-19). These malposed teeth can be returned to their proper position and held there until permanent teeth erupt.

The ideal management of a child's developing oc-

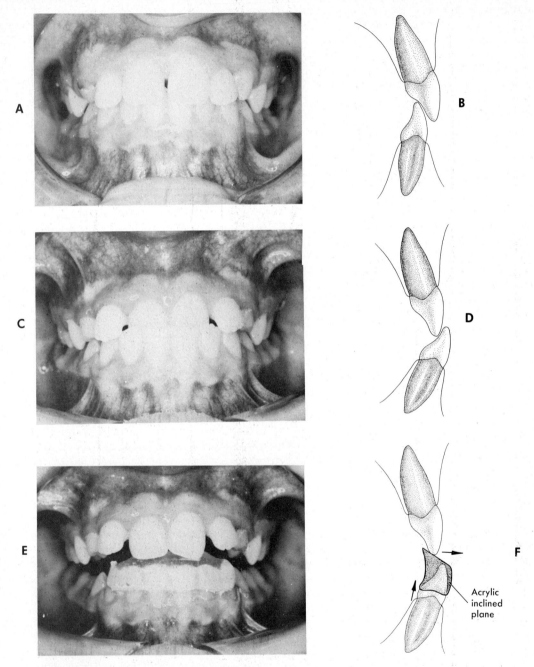

Fig. 24-20. A and **B,** Incisors in normal occlusion (anterior and lateral views). **C** and **D,** Anterior crossbite of maxillary central incisors. **E** and **F,** Acrylic inclined plane in place (anterior and lateral views). (**A, C,** and **E** courtesy Dr. D.R. Balbach, Ann Arbor, Mich.)

clusion is to preserve the primary teeth by vigorous caries prevention. Restoration of carious primary teeth is the second best approach to preservation of the primary teeth. If a primary tooth is lost prematurely, the third best procedure is use of space-maintainer appliances to prevent drifting and space loss. Finally, the least desirable management procedure is to regain the lost space caused by drifting.

Typically the mixed dentition stage ends when the child is approximately 11 or 12 years old, with the eruption of the permanent maxillary canines that replace the remaining primary canines.

Crossbite correction. Normal occlusion calls for the facial aspects of the maxillary teeth to be located labial to the mandibular teeth when the jaws are brought together (Fig. 24-20, *A* and *B*). Maxillary teeth that are located lingual to mandibular teeth when the jaws are closed are said to be in crossbite (Fig. 24-20, *C* and *D*).

Simple anterior crossbites that are present in children with normal jaw relationships can often be easily treated without extensive orthodontic treatment. One method of treatment is the use of the acrylic inclined plane (Fig. 24-20, *E* and *F*). The patient must have space for the malposed teeth to be moved into proper position. Once this is accomplished, an inclined plane of acrylic is cemented on the mandibular anterior teeth. Only the teeth in crossbite contact the inclined plane when the jaws are closed. The force applied to the teeth plus the direction of the inclined plane will guide the teeth into proper position. This process may require only a few days to a few weeks. Once the incisal edges of the maxillary teeth are located labial to the incisal edges of the mandibular anterior teeth, the inclined plane can be removed.

Habit control. Oral habits such as thumb-sucking and tongue thrusting involve abnormal muscle behavior that can have a damaging effect on the growth of the jaws, the developing occlusion, facial contour, and speech. The forces produced by normal action of the muscles in the tongue, lips, and cheeks aid in the proper growth of the orofacial region. Likewise, abnormal muscle behavior can generate forces that alter normal growth. Malposed teeth, jaw malformation, and speech defects are common examples of the ill effects of abnormal muscle behavior.

Although there are many mechanical devices used to discourage undesirable oral habits, the real treatment lies in retraining muscles to function properly. Habit control is a process of retraining muscles to create normal forces on the teeth and jaws.

Thumb-sucking (and finger-sucking). There are many theories as to the origin of a thumb-sucking habit. Most of the theories relate to the behavior pattern of the infant's need to suckle to feed himself and to gain comfort and warmth from the mother. The persistence of a child's desire to suckle after infancy is often viewed as a regression to duplicate the comfort and security derived from suckling as an infant.

From a clinical point of view, this type of habit can cause malocclusion but will not do so in every instance. Some patients develop a profound malocclusion from thumb-sucking, but others experience only mild effects from the habit or none at all. This variation depends on the individual's skeletal makeup, the frequency and vigor of the habit, and the method the child uses to suck the thumb or fingers.

When malocclusion occurs as a result of thumb-sucking, it is frequently expressed in the form of an anterior open bite (Fig. 24-21). The maxillary incisors are tipped labially by the force applied by the thumb on the teeth, while the mandibular teeth may be tipped lingually (Fig. 24-22).

Thumb-suckers are often tongue-thrusters as well. The open bite that results from this habit causes the tongue to be thrust forward to create a seal behind the anterior teeth during swallowing (Fig. 24-23).

Vigorous thumb-sucking creates forces against the buccal aspects of the posterior teeth resulting from suction pulling the cheeks against these teeth. This can result in narrowing of the arch form of the jaws.

There is varied opinion on treatment of a thumb-sucking problem. Psychologists tend to endorse a "let it run its course" approach, at least until the perma-

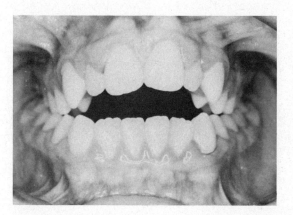

Fig. 24-21. Open bite in anterior area. (Courtesy Dr. D.R. Balbach, Ann Arbor, Mich.)

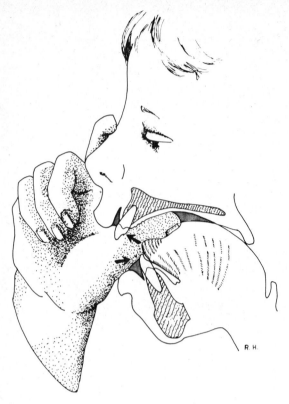

Fig. 24-22. Forces applied to anterior teeth during thumb-sucking.

nent anterior teeth erupt. It is hoped that the habit will disappear before then. Thumb-sucking is looked on by certain psychologists as a means by which a child can satisfy some basic emotional needs. Any interference with this activity by the well-meaning dentist or parents can possibly result in some form of emotional upset that may persist for many years. On the other hand, many dentists feel that once the thumb-sucking habit extends beyond 4 years of age, some corrective measures should be taken. This is the age when the habit can affect the permanent dentition. The habit itself may be a sign of a significant psychological problem in a child over 4 years of age. In either case, the child may be benefit emotionally and dentally from joint treatment from both the dentist and psychologist.

Moyers* suggests that the following be incor-

*Moyers, R.E.: Handbook of orthodontics for the student and general practitioner, ed. 2, Chicago, 1963, Year Book Medical Publishers, Inc.

porated into the approach to treatment of thumb-sucking:

1. Sincerely discuss the problem directly with the child without the presence of the parents.
2. Educate the child as to the ill effects of the habit.
3. Avoid shaming the patient and create a sincere attitude of cooperation between him and the dentist to eliminate the habit.
4. Have the child try to end the habit on his own by keeping a record of whether he sucked his thumb each day. The record is presented to the dentist at each appointment.
5. Encourage the parents to avoid any discussion of the habit with the child during treatment.
6. If this approach is unsuccessful, habit correction appliances can be inserted in the patient's mouth as a reminder to keep the thumb out. These appliances are usually arch-wire devices placed across the anterior palatal region, with small projections extending from them to discourage the placement of the thumb in this region.
7. A cooperative effort with a child psychologist or psychiatrist is indicated in severe cases.
8. Appliances should serve only as reminders to keep the thumb out of the mouth. The design of the appliance should allow normal oral function and not create embarrassment to the child.

Tongue thrusting. The tongue thrust is a habit that involves a forceful movement of the tongue against the anterior teeth during swallowing. Normal swallowing patterns involve contact of the tip of the tongue against the hard palate just lingual to the incisors (Fig. 24-23, *A*). As the swallow progresses, the tongue is elevated against the palate, forcing the contents of the mouth into the throat area, where it enters the esophagus.

An abnormal swallowing pattern or tongue thrust may be caused by discomfort in the throat area (tonsillitis, pharyngitis), or it may be a result of thumb-sucking. If a child has a chronic sore throat, the tongue will press against the painful area at the completion of the normal swallow. As the tongue stimulates the painful throat area, the mouth opens slightly, and the tongue is thrust forward away from the tender tissues. The force from the tongue being thrust forward can result in an open bite (Fig. 24-23, *B*). If the chronic irritation in the throat area persists, the child will continue tongue thrusting even after the irritation has been eliminated, because it has become a habit. Enlarged pharyngeal tonsils (adenoids) and palatine tonsils are considered by some orthodontists to be possible causes of tongue thrusting. These enlarged tissues reduce the size of the patient's airway. It is believed that patients with this condition tend to posi-

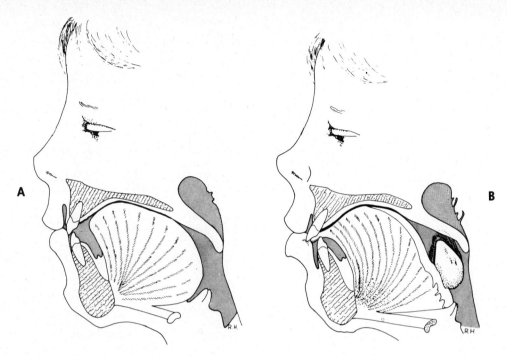

Fig. 24-23. A, Normal tongue position during swallowing. **B,** Tongue thrusting during swallowing forces maxillary anterior teeth labially.

tion their tongue more forward than normal to improve their ability to breathe.

As was noted previously, an open bite can be caused by persistent thumb-sucking. In these cases, the tongue is thrust forward to form a seal behind the anterior teeth during swallowing. This thrusting action helps to maintain the undesirable open bite.

Tongue thrusting can be observed by having the patient swallow. During the swallow, part the lips with the fingers and see whether the tongue is being thrust forward. Difficulty in keeping the lips parted during the swallow may be encountered because the muscles around the mouth and chin contract vigorously to contain the tongue within the mouth. The contraction of these muscles is helpful in the diagnosis of tongue thrusting.

There are different opinions among orthodontists regarding the treatment of tongue thrusting. Some believe that the problem can be eliminated by retraining the patient to position the tongue properly through exercises designed to develop more favorable control of the muscle tissue of the tongue. These exercises are one type of myofunctional therapy. Other orthodon-

tists view myofunctional therapy of the tongue musculature as futile and prefer to use orthodontic appliances on a long-term basis to counteract the forces put on the teeth by tongue thrusting.

CORRECTIVE ORTHODONTICS

Corrective orthodontic procedures are designed to reduce the severity of an existing malocclusion or to eliminate it entirely. Sometimes it is necessary to carry out both interceptive and corrective procedures simultaneously.

No attempt will be made to discuss this subject in detail, for the subject is so vast that it would require several volumes to do so. However, it will be helpful for an orthodontic assistant to be familiar with some of the principles employed in corrective orthodontics, as well as with the appliances, instruments, and materials that are used.

Considerations before treatment

The ultimate goal of corrective orthodontics is to establish a favorable functional occlusion. Secondarily, orthodontic treatment generally improves the pa-

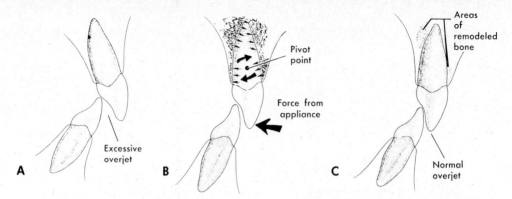

Fig. 24-24. Tooth movement when tipping forces are applied to crown of tooth. **A,** Excessive overjet in anterior region. **B,** Force from orthodontic appliance causes tooth to be tipped lingually around imaginary pivot point. Alveolar bone is remodeled by cellular action as force is maintained. **C,** When teeth are in desired position, retainer is used to maintain position until bone remodeling is complete.

tient's appearance by repositioning the teeth and altering facial profiles within certain limits.

The orthodontist must have the cooperation of the patient and the patient's parents if treatment is to achieve maximum success. This is a critical factor, since corrective orthodontic treatment is often a long-term procedure that may require several years to complete. The patient's willingness to wear appliances as directed by the orthodontist and to maintain a high level of oral hygiene will help to ensure a favorable treatment outcome.

Principles of tooth movement. Orthodontic appliances are devices that apply forces to a tooth or set of teeth to cause them to move to a specific position in the jaw. Orthodontic appliances can also be used to hold or retain teeth in a specific position in the dental arch. Orthodontic appliances move teeth by applying force to the crown of the tooth that is transmitted down the root to the periodontium. A tooth moves in response to force according to the following theory.

Tooth movement is a result of a remodeling process of the alveolus, or socket, in which the tooth rests. When force is applied to the tooth, some portions of the periodontal ligament are compressed, as are the capillaries in the ligament. This compression causes the bone in the area to resorb (break down) through the action of bone-removing cells called osteoclasts. At the same time some areas of the periodontal ligament are stretched, which stimulates another type of

cell, called osteoblasts, to produce new bone in these areas. As the areas of the alveolus under compression resorb, the tooth moves. The areas under tension produce new bone behind the moving tooth. Thus the alveolus is remodeled as the tooth is being moved (Fig. 24-24).

This is a simplified example, but the principle is the same in more complex tooth movements. The key to successful tooth movement is related to the following factors:

1. *Magnitude of force.* The optimum amount of force required to move a tooth is unique to the patient and individual tooth. Too much force can be destructive to the root of the tooth or inhibit tooth movement. Reassessment of the force applied to a tooth is a continuing concern of the orthodontist.

2. *Duration of application.* The length of time force is applied influences the rate of tooth movement. Orthodontists vary in opinion about how long force should be applied to teeth.

3. *Direction of force.* Appliance design is carefully accomplished so that force can be directed properly to cause a tooth to move into the intended position.

4. *Distribution of force.* Some teeth, such as small single-rooted teeth, move more readily in response to force than other larger or multirooted teeth. In complex cases the orthodontist uses this principle to distribute forces to smaller teeth, using multirooted teeth for anchorage for the orthodontic appliance.

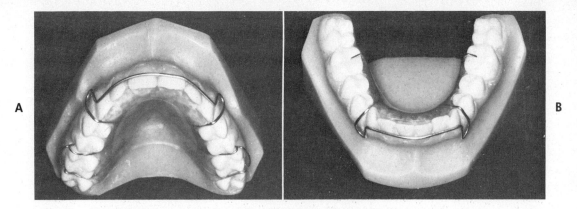

Fig. 24-25. Hawley appliance (removable). **A,** Maxillary. **B,** Mandibular.

ORTHODONTIC APPLIANCES
Removable appliances

Orthodontists have access to a multitude of orthodontic appliances that can reposition teeth. These appliances are generally divided into removable and fixed appliance categories.

Removable appliances can be removed and reinserted by the patient. They are generally used for more simple tooth movements, such as tipping teeth. Although they do not offer the precise control that fixed appliances offer, they are effective if the patient will wear them according to directions.

The Hawley appliance is a very popular removable appliance because it can be designed in various ways to accomplish a variety of functions (Fig. 24-25). After the desired tooth movement is accomplished, the Hawley appliance can be used as a retainer by deactivating the appliance. No further force is placed on the teeth by the appliance, yet it holds the teeth in the desired position until the teeth become stable in the newly remodeled alveolus.

Fixed appliances (nonremovable)

Fixed orthodontic appliances are attached to the patient's teeth with a dental cement and circumferential bands or by direct bonding (Fig. 24-26). These appliances cannot be removed by the patient. Fixed appliances offer the orthodontist the advantage of a more positive control over tooth movement than is possible with removable appliances. Since the patient cannot remove the appliance, treatment is less likely to be interrupted by the patient. With removable appliances, interruptions in treatment can result from

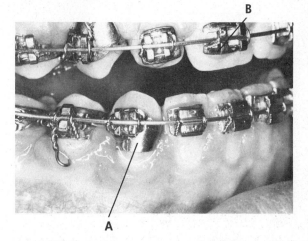

Fig. 24-26. Attachments for fixed orthodontic appliances. **A,** Circumferential band. **B,** Direct bonded bracket.

the loss of the appliance or from the patient not wearing it.

Severe orthodontic cases are often treated with a variety of appliances, such as removable appliances, intraoral fixed appliances, and combination extraoral headgear appliances (Fig. 24-27).

Common elements of fixed appliances. Since orthodontic appliances are tailored to the individual patient's needs, a complete description of all appliances and their variations cannot be presented within the confines of this chapter. However, some of the basic elements of some common fixed appliances will be described here.

Orthodontic bands (Fig. 24-28) are circumferential

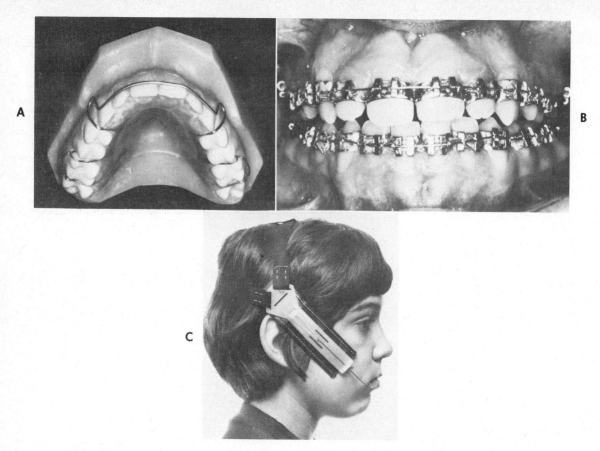

Fig. 24-27. Common orthodontic appliances. **A,** Removable appliance. **B,** Fixed appliance. **C,** Extraoral appliance.

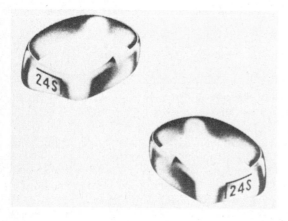

Fig. 24-28. Molar bands with number code for identification. (Courtesy Rocky Mountain Orthodontics, Denver, Colo.)

stainless steel bands that are fitted to individual teeth. They serve to connect the appliance to the teeth when cemented into place. Orthodontic bands are available in a variety of sizes for each tooth in the dental arches.

Brackets (Fig. 24-29) are attachments that are welded to the orthodontic bands. Brackets hold the arch wire in place and transmit the force of the arch wire to the teeth. Some brackets are designed to be bonded directly to the teeth using an acid etch composite material, thus eliminating the need for an orthodontic band.

Arch wires (Fig. 24-30) are the principal guide portions of the fixed appliance. The arch wire is attached to the brackets by wire ligatures or elastic ligatures on either the facial or lingual aspect of the teeth, depending on the task to be performed by the wire. Arch

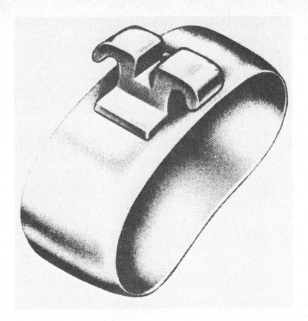

Fig. 24-29. Circumferential band with edgewise-style bracket. (Courtesy Rocky Mountain Orthodontics, Denver, Colo.)

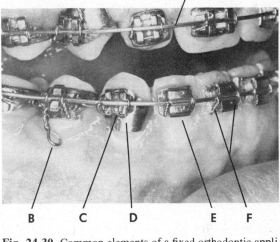

Fig. 24-30. Common elements of a fixed orthodontic appliance. **A,** Arch wire. **B,** Loop for elastics. **C,** Bracket. **D,** Circumferential band. **E,** Direct bonded bracket. **F,** Ligature.

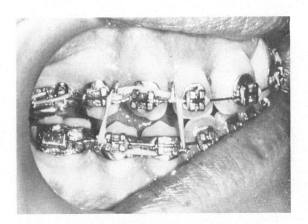

Fig. 24-31. Elastics (intermaxillary).

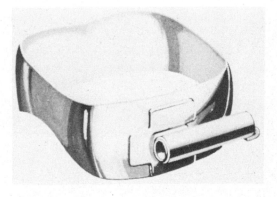

Fig. 24-32. Buccal tube. (Courtesy TP Laboratories, Inc., La Porte, Ind.)

wires function either to move individual teeth or to hold them in a desirable fixed position. Forces from the arch wire are transmitted to the teeth through the brackets.

Ligatures (Fig. 24-30) are fine wires that are used to tie, or ligate, the arch wire to the brackets. There are elastic ligatures available that can be used in conjunction with lighter gauge arch wires.

Elastics (Fig. 24-31) are rubber bands that are used to exert force on teeth. These elastics are available in different lengths and thicknesses. They are frequently used to exert force between the upper and lower teeth to improve occlusal relationships. Special buttons or hooks are attached to orthodontic bands and serve as connectors for the elastics.

Buccal tubes (Fig. 24-32) are essentially hollow-

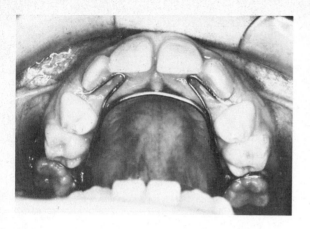

Fig. 24-33. Finger springs attached to fixed appliance.

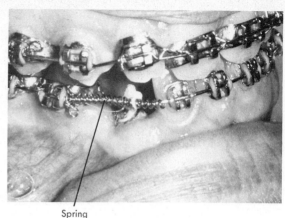

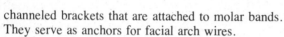

Spring

Fig. 24-34. Coil spring.

channeled brackets that are attached to molar bands. They serve as anchors for facial arch wires.

Finger springs (Fig. 24-33) are used to apply forces to individual teeth. They can be soldered to the main arch wire or used on removable appliances.

Coil springs (Fig. 24-34) are attached to the arch wire. They are available in two types. Open coil springs are compressed between teeth and exert a pushing force on these teeth when the coil attempts to return to its normal length. Closed coil springs are stretched between teeth and exert a pulling force on selected teeth.

Extraoral devices

Orthodontists can use extraoral devices such as shown in Fig. 24-27, *C,* either to hold teeth in a specific position or to move the maxillary molar teeth in a distal direction. Forces from these devices are transmitted through a face-bow or headgear to an intraoral appliance. The force to be applied to the teeth can be adjusted by altering the tension of the adjustment straps on the extraoral device.

COMMON ORTHODONTIC HAND INSTRUMENTS

Although a wide variety of hand instruments is used in orthodontic treatment, only a few of the most common ones are shown in Fig. 24-35.

SPECIAL DUTIES FOR THE ORTHODONTIC ASSISTANT

Many states permit dental assistants to perform certain tasks that are unique to orthodontic treatment.

Regardless of whether the assistant can or cannot actually perform these tasks, it is helpful for dental assistants to be familiar with the techniques described here.

Separator placement

Orthodontic separators are devices that are placed between the teeth to cause them to move apart. This creates space between teeth so that orthodontic bands can be fitted properly.

Latex separators are commonly used today because they apply a constant force as the teeth move apart and are the most comfortable for the patient. Latex separators also cause less trauma to soft tissue. Following is the technique for placing these separators:

1. Place a latex separator on a separating plier and squeeze the plier handles to stretch the separator to a length of approximately ½ to ¾ inch.
2. Using a buccolingual sawing movement similar to that used in the placement of dental floss, carefully pass the cervical aspect of the separator through the contact area (Fig. 24-36).
3. While the cervical aspect of the separator is placed under the contact area, the occlusal aspect is allowed to remain above the contact area. Relax the tension on the separator and remove the separating plier. The latex separator relaxes and exerts a mild force between the teeth to cause them to move apart over a period of 1 to 3 weeks (Fig. 24-36, *C*).

An alternative technique that can be used to place latex separators without the use of separating pliers is as follows:

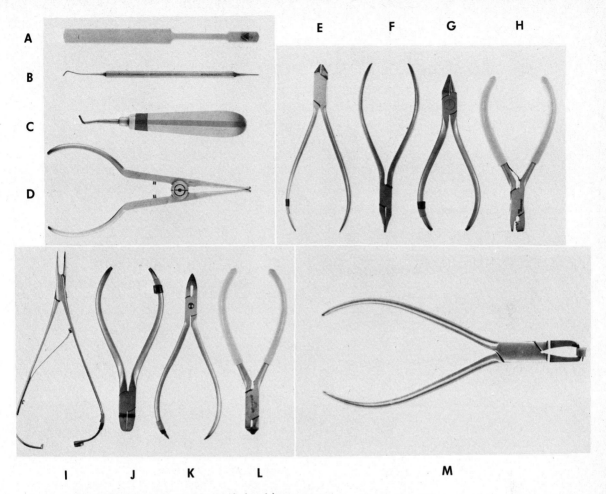

Fig. 24-35. Common orthodontic hand instruments.

Instrument	Principle use
A Band seater	Seat posterior circumferential bands
B Ligature director	Tuck twisted ends of ligature wire into embrasure areas
C Band adaptor	Seat and adapt circumferential bands to teeth
D Ligature tying pliers (Coons)	Tying stainless steel ligature wires
E Three-jaw (prong) pliers	Wire and clasp bending and adjusting
F Tweed loop pliers	Forming loops and springs in wire
G "Bird beak" pliers	Most common pliers for small wire and spring forming
H De La Rosa pliers	Contouring wire loops and molar band material
I Mathieu needle holder	Tying stainless steel ligatures and placng elastic ligatures
J Tweed arch-bending pliers	Forming and shaping square or rectangular arch wires
K Ligature cutter	Removing or trimming stainless steel ligatures
L Distal-end cutter	Cutting distal ends of arch wires
M Posterior-band removing pliers	Removing posterior circumferential bands

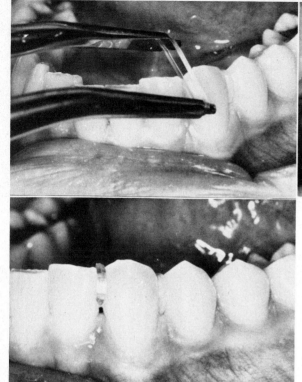

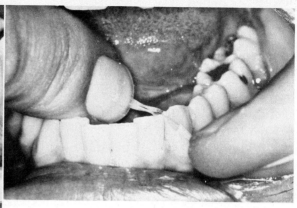

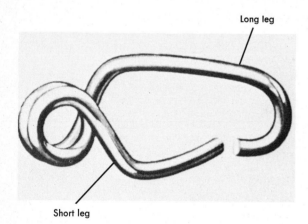

Fig. 24-36. Placement of elastic separators. **A,** Use of separating pliers. **B,** Use of floss handles. **C,** Separators in place.

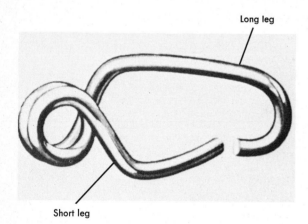

Long leg

Short leg

Fig. 24-37. Separating spring. (Courtesy TP Laboratories, Inc., La Porte, Ind.)

1. Cut two strands of dental tape or floss into lengths of approximately 20 inches.
2. Thread each strand of floss through the separator (Fig. 24-36, *B*). The floss strands serve as handles for the assistant to stretch the separator while it is placed between the teeth as described previously. This technique is safer because it offers more control of the ligature as it passes through the contact area.

In some patients with very tight contacts it is difficult to place latex separators. In these instances a separating spring (TP brand) can be used (Fig. 24-37). These separators are placed as follows:

1. Grasp the shortest leg of the spring with No. 139 pliers. Place the opening of the spring over the contact area (Fig. 24-38, *A*).
2. Twist the pliers to force the longest leg of the spring to slip under the contact. Release the short leg and allow it to move under the contact (Fig. 24-38, *B*). To remove the separating springs, simply grasp either the coiled portion of the spring or its longest leg and lift the spring in an occlusofacial direction.

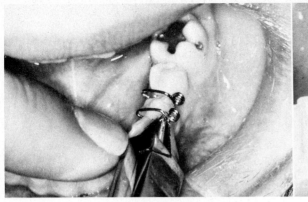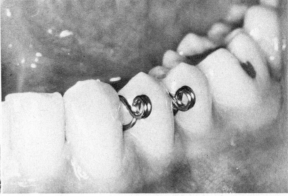

Fig. 24-38. Placement of separating springs. **A,** Use of the No. 139 plier. **B,** Springs in place.

Trial sizing of orthodontic bands

Orthodontic bands are available in a large assortment of sizes for each tooth in the dental arches. Most manufacturers label the bands on the mesial aspect for easy orientation and identification.

As an example, a Unitek brand of band might have a code RL 36 printed on the mesial aspect of the band. This band is selected from the lower molar section of a complete kit of orthodontic bands. The code RL 36 simply means that it is a right lower molar band, size 36. This band could be placed on the appropriate tooth of the patient's study model to determine the approximate size range. If the band appears to be close in size, the following steps are taken to select the appropriate band:

1. Remove the elastic separators around the tooth to be banded. This is accomplished by pulling the separator through the contact using a curved explorer.
2. Orient the selected band properly over the tooth with the mesial aspect toward the midline. Push the band cervically, using finger pressure initially.
3. If the band will not move cervically at all, select a larger size.
4. Once a band is selected that will move cervically on the tooth, a band pusher (seater) is used to push the band into place. The band pusher is carefully placed alternately on each corner of the band, and slight pressure is applied in a cervical direction to push the band slowly into place. The patient can assist by gently biting on the band pusher to drive the band into place a little at a time as the band pusher is moved from one corner to another (Fig. 24-39).

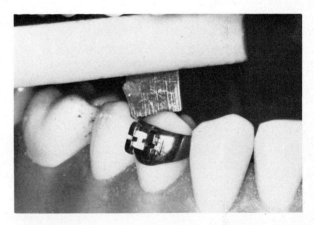

Fig. 24-39. Trial sizing orthodontic band. Band pusher is used to seat band.

5. A properly fitted band should fit tightly around the tooth so that it does not rock when buccal and lingual forces are applied to the band.
6. The band can be removed with band-removing pliers. The Teflon beak of the pliers is placed on the occlusal surface on the buccal aspect of the tooth. The other beak engages the cervical edge of the band. The plier handles are squeezed, and the band is lifted from the tooth (Fig. 24-40).
7. The band is stored and identified. The dentist can make final adjustments in the adaptation of the band once all the bands have been selected. The same procedure is repeated for each tooth to be banded.
8. The separators are reinserted until the cementation appointment.

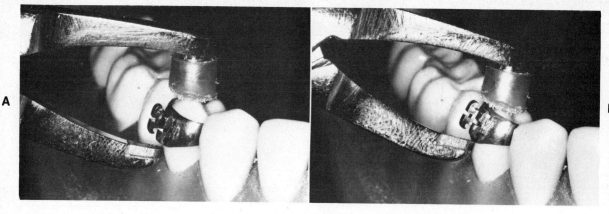

Fig. 24-40. Use of the band-removing pliers. **A,** Correct placement. **B,** Lifted band.

Cementation of orthodontic bands

After all orthodontic bands have been finally adjusted to each tooth that is to be banded, brackets, buccal tubes, or other attachments are spot welded to the bands.

At the band cementation appointment the following steps are carried out:

1. The separators are removed, the teeth are polished with a rubber cup and pumice, and a fluoride treatment is given.
2. Utility wax is placed over the attachments (brackets, etc.) to prevent cement from becoming lodged in them during cementation.
3. The teeth to receive bands are isolated with cotton rolls by segments and dried thoroughly.
4. Zinc phosphate cement is mixed according to the technique described on p. 233. The final consistency should be thicker than that used to cement gold restorations, although not the doughlike consistency required for a cement base. The cement should be a very thick, sticky, creamlike consistency. Some orthodontists use a "frozen slab" technique to mix the cement. The glass mixing slab is stored in a freezer and wiped dry just before mixing the cement. The cold slab helps to slow down the set of the cement so that more bands can be cemented at a time from one mix of cement.
5. Several bands can be cemented at a time. Fill the interior of the bands completely with cement and deliver to the orthodontist on the glass slab for placement on the teeth.
6. The band pusher is used to seat the bands completely, as previously described. The cement is allowed to set completely before removing excess cement.
7. After the cement has set, scalers can be used to scrape off excess cement. An explorer is used to remove cement that may be lodged between the teeth.

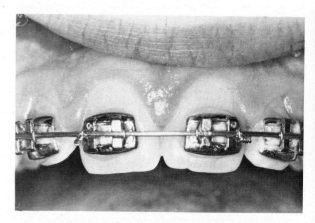

Fig. 24-41. Direct bonded brackets.

This same procedure is repeated until all bands are in place. After all excess cement is removed, the protective wax can be removed from the brackets. The role of the assistant in the cementation procedure will vary according to state laws and the preference of the orthodontist.

Direct bonding of orthodontic brackets (Fig. 24-41)

In recent years the direct bonding of orthodontic brackets to the teeth has become rather popular. This technique eliminates the need for an orthodontic band in cases that are suitable for this technique. Direct bonding offers the advantage of not having bands pass between the teeth. This consumes space that could be used for tooth movement.

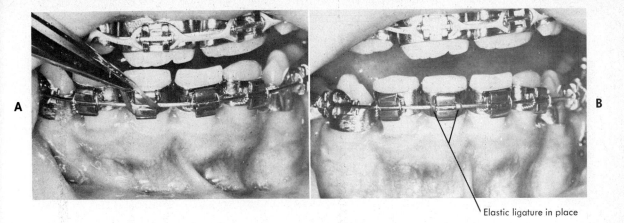

Elastic ligature in place

Fig. 24-42. Placement of elastic ligature. **A,** Stretching elastic over bracket. **B,** Elastic in place.

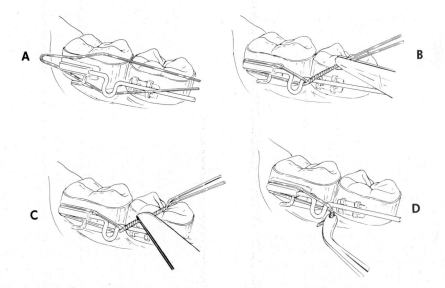

Fig. 24-43. Tying in arch wire to buccal tube. **A,** Ligature wire is looped around buccal tube and under omega loop. **B,** The needle holder is used to pull ligature wire mesially as it is twisted in front of loop. **C,** The twisted ligature is cut to length of 3 to 4 mm with straight wire cutters. **D,** Cut ligature is tucked into embrasure area with either ligature-tucking instrument or serrated amalgam condenser.

Special brackets are used for direct bonding. The procedure for direct bonding of brackets is as follows:

1. The teeth to be bonded are polished with a rubber cup and pumice.
2. The surfaces of the teeth to receive brackets are acid etched with the etching agent provided in the bonding agent kit. Cotton roll isolation is used.

3. The etching agent is rinsed away, and the teeth are dried thoroughly and again isolated with cotton rolls.
4. The bonding adhesive is mixed according to the manufacturer's directions.
5. The bonding agent is either applied to the bracket or placed on the etched areas of the teeth. The brackets are then positioned on the teeth and held in place until the bonding agent sets completely.

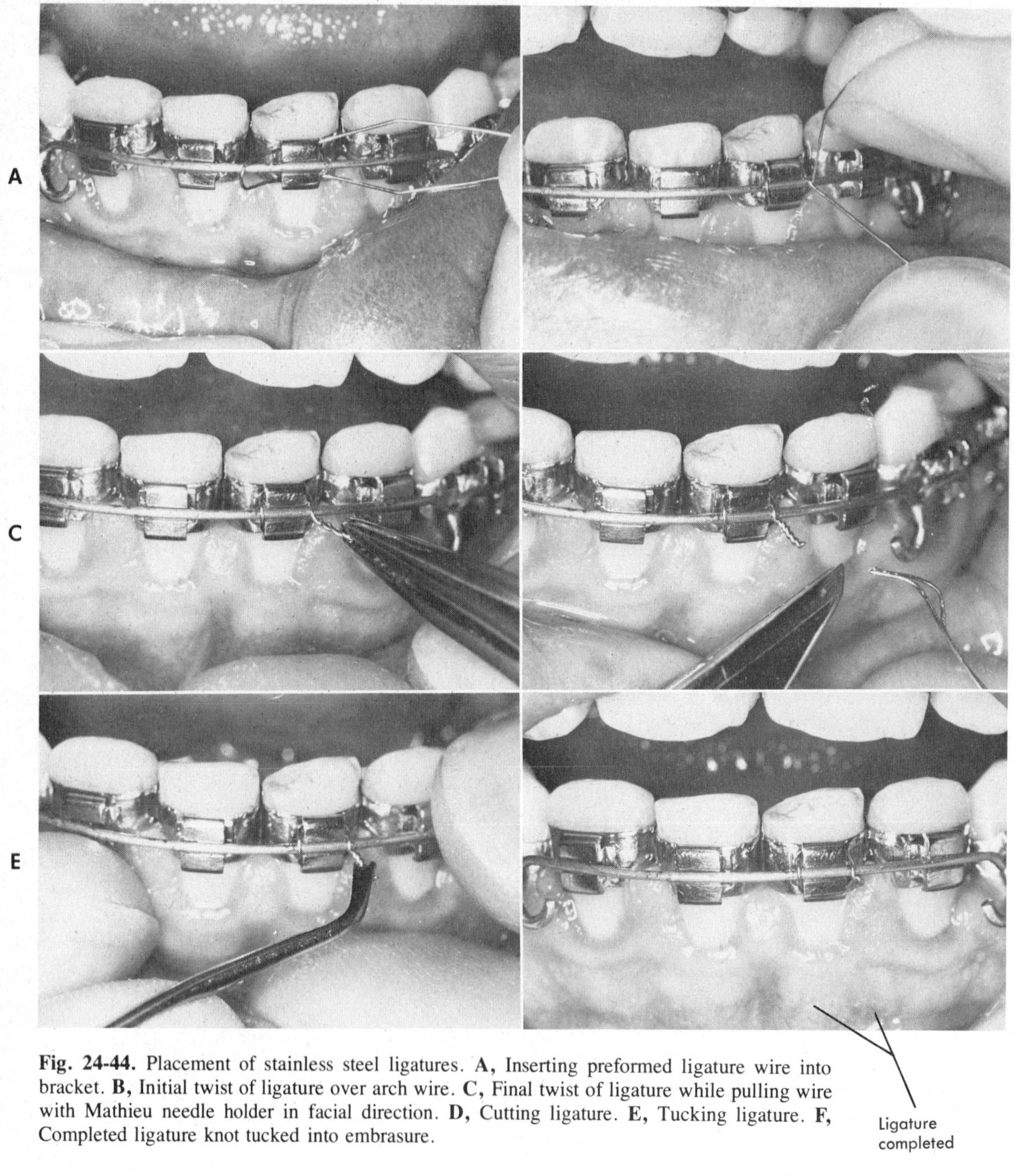

Fig. 24-44. Placement of stainless steel ligatures. **A,** Inserting preformed ligature wire into bracket. **B,** Initial twist of ligature over arch wire. **C,** Final twist of ligature while pulling wire with Mathieu needle holder in facial direction. **D,** Cutting ligature. **E,** Tucking ligature. **F,** Completed ligature knot tucked into embrasure.

Ligature
completed

Placement of arch wires

Some states permit the dental assistant to place the arch wire in the attachments on the bands and ligate them in place after the orthodontist has fabricated the appropriate arch wires. When the very popular edgewise-style arch wire technique is being used, the procedue is as follows:

Elastic ligature method

1. Insert the ends of the arch wire into the buccal tubes that are attached to bands on the last molars on both sides of the arch.
2. Press the arch wire into the horizontal slots in the brackets along the entire arch.
3. Start on the anterior teeth and work toward the posterior. Loop the elastic over the cervical portion of the bracket using a Mathieu needle holder to grasp the ligature. The elastic is pulled over the arch wire and looped around the occlusal aspect of the bracket (Fig. 24-42).
4. This same procedure is continued until all brackets are ligated to the arch wire.
5. The arch wire is "tied in" to the buccal tubes using stainless steel ligature wire. The wire is threaded around the loop (or a helix) located anterior to the buccal tube. The wire is placed around the distal end of the tube and twisted as shown in Fig. 24-43. The needle holder is used to grasp the twisted ligature wire. The beaks of the needle holder are locked and the ligature is pulled anteriorly as the wire is twisted four to six times. This tightens the ligature to hold the arch wire in the buccal tube. End-cutting pliers are used to cut the excess ligature wire off to the desired length. Usually 3 to 4 mm of twisted ligature wire is sufficient to hold the wire in place. A large serrated amalgam condenser or a special ligature-tucking instrument can be used to bend the cut wire into the embrasure area.
6. Distal end cutters are used to cut off any excess arch wire that extends beyond the distal ends of the buccal tubes.

Stainless steel ligature method

1. Insert the ends of the arch wire into the buccal tubes that are attached to the bands on the last molars on both sides of the arch.
2. Press the arch wire into the horizontal slots in the brackets along the entire arch.
3. Start on the anterior teeth and work posteriorly. Bend a ligature wire to about a 45-degree angle. Slide the narrow preformed portion of the wire into the occlusal and cervical channels of the bracket from the distal toward the mesial. Cross the ends of the ligature wire facial to the arch wire (Fig. 24-44, *A*).
4. If a Mathieu needle holder is used, grasp the crossed ligature wire and lock the beaks together. Pull on the ligature wire in a mesial direction as the needle holder is

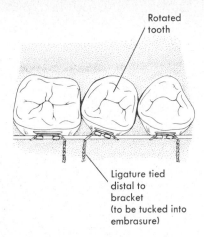

Fig. 24-45. Ligature tied on end of bracket farthest away from arch wire to aid in aligning malposed tooth.

rotated to twist the ends of the ligature wire together (Fig. 24-44, *B*). CAUTION: The patient's eyes should be closed while the wire is being twisted to avoid injury to the eye from the long strands of ligature wire.
5. All ligatures are placed in the same manner, cut to a length of 3 to 4 mm, and bent into the embrasure area.
6. The arch wire is tied in using the technique described previously.

Usually wire ligatures are tied mesial to the bracket because of better access. However, if a tooth is malposed so that the distal end of the bracket is located further away from the arch wire than the mesial, the tie should be placed on the distal. The force applied by the ligature helps to move the tooth into alignment with the arch wire (Fig. 24-45).

It is well recognized that orthodontists use a wide range of appliances, techniques, and instruments to accomplish the same task. The procedures described here should only serve as examples for the orthodontic assistant and not as the last word on how these procedures must be done.

SUMMARY

The role of the dental assistant in orthodontic treatment will at the very least require proficiency in the performance of standard chairside duties. Additional duties such as recording clinical information on dental records, taking impressions, photography, and radiography are frequently delegated to the dental assistant. Some of the other intraoral tasks described in this chapter may be delegated to the assistant, depending on the dental practice act in individual states, the willingness of the orthodontist to delegate, and the ability of the individual dental assistant to perform the tasks.

BIBLIOGRAPHY

Cohen, M.M.: Minor tooth movement in the growing child, Philadelphia, 1977, W.B. Saunders Co.

De Angelis, V.: Dental auxiliary practice. Module 2. Dentofacial growth and development—orthodontics, Baltimore, 1975, The Williams & Wilkins Co.

Graber, T.M., editor: Current orthodontic concepts and techniques, vol. 1, Philadelphia, 1969, W.B. Saunders Co.

Moyers, R.E.: Handbook of orthodontics for the student and the practitioner, ed. 2, Chicago, 1963, Year Book Medical Publishers, Inc.

Proffit, W., and Mason, R.: Myofunctional therapy for tongue thrusting: background and recommendations, J. Am. Dent. Assoc. **90:**403-411, 1975.

CHAPTER 25

ORAL SURGERY

The American Board of Oral Surgery defines oral surgery as follows:

Oral surgery is that part of dental practice which deals with the diagnosis, the surgical and adjunctive treatment of the diseases, injuries, and defects of the human jaws and associated structures.

The oral surgeon is a dentist who has had extensive graduate training in surgery that involves the orofacial region. The practice is limited to these tasks. As is the case with other dental specialities, oral surgery is a vast, complicated subject. This is particularly true of oral surgery because of the complex anatomy of the orofacial region and the proximity of the oral region to vital structures.

The amount of oral surgery that is done in a general dental practice is dictated by the interest and training of the general practitioner. Some dentists devote a great deal of their practice to surgery, whereas others prefer to refer all their surgery patients to the oral surgeon.

The purpose of this chapter is to introduce the dental assistant to some of the common surgical instruments and procedures that are most likely to be encountered in a general practice.

COMMON SURGICAL INSTRUMENTS

Scalpel. The surgical scalpel is a time-honored instrument used by all surgeons. Its sharp blade allows the dentist to make a precise incision into soft tissue with the least amount of trauma to the tissue.

Scalpels with disposable blades are the most popular. They assure the dentist of a new sharp blade and eliminate the possibility of cross contamination between patients. The scalpel handle and the common blade styles are shown in Fig. 25-1.

Surgical curette (Fig. 25-2). The surgical curette is an instrument of many uses. It is rather scoop-shaped with sharp edges, and looks somewhat like a large spoon excavator. This design makes it an ideal instrument for scraping the interior of cavities in bone or other tissues. This curettage of such cavities is done to remove abnormal tissue or to obtain material for diagnostic purposes. The curette is also commonly used to sever the epithelial attachment of the gingiva around the tooth during the first step in the extraction of a tooth.

Surgical curettes are available in different sizes, as shown in Fig. 25-2.

Periosteal elevator (Fig. 25-3). Periosteal elevators are varied in design, yet they all have the same basic function. They are used to separate the periosteum (fibrous covering of bone) from the bone surface. A secondary function of these instruments is to retract the mucoperiosteum so that access can be maintained to the underlying bone (Fig. 25-31, *B*). The mucoperiosteum is the soft tissue covering of the jaws that consists of both the mucosa and the periosteum. The assistant is often called on to perform this retraction for the surgeon.

Surgical mallet and chisels (Fig. 25-4). There is frequently the need for removal of some bone to facilitate removal of a tooth or to reshape the jaws. This can be accomplished with sharp surgical chisels tapped lightly with a mallet.

An alternate method of removing bone is through the use of a conventional-speed straight handpiece with a surgical bur. Irrigation of the surgical site with an irrigation syringe filled with sterile saline solution is necessary to remove the loosened bone fragments. The syringe is used along with the suction tip to jointly flush and evacuate the surgical site. This procedure maintains the visibility for the operator.

If the handpiece is used for bone removal, continuous drops of saline solution should be allowed to drop from the syringe onto the bur. This prevents the bur from clogging and reduces frictional heat that can damage the remaining bone.

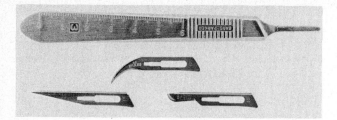

Fig. 25-1. Surgical scalpel and disposable blades. *Left to right:* No. 11, No. 12B, No. 15.

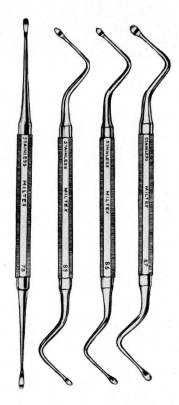

Fig. 25-2. Surgical curettes. (Courtesy Miltex Instrument Co., New York, N.Y.)

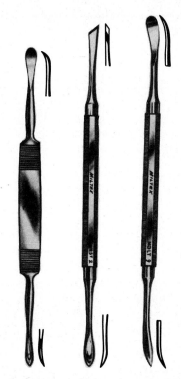

Fig. 25-3. Periosteal elevators. (Courtesy Miltex Instrument Co., New York, N.Y.)

Suction tips and irrigation syringes (Fig. 25-5). These instruments are used jointly to clear the surgical site in the manner just described.

The smaller-size suction tips are more favorable for the removal of blood from the surgical site than the larger sizes used in operative and restorative dentistry.

The suction tip should be dipped in a container of sterile saline solution periodically during a procedure to prevent it from clogging with clotted blood.

Rongeur forceps (Fig. 25-6). The rongeur is a nipperlike instrument that is used to trim alveolar bone. It is widely used after multiple extractions to shape the edentulous ridge (alveoloplasty).

Several styles and sizes are available.

Bone files. Whenever an alveoloplasty is needed

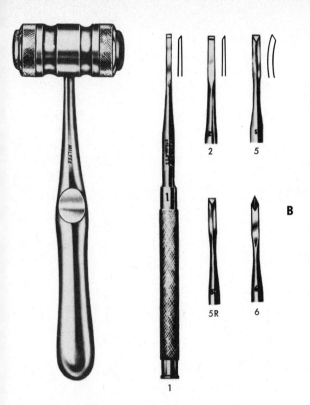

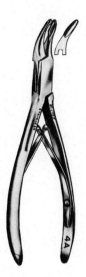

Fig. 25-6. Rongeur forceps. (Courtesy Miltex Instrument Co., New York, N.Y.)

Fig. 25-4. A, Surgical mallet. **B,** Surgical chisels. (Courtesy Miltex Instrument Co., New York, N.Y.)

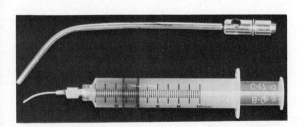

Fig. 25-5. Surgical suction tip and irrigation syringe.

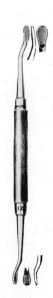

after the extraction of teeth or in the correction of poorly shaped edentulous ridges, the rongeur is most often used to remove the majority of the undesirable bone. Bone files are used to accomplish minor bone removal and to smooth the surface of the bone before wound closure.

The instruments are available in different shapes and sizes (Fig. 25-7).

Fig. 25-7. Bone file. (Courtesy Miltex Instrument Co., New York, N.Y.)

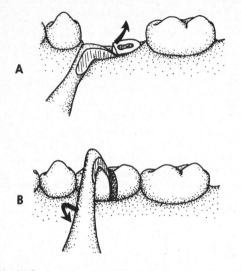

Fig. 25-8. A, Extraction of root fragments using elevator. **B,** Sectioning tooth.

Extraction elevators. Extraction elevators are leverlike instruments that are used to apply controlled force against a tooth to loosen (luxate) it in its alveolus (Fig. 25-31, *D*). It is not uncommon for certain teeth to be completely removed with only an elevator.

Other uses of extraction elevators include the removal of residual root fragments (Fig. 25-8, *A*) and sectioning of teeth (Fig. 25-8, *B*). It is sometimes necessary to divide or section a tooth into two or more parts to remove it. The tooth to be sectioned can be cut part way with an ultraspeed handpiece and No. 557 bur. The elevator is inserted in the bur cut and twisted to complete the section.

Elevators are available in different styles and sizes as shown in Fig. 25-9.

Extraction forceps. Extraction forceps are plierslike instruments that are used to grasp the tooth and deliver it from its alveolus. As with most other instruments, the individual dentist has a preference for certain forceps designs. The many choices available are divided into two basic groups. One group of for-

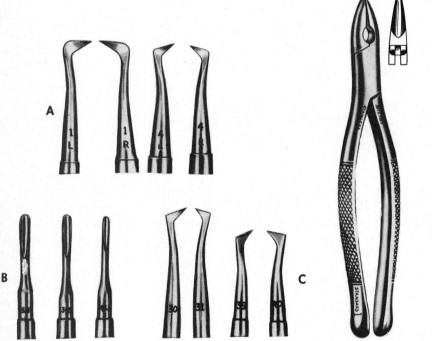

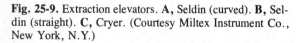

Fig. 25-9. Extraction elevators. **A,** Seldin (curved). **B,** Seldin (straight). **C,** Cryer. (Courtesy Miltex Instrument Co., New York, N.Y.)

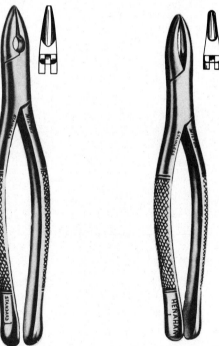

Fig. 25-10. Standard No. 1 forceps for upper incisors and canines. (Courtesy Miltex Instrument Co., New York, N.Y.)

ceps is designed for use on a specific group of teeth on one side of the mouth, (for example, right maxillary molars). The other group is referred to as "universal forceps." These forceps are designed for a specific group of teeth on either side of the same arch, (for example, right and left maxillary molars).

Some of the most common extraction forceps in use today are listed as follows according to their area of use.

Maxillary teeth

1. Anterior—standard forceps No. 1 (Fig. 25-10); a universal forceps for incisor and canine teeth.
2. Premolars—standard forceps No. 150 (Fig. 25-11); a universal forceps principally used for maxillary premolars but which can be used for incisor teeth.
3. First and second molars—standard forceps No. 18R and No. 18L (Fig. 25-12); forceps specifically used for the

maxillary first and second molars. The R indicates that this forceps is used on the patient's right side, and L indicates usage on the left side.
4. Third molars—standard forceps No. 210 (Fig. 25-13); a universal forceps used for maxillary third molars. The bayonet design assists in gaining access to the third molar area.

Mandibular teeth

1. Anterior and premolar—standard forceps No. 151 (Fig. 25-14); a universal forceps convenient for use on both anterior and premolar teeth. The design is similar to that of the No. 150, except the beaks are bent at a greater angle to the handles for better access to the lower teeth.
2. First and second molars—standard forceps No. 15 (Fig. 25-15) and No. 16 (Fig. 25-16); universal forceps designed for mandibular first and second molars. The No. 16 forceps is often referred to as the "cowhorn" because of the design of the beaks. The beaks of the No. 16 slide

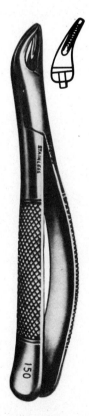

Fig. 25-11. Standard No. 150 forceps used primarily for maxillary premolars. (Courtesy Miltex Instrument Co., New York, N.Y.)

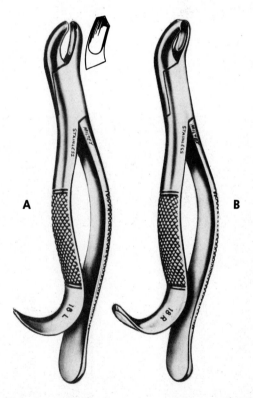

Fig. 25-12. Standard No. 18R and No. 18L forceps. **A,** No. 18L for upper left first and second molars. **B,** No. 18R for upper right first and second molars. (Courtesy Miltex Instrument Co., New York, N.Y.)

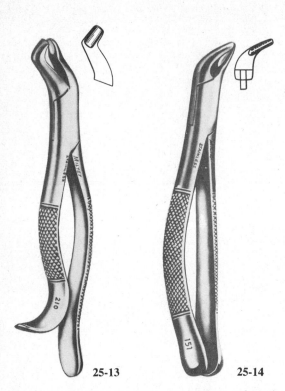

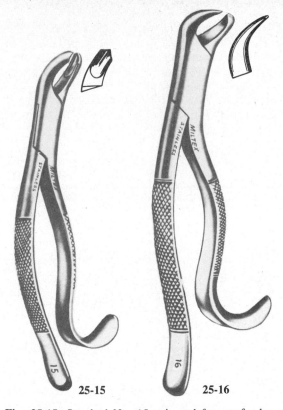

25-13 25-14 25-15 25-16

Fig. 25-13. Standard No. 210 universal forceps for upper third molar. (Courtesy Miltex Instrument Co., New York, N.Y.)

Fig. 25-14. Standard No. 151 universal forceps for lower incisor, premolar, and large root fragments. (Courtesy Miltex Instrument Co., New York, N.Y.)

Fig. 25-15. Standard No. 15 universal forceps for lower first and second molars. (Courtesy Miltex Instrument Co., New York, N.Y.)

Fig. 25-16. Standard No. 16 forceps used for lower first and second molars. (Courtesy Miltex Instrument Co., New York, N.Y.)

into the bifurcation area, which permits a positive grasp of the tooth. The tooth is lifted somewhat from the alveolus as the beaks are squeezed into the bifurcation area.

3. Third molars—standard forceps No. 222 (Fig. 25-17); a universal forceps that can be used for mandibular third molars. Since these teeth often differ in their anatomical positions because of lack of arch space, they are frequently extracted with a variety of elevators and forceps. The No. 222 is generally used when the tooth is in a normal vertical position in the dental arch.

Some forceps manufacturers make forceps with both plain and serrated beaks (Fig. 25-18). The style desired must be designated when these instruments are ordered.

Root picks (Fig. 25-19). Root picks are surgical probes used to remove root fragments that may break away from the tooth during the extraction. A variety of shapes and sizes are available.

Surgical scissors (Fig. 25-20). A wide variety of scissors styles are available for surgical use. Many are available with smooth and serrated blades. Most of the scissors styles have handles that range in length from approximately 3½ to 6¼ inches.

Scissors are used to trim soft tissue and cut suture material. Maintaining sharpness is important for the maximum effectiveness of these instruments. Surgical scissors should never be used for nonsurgical tasks that would dull the cutting blades.

Tissue forceps (Fig. 25-21). An important prin-

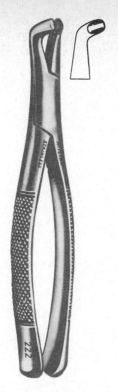

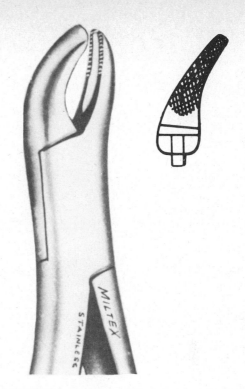

Fig. 25-17. Standard No. 222 universal forceps for lower third molar. (Courtesy Miltex Instrument Co., New York, N.Y.)

Fig. 25-18. Forceps of serrated-beak design. (Courtesy Miltex Instrument Co., New York, N.Y.)

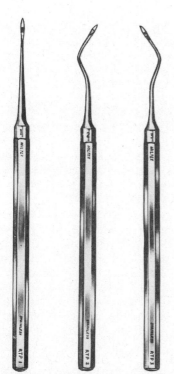

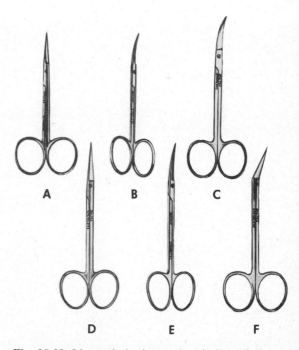

Fig. 25-19. Root picks. (Courtesy Miltex Instrument Co., New York, N.Y.)

Fig. 25-20. Iris surgical scissors. **A,** 4-inch, straight, very delicate. **B,** 4-inch, curved. **C,** 4½-inch, curved sideways, delicate. **D,** 4½-inch, straight delicate. **E,** 4½-inch, curved delicate. **F,** 4½-inch, angular delicate. (Courtesy Miltex Instrument Co., New York, N.Y.)

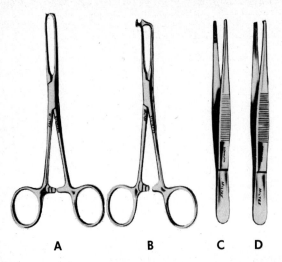

Fig. 25-21. Allis tissue forceps, stainless steel. **A,** 6-inch, straight. **B,** 6-inch, angular jaws. **C,** Serrated jaws. **D,** Mouse tooth. (Courtesy Miltex Instrument Co., New York, N.Y.)

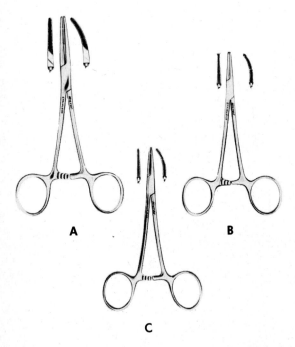

Fig. 25-22. Hemostats, stainless steel. **A,** Kelly, 5½-inch, straight and curved. **B,** Mosquito, 5-inch, straight and curved. **C,** Mosquito, 5-inch, straight and curved. (Courtesy Miltex Instrument Co., New York, N.Y.)

ciple of surgery is to handle soft tissue as carefully as possible to avoid trauma that may delay healing. The use of tissue forceps assists the dentist in handling soft tissue with care during trimming and suturing procedures. They provide a positive grasp of tissue for maximum control during these procedures.

Hemostat (Fig. 25-22). The hemostat is a multipurpose instrument. Its principal use in surgery is to clamp blood vessels that may be severed during a surgical procedure. The narrow beaks are serrated, and the handles have locks on them to hold the beaks in a closed position without force being applied by the operator.

The hemostat is a popular instrument used to grasp unwanted tissue that will be removed during a surgical procedure. Bone and tooth fragments are conveniently removed from the surgical site with a hemostat.

These instruments are available in a variety of sizes, with straight and curved beaks, and with different handle lengths.

Suture needles and holders (Fig. 25-23). Surgical wounds that involve significant soft tissue incisions must be sutured to control hemorrhage and promote proper healing. Suturing is accomplished using suture needles attached to silk thread. The needle is guided through the tissue while it is held in the beaks of a needle holder. The needle holder is also used to handle the needle and surgical thread while it is tied to secure the suture. Surgical scissors are then used to cut the silk thread to proper length.

Probably the most popular suture material used in dentistry is black silk of 3-0 size. Although it is available in spools and can be threaded into suture needles with eyelets, a far more convenient method is to purchase the material already sterilized and attached to the end of a suture needle, with the whole assembly packaged in a sterile wrap (Fig. 25-24). The needle is discarded after use.

A variety of needle sizes are available. Intraoral suturing generally requires the use of the curved-style needles shown in Fig. 25-24.

Needle holders look and operate much like a hemostat. The beaks are straight with fine serrations. There is a groove on the serrated surface of the beaks for certain styles of suture needles. The handle design allows the dentist to tie the suture material using the needle holder without snagging it in the joint of the instrument.

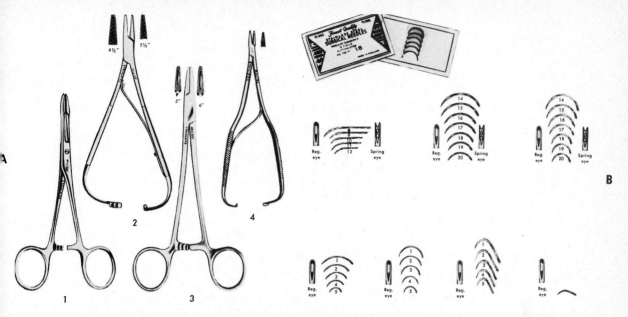

Fig. 25-23. A, Suture needle holders, stainless steel. **B,** Resealable suture needle assortment. (Courtesy Miltex Instrument Co., New York, N.Y.)

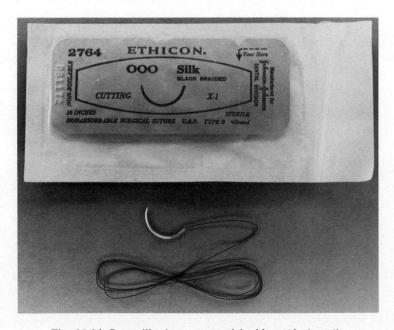

Fig. 25-24. Presterilized suture material with attached needle.

BIOPSY

A biopsy is the examination of tissues and cells that have been removed from a living patient. This examination may be a gross evaluation (with the naked eye), or a microscope may be used. The information obtained from a biopsy procedure assists the dentist in arriving at a diagnosis and ultimately predicting the outcome of the disease (prognosis).

It is common in dentistry to remove both normal and abnormal tissue from the surgical site for purposes of comparison. The three most common biopsy procedures used in dentistry are the incisional biopsy, the excisional biopsy, and surface scraping (for exfoliative cytology).

Incisional biopsy

A localized site of abnormal tissue is referred to as a lesion. Incisional biopsy procedures involve the removal of a sample of the lesion for examination. A common method used is to cut a wedge of tissue from the lesion, along with some normal adjacent tissue for comparison (Fig. 25-25). The sample tissue is placed immediately in a small bottle of 10% formalin solution to preserve it. The wound is sutured, and the patient is dismissed. The biopsied tissue is sent to a pathology laboratory for analysis.

The incisional biopsy is generally used when the lesion is rather large or in a strategic area where complete removal of the lesion would create significant esthetic or functional impairment. For example, a large ulcerated lesion on the lip is biopsied with the incisional method. Complete surgical removal of the lesion is not indicated until a final diagnosis is made, since the lesion may not be malignant and may heal in time on its own without further surgery. Complete surgical removal before a final diagnosis is made may create unnecessary alteration of the lip, caused by loss of tissue and scarring. On the other hand, if the incisional biopsy leads to a diagnosis that warrants complete surgical removal, the surgery is done with good reason.

Excisional biopsy

Excisional biopsy involves removal of the entire lesion plus some adjacent normal tissue (Fig. 25-26). This procedure is done on small lesions where complete excision (removal) would not create significant esthetic or functional impairment. For example, a small, nonhealing sore on the buccal mucosa may be completely removed during the biopsy, since only a small volume of tissue in a nonstrategic area is being

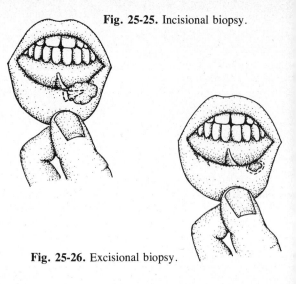

Fig. 25-25. Incisional biopsy.

Fig. 25-26. Excisional biopsy.

excised. Neither functional nor esthetic impairment is involved.

Exfoliative cytology

Another method that is helpful in diagnosing oral lesions is the nonsurgical technique of wiping or scraping the surface of the lesion to gather a sample of cells for microscopic examination. The science of examining cells that are shed (exfoliated) during the scraping process is called exfoliative cytology.

This procedure has limitations in value and is viewed as an adjunct to the surgical techniques just described. The collected cells must be placed on a glass slide and spread out for examination under the microscope. This slide setup is called a smear. Probably the best known exfoliative biopsy is the Papanicolaou smear (Pap smear) that is used to detect disease of the vaginal area.

Biopsy report

After the tissue is removed from the patient, it is sent to a pathology laboratory for analysis. The sample tissue must be carefully handled with tissue forceps and placed immediately in a container of 10% formalin solution. There should be at least 20 times the volume of the specimen in the container to ensure proper preservation. Formalin can be obtained from a pharmacy along with suitable tight-sealing bottles.

The specimen bottle should be labeled with the following information on a stick-on label: (1) patient's name, (2) patient's address, (3) patient's age, and (4) date of biopsy.

A short biopsy report should be included with each specimen to be sent. The report should include the following information:

1. Patient's name
2. Patient's age
3. Description of lesion (size, shape, location, color, etc.)
4. History of lesion (time present, enlargement, pain, etc.)
5. Tentative diagnosis (the dentist's impression of what the disease might be)

Sometimes a small sketch of the lesion is helpful to the pathologist to clarify its description and location.

The specimen bottle and biopsy report should be carefully packed and sent to the laboratory immediately. The laboratory will return a report of the pathologist's findings on completion of the analysis of the biopsy specimen.

EXODONTIA

Exodontia is the area of dental practice that deals with the removal, or extraction, of teeth. Although modern dental practice is geared toward the preservation of teeth, the fact remains that it is necessary to remove teeth under certain circumstances as a part of treatment planning.

Extractions are often thought of as the end result of severe dental caries, periodontal disease, and tooth fracture. Various studies indicate that from 50% to 89% of all extractions result from these disease processes. Preventive and restorative procedures can play a major role in the reduction of this needless tooth loss. However, other circumstances may make the extraction of teeth necessary: impactions, orthodontic therapy, and involvement in surgical procedures such as treatment of neoplasms and jaw fracture. Although dentists agree that they would prefer to reduce needless loss of teeth, exodontia will always be a necessary dental service.

Since surgical procedures influence several systems of the body, it is imperative that a thorough medical-dental history be taken as described in Chapter 3. Since most surgical procedures are irreversible, an accurate diagnosis and treatment plan are mandatory. Accurate clinical records and radiographs are essential parts of any oral surgical treatment.

Patient preparation for surgery begins with consideration for necessary premedication and medical precautions that are revealed in the health history. Once seated in the operatory, the patient must be prepared for the procedure. Dentists vary in their opinion on how a patient should be prepared for surgery. The oral cavity is a heavily contaminated surgical site. The saliva is teeming with the organisms that normally inhabit the mouth. Because of the presence of organisms in the oral cavity, some operators feel little need for much patient preparation. However, studies indicate that most patients tolerate their own organisms quite well but do not tolerate organisms from other sources. Therefore preparation of the patient for surgery should be geared to minimizing contamination of the mouth with organisms foreign to the patient's oral cavity.

Some of the following common methods of controlling the operating field have been recommended.

1. Use full-length patient drapes.
2. Wrap the patient's head with sterile towels to cover the hair.
3. Place a sterile towel over the patient's chest on top of the drape.
4. Shave facial hair before the appointment.
5. Scrub the oronasal area with a disinfectant soap, using a sterile 4 × 4 inch gauze sponge.
6. The surgical site can be swabbed with a disinfectant solution before the procedure.

In addition to patient preparation, the environment around the patient should be prepared. This includes disinfecting and sterilizing everything possible that comes in contact with the patient: light handles, evacuator tips and hose connectors, handpieces, and control switches on the chair. Surgical instruments should be kept in sterile wraps until they are set up on a sterile towel for the procedure. The surgical setup should be kept covered with a sterile towel until the procedure begins.

It is recommended that the surgical team wear rubber gloves and face masks. Although sterile rubber gloves are ideal, they are not absolutely essential. After the rubber gloves are on the hands, they can be thoroughly scrubbed with a disinfecting soap and dried with a sterile towel.

Dentists who perform surgical services will establish their own method of patient preparation. The assistant will be required to prepare the patient for surgery and maintain the environment for the procedure.

For purposes of discussion, extractions can be divided into three categories: (1) routine, (2) complex, and (3) multiple.

Routine extractions

It has often been said by many dentists that there are no routine or simple extractions. Each extraction presents a new challenge for the dentist. The term routine is meant to imply that the extraction can be done without extensive instrumentation or complication during surgery. These extractions are often referred to as forceps extractions, since they can be done with a standard forceps without removing bone or sectioning the tooth.

Armamentarium. A typical armamentarium for a routine extraction is shown in Fig. 25-27.

Procedure. The steps involved in a routine extraction include the following:

1. Local anesthetic is administered.
2. The anesthesia is checked by gently probing the gingiva surrounding the tooth to be extracted with the surgical curette.
3. The epithelial attachment is severed around the tooth with the surgical curette to free the gingiva from the tooth (Fig. 25-28, *A*).
4. The beaks of the forceps are placed on the tooth and seated firmly so that the tips of the beaks grasp the tooth around the cementoenamel junction (Fig. 25-28, *B*).
5. The operator moves the tooth in the alveolus to sever the attachment of the periodontal ligament around the tooth and to expand the size of the alveolus (Fig. 25-28, *B* and *C*). This is called luxation. In addition to luxation with the forceps, extraction elevators are helpful in luxating certain teeth.
6. After luxation, the tooth is lifted from the alveolus (Fig. 25-28, *D*).
7. The suction tip is used to debride the surgical site. Often tooth fragments, carious tooth structure, and broken restorative material are left around the open alveolus after the tooth is removed. It is important to remove this debris so that it does not become incorporated in the wound.
8. After debridement, the wound is covered with a compress made of one or two 2 × 2 inch moistened gauze sponges. The sponges should be folded so that the patient can bite down on the compress to apply pressure over the open alveolus. This aids in control of bleeding.
9. Usually, routine extraction sites do not require suturing. The patient should be allowed to sit up for a few minutes while being given postoperative instructions, and then the patient can be dismissed.

The operator must use both hands during extractions. The right hand operates the forceps while the left hand stabilizes the patient's head and palpates the movement of the tooth while it is being luxated (assuming the dentist is right-handed).

The assistant can deliver surgical instruments using a two-handed exchange, out of the line of sight of the patient. The unwanted instrument is picked up from the dentist with one hand and the next instrument is delivered with the other (Fig. 25-29). Most surgical instruments are rather heavy to exchange effectively using the one-handed transfer technique. Rubber gloves also inhibit an effective one-handed transfer. The choice of a one- or two-handed transfer is left to the operating team.

The small suction tip should be used as needed during the extraction. It does not have to be held constantly in the surgical site during a routine extraction.

The assistant should be constantly aware of the need for retraction of soft tissue during a surgical procedure. The dentist should offer some guidance in this regard so that the well-intentioned assistant does not interfere with the operator's access while trying to improve visibility.

Once the tooth is lifted from the alveolus, the assistant should take the extracted tooth in the forceps by grasping the beaks of the forceps in the palm of the hand.

It is good for the assistant to observe a patient before dismissal until the assistant is reasonably certain the patient is able to stand and walk from the operatory. It is not uncommon for a patient to feel dizzy or even faint after a surgical procedure. The assistant should stand near the patient, as a precautionary measure, when he or she first stands and walks from the operatory.

Complex extractions

The term *complex extraction* implies that a more extensive effort is needed to extract a tooth. There is no precise definition of a complicated extraction because extractions can be complicated for one or more reasons. Complex extractions may involve one or more of the following procedures during or after the extraction:

1. Mucoperiosteal flap retraction
2. Ostectomy (bone removal)
3. Alveoloplasty (bone shaping)
4. Tooth sectioning
5. Root recovery
6. Soft tissue resection

A classic example of a complex extraction is the removal of an impacted (unerupted) mandibular third molar. It often involves several of the procedures just mentioned.

Armamentarium. A suggested basic armamentarium for a complicated extraction is shown in Fig. 25-30.

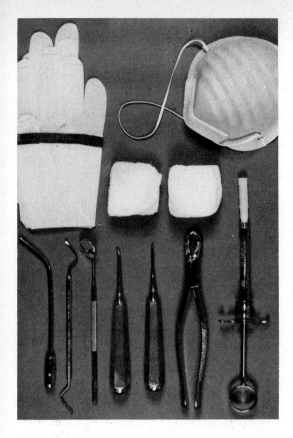

Rubber gloves (two pair)
Sterile gauze sponges, 2 × 2 inch
Face masks (two)
Surgical evacuator tip
Surgical curette
Mouth mirror, No. 4
Extraction elevators
Extraction forceps
Anesthetic syringe, loaded

Fig. 25-27. Armamentarium for routine extraction.

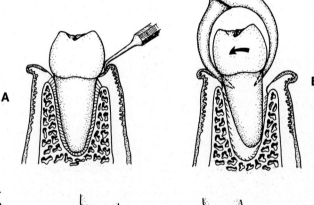

Fig. 25-28. Routine extraction sequence. **A,** Severing epithelial attachment with curette. **B,** Beaks of forceps grasp tooth at cementoenamel junction. Tooth is tipped in buccal direction. **C,** Tooth is tipped in lingual direction. **D,** Tooth is lifted from alveolus.

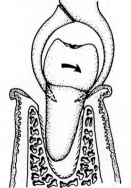

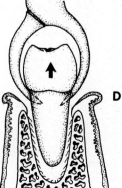

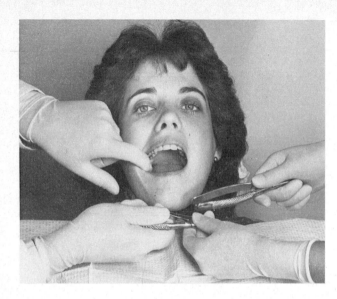

Fig. 25-29. Two-handed instrument transfer.

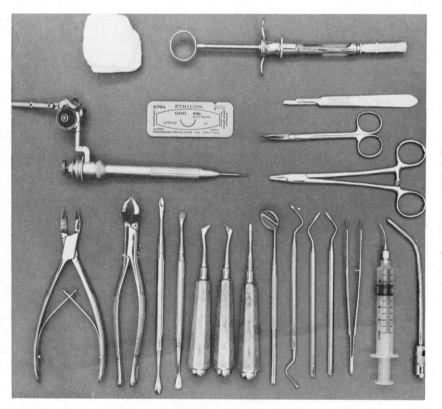

Sterile gauze sponges, 2 × 2 inch
Anesthetic syringe, loaded
Conventional speed handpiece
  with surgical bur
Suture material
Scalpel, No. 15 blade
Suture scissors
Needle holder
Rongeur forceps
Extraction forceps
Periosteal elevator
Bone file
Extraction elevators
Mouth mirror, No. 4
Surgical curette
Root picks
Cotton pliers
Irrigation syringe
Surgical evacuator tip

Fig. 25-30. Armamentarium for complicated extraction.

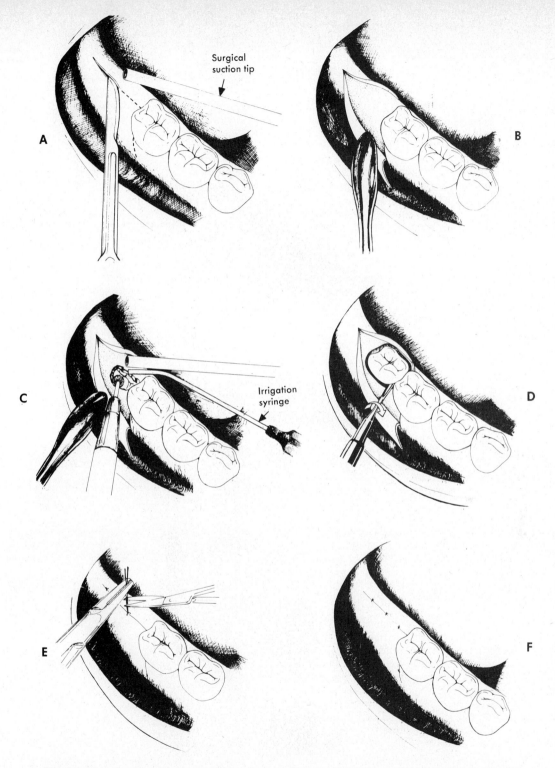

Fig. 25-31. Extraction of impacted third molar with the help of chairside assistant. **A,** Evacuation of incision. **B,** Retraction of both mucoperiosteal flap and cheek with periosteal elevator. **C,** Simultaneous irrigation and evacuation during bone removal. **D,** Luxation with extraction elevator. **E,** Assistant cutting sutures. **F,** Closed incision.

Procedure. Following is a summary of the principal steps involved in the extraction of an impacted mandibular third molar:

1. Local anesthetic is administered.
2. Test for anesthesia by probing the surgical area with the surgical curette.
3. An incision is made along the superior surface of the ridge distal to the second molar and extended down the buccal aspect of the ridge (Fig. 25-31, *A*). The incision is made through both the gingival mucosa and the periosteum that covers the underlying bone.
4. The combination mucosa and periosteum (mucoperiosteum) is lifted from the surface of the underlying bone with a periosteal elevator. This "mucoperiosteal flap" is retracted with the elevator to allow the operator access to the bony covering over the impacted tooth (Fig. 25-31, *B*). The assistant has to constantly evacuate blood from the surgical site once the incision is made and the flap is retracted.
5. The bony covering over the impacted tooth has to be removed to gain access to the tooth (Fig. 25-31, *C*). This bone removal (ostectomy) can be accomplished with either a surgical mallet and chisels or a straight handpiece with surgical burs. If a surgical mallet and chisels are used, the assistant may be required to retract the mucoperiosteal flap while the operator holds a chisel in one hand and the surgical mallet in the other. Some dentists prefer to retract the flap with one hand and hold the chisel in the other while the assistant gently taps the end of the chisel with the surgical mallet.

   The surgical site should be irrigated with saline solution and evacuated to remove bone fragments and improve visibility.

   If a surgical bur in a handpiece is used to remove bone, the assistant must continually drop saline solution on the bur while it is cutting. This keeps the bur from clogging and reduces frictional heat on bone. The suction tip is held in the assistant's right hand, and the irrigating syringe is held in the left hand. Thus the surgical site can be constantly irrigated and evacuated during bone removal with the surgical bur. The dentist retracts the mucoperiosteal flap with the left hand while operating the handpiece with the right hand.
6. Once the impacted tooth is uncovered, it can be luxated and lifted from the alveolus with extraction elevators (Fig. 25-31, *D*). These are leverlike instruments that are wedged between alveolar bone and the tooth to be extracted. They are activated by twisting the large handle so that the tooth is forced in a disto-occlusal direction. On occasion, an impacted third molar is lodged between the ramus of the mandible and the distal surface of the second molar so that there is no pathway to lift the tooth from the alveolus. In these cases the crown of the tooth may have to be divided, or

sectioned, into two or more parts to allow room for luxation and removal of the tooth. Sectioning is done with either the mallet and chisel or the surgical bur.
7. After the tooth is delivered from the alveolus, the surgical site should be irrigated and evacuated and then examined to see that all loose debris has been removed.
8. In young developing third molars the dental sac still exists around the tooth and should be removed from the alveolus with the curette.
9. If the bony edges of the opening into the alveolus are sharp or rough, they should be trimmed and smoothed with the rongeur and the bone file, respectively.
10. After thorough debridement, the mucoperiosteal flap is returned to its normal position over the wound and sutured to the undisturbed gingiva (Fig. 25-31, *E* and *F*). The assistant can be of great assistance to the dentist during suturing by retracting soft tissue, supporting the suture material with the left hand so that it does not drag over the patient's face when it is pulled through the tissues, and cutting the suture after it is tied (Fig. 25-32).
11. Postoperative instructions are given, and the patient is allowed to remain seated upright until he or she is comfortable enough to move. Some dentists like to give the patient a cold pack to apply to the face over the surgical site to reduce postoperative swelling. There are commercial cold packs available.

    Patients must be instructed as to when to return for removal of the sutures and postoperative evaluation.

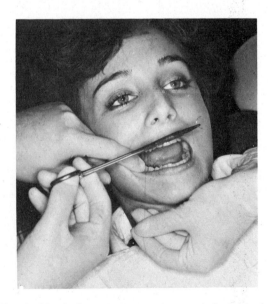

Fig. 25-32. Assistant supports suture as it is drawn into surgical site.

Multiple extraction

The extraction of several teeth in preparation for complete or removable partial dentures presents the dentist with a special type of complicated exodontia. The operator has to not only remove teeth but also surgically contour the remaining bone and soft tissue. This is necessary to provide a favorably shaped edentulous ridge on which the denture will rest. A properly contoured ridge is essential to achieve maximum comfort and function for the denture wearer.

Armamentarium. The same basic armamentarium that was used for a single complex extraction can be used for multiple extractions. Additional extraction forceps must be added for each additional type of tooth to be extracted (anterior, premolar, molar).

Procedure. Following is a description of the extraction of the mandibular right premolars and molars in preparation for a complete denture:

1. Local anesthetic is administered.
2. The surgical curette is used to test for anesthesia by probing around the teeth to be extracted.
3. If contouring of the edentulous ridge after the removal of the teeth is anticipated, an incision is made, and then a mucoperiosteal flap is reflected away from the teeth on the buccal aspect of the alveolar ridge (Fig. 25-33, *A* and *B*). Contouring is almost always required to some degree.
4. Removal of the teeth generally starts with the most posterior tooth and moves anteriorly. This gives the dentist some mechanical advantage in luxating the remaining teeth after the last molar in the arch has been removed. The teeth are luxated with extraction elevators and forceps. The forceps are then used to lift the teeth from their alveoli.
5. After the teeth have been removed and all root tips recovered (if necessary), the alveolar bone is contoured with rongeur forceps and the bone file (Fig. 25-33, *B* and *C*). All sharp edges of bone are smoothed with the file. This contouring of the alveolar process is called an alveoloplasty.
6. After the alveoloplasty the border of the mucoperiosteal flap and remaining attached gingiva are often trimmed with surgical scissors. This removes any soft tissue that may have been damaged during the extraction procedure and, by eliminating excess soft tissue, provides for a smoother surface of the edentulous ridge. The surgical site should be irrigated and evacuated before suturing is done.
7. The mucoperiosteal flap is repositioned and sutured to the remaining attached gingiva on the lingual aspect of the ridge (Fig. 25-33, *D*).
8. A moist compress of several 2 × 2 inch sterile gauze sponges is placed over the surgical site, and the patient is instructed to bite on the compress.
9. The patient is allowed to sit upright while postoperative instructions are given and is then escorted out of the operatory. An appointment is made for postoperative evaluation and suture removal.

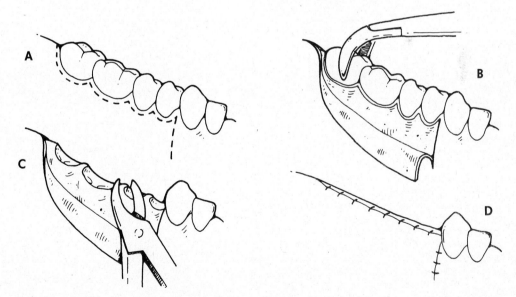

Fig. 25-33. Multiple-extraction sequence. **A,** Gingival incision. **B,** Retraction of mucoperiosteal flap and extraction of teeth. **C,** Alveoloplasty using rongeur. **D,** Sutured wound.

Immediate complete dentures are dentures that are made before the removal of the anterior teeth in a patient. When the patient has the anterior teeth removed, the denture is placed over the sutured wound, and the patient is dismissed. This patient should return the next day after surgery for postoperative evaluation and cleaning of the surgical site. The immediate denture technique will be described in detail in Chapter 26.

Root recovery

Portions of the root structure of a tooth may have to be recovered separately either because the crown portion of the tooth is missing as a result of extensive caries or because the tooth is fractured during luxation by the dentist. Such root recovery is a necessary part of an extraction procedure. In most instances, root fragments should be removed because of the rather high potential for infection in the future.

Several techniques are used to recover root fragments. The dentist selects the technique that is suitable for the specific problem the patient presents at the time. A brief description of various root recovery methods follows.

Root pick technique (Fig. 25-34, *A*). The alveolus is rinsed and evacuated. The root pick is forced between the wall of the alveolus and the root tip to remove it.

Forceps technique (Fig. 25-34, *B*). Special root-extraction forceps are available with long, narrow beaks that are convenient for recovering root fragments of one third the root length or larger. Usually a mucoperiosteal flap is reflected, and buccal or labial bone is removed to gain access to the root. These forceps are often used alternately with root picks to remove the root fragment.

Elevator technique (Fig. 25-34, *C*). This is a helpful method of removing roots of multirooted teeth. The teeth are sectioned through the bifurcation or trifurcation of the roots with a surgical bur or chisel. An elevator is inserted in either the cut area of the interdental area and twisted to luxate and elevate the roots from the alveolus.

Bur technique (Fig. 25-34, *D*). This method is

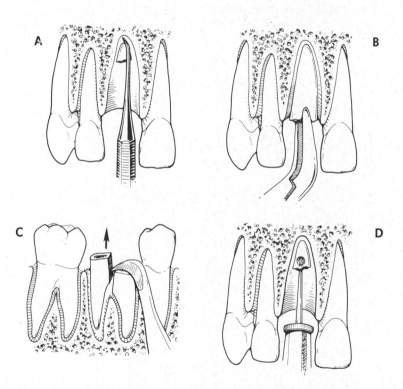

Fig. 25-34. Root recovery technique. **A,** Root-pick method. **B,** Forceps method. **C,** Elevator method. **D,** Bur method.

helpful in the anterior and premolar areas. A straight handpiece with a No. 4 to No. 6 round bur (HP) is used to bore into the root canal of the fragment. The handpiece is tipped so that the bur locks in the canal, and the fragment is lifted from the alveolus with the handpiece. This method is usually limited to small root tips.

Postoperative instructions

Postoperative instructions to the patient are important guidelines the patient should follow to avoid complications and unnecessary discomfort. It is advisable to go over these instructions verbally with the patient after surgery to avoid confusion. However, the patient should be given a printed copy of the instructions to review after leaving the office. Patients tend to forget verbal instructions, especially when they are given right after surgery. The verbal instructions should be given only to emphasize the important written guidelines.

Healing of an extraction site begins with blood clot formation in the empty alveolus. This clot is the first step in the healing process. The formation and preservation of the clot in the alveolus is the principal goal of postoperative care. Anything that interferes with this process can lead to complications such as prolonged bleeding, infection, "dry socket," and delayed healing. Table 25-1 lists typical postoperative instructions and the reason for each instruction.

POSTOPERATIVE COMPLICATIONS

Careful diagnosis, treatment planning, and surgical technique can prevent many unnecessary postsurgical complications. Among the more common complications that occur after surgery are prolonged bleeding, infection, and alveolitis (dry socket).

Prolonged bleeding

Prolonged bleeding is the most common postoperative complication. Patients may call after removing

Table 25-1. Postoperative instructions for the surgical patient

Instruction	Rationale
1. Maintain biting pressure on gauze compress for 30 minutes. Repeat for 30 more minutes if bleeding continues.	Compression of wound is one of the best ways to stop bleeding and promote clot formation.
2. Place a cold pack on face over surgical site for 5 to 10 hours after surgery. This should be started as soon as possible.	Cold packs help to reduce swelling in surgical area. Excessive swelling can delay healing and create esthetic problems for the patient.
3. Avoid rinsing mouth until the day after surgery. Small sips of water are permitted after gauze compress is removed and bleeding has stopped.	Rinsing can dislodge newly formed clot from alveolus, causing additional bleeding and delayed healing.
4. On the day after surgery, *gentle* rinsing of mouth is permitted using ½ tsp of salt in 8 oz drinking glass of very warm water	This freshens mouth for patient. Salt water is more compatible with tissue cells, since it is similar to salty nature of tissue fluid. Warmth of rinse enhances circulation to oral cavity, which promotes healing.
5. Remaining teeth should be brushed gently with soft-bristle toothbrush beginning day after surgery.	This freshens patient's mouth as well as removing bacterial plaque accumulation, which can increase possibility of infection.
6. Diet should be limited to very soft foods for 24 hours; continue this as necessary for comfort. Drink lots of liquids by sipping. Do not use a straw.	Heavy-textured foods can bruise the surgical site and even dislodge clot. Sucking on a straw can also draw clot from alveolus. Liquid consumption helps to replace lost fluids during surgery and maintain favorable fluid and electrolyte balance in body.
7. Take any prescribed medication as directed after compress is removed.	Medications are prescribed for pain and prevention of infection in some cases.
8. If prolonged bleeding continues after 1 hour, contact dentist for further instructions.	Prolonged bleeding may require additional treatment by dentist.
9. Elevate head with pillows when sleeping during first 24 hours.	This helps to avoid additional bleeding and swelling.

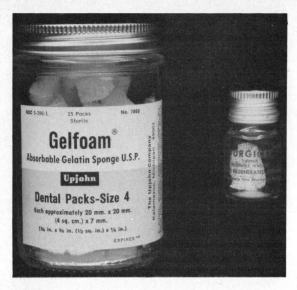

Fig. 25-35. Two common materials used to pack alveolus to control hemorrhage.

the gauze compress and complain of continued bleeding. It is common for the saliva to be tinted with a small quantity of blood for several hours after surgery. However, if the patient has a deep red discoloration to the saliva, a bleeding problem exists.

Prolonged bleeding should be treated initially by instructing the patient to pack a moist, folded gauze compress over the extraction site and apply biting pressure for another 20 to 30 minutes. If no gauze is available, a moistened tea bag can be used for the same purpose. If bleeding continues after this procedure, the patient should return to the office for further treatment.

Once the patient arrives, anesthesia is administered and the surgical wound is irrigated and inspected. A common method to control hemorrhage is to pack the alveolus with absorbable Gelfoam or oxidized cellulose (Fig. 25-35). Some dentists prefer to saturate oxidized cellulose with a topical thrombin solution to further enhance clotting. These agents form a network around which blood can clot. They need not be removed, since they are absorbed by the body as healing takes place. Sutures are sometimes placed across the opening of the alveolus to hold the pack in place. The patient is instructed to bite on a new moist gauze compress for another 30 minutes. This procedure solves the majority of bleeding problems.

Infection

Whenever any type of surgery is performed, there is a possibility of infection developing in the open wound. Considering the bacteria-laden environment of the oral cavity, it is somewhat amazing that postoperative infection does not occur more often than it does.

Postsurgical infections generally develop 2 to 4 days after surgery. Some common characteristics of oral infection are (1) pain, (2) swelling, (3) muscle spasm, (4) elevated body temperature, and (5) accumulation of pus in the surgical wound.

Treatment for infection is divided into two categories: local treatment and systemic treatment.

Local treatment

1. The wound is irrigated with warm saline solution.
2. The patient is instructed to rinse the mouth every hour with ½ tsp of salt in an 8 oz glass of very warm water.
3. Hot moist compresses are applied to the face over the surgical site to localize the infection to one area. A washcloth folded into fourths is moistened under the hot water tap. (Make it as hot as can be tolerated by the skin on the arm.) The moist washcloth is applied to the face and covered by a dry hand towel, and a hot water bag is laid on top. This should be maintained for 30 minutes, removed for 30 minutes, and then reapplied throughout the day. A cold cream applied to the skin will help prevent drying of the facial skin.
4. Once the localization of pus occurs under the mucosa, the mucosa can be incised, and the pus drained away. Often the pus will drain on its own from the extraction site.

Systemic treatment

1. Bed rest is encouraged.
2. High fluid intake is helpful to promote recovery.
3. Drugs are administered as needed.
   a. Antibiotics to combat infection
   b. Analgesics to relieve pain
   c. Sedative-hypnotics to relax the patient

Since orofacial infections are close to vital anatomical structures, the patient's progress should be followed closely to avoid more serious complications.

Alveolitis (dry socket)

After the extraction of a tooth from its alveolus, healing begins immediately with blood oozing into the alveolus and clotting. The clot is later replaced by scar tissue and ultimately bone as healing progresses. Unfortunately, some extraction sites do not undergo this favorable progression. The blood clot that normally fills the alveolus either does not form or forms and is lost from the alveolus. The reason for this phenomenon is still not clear; however, there seem to be several causative factors involved. Some of these are the following:

1. Anatomical deficiencies resulting in inadequate blood supply to the surgical site
2. Excessive trauma to the alveolus during the extraction
3. Vasoconstriction of vessels from the local anesthetic, diminishing the blood supply to the surgical site
4. Preoperative or postoperative infection interfering with the normal healing process
5. Carelessness on the part of the patient, dislodging the clot from the alveolus by vigorous rinsing or sucking on a straw after surgery
6. Existing nutritional deficiencies in the patient
7. Foreign debris contaminating the alveolus either during surgery or immediately afterward

Although the exact cause is still unclear, patients present themselves 2 to 4 days after the extraction complaining of mild to severe dull pain and a foul odor and taste. When the alveolus is inspected, the clot is found to be missing and bone is exposed. The wound is then irritated by the oral environment.

Treatment of this condition is strictly geared to making the patient comfortable while the wound heals. This is called palliative therapy. Healing can take from 10 to 40 days.

Armamentarium. The armamentarium for this procedure includes the following:

Mouth mirror   Warm saline solution
Cotton pliers   Iodoform gauze
Scissors   Dentalone solution
Irrigation syringe   Oral evacuator tip

Procedure. Although treatment varies between dentists, a typical regimen is as follows:

1. The alveolus is gently irrigated with warm saline solution and dried.
2. A narrow strip of iodoform gauze is cut to a length that will fill the alveolus (Fig. 25-36).
3. The gauze is dipped in Dentalone solution and gently packed into the alveolus.

The patient is dismissed and asked to return every 1 to 2 days initially to repeat this procedure.

The rationale behind this treatment is as follows:

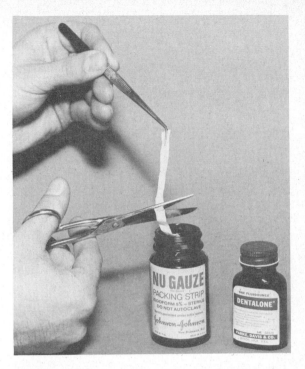

Fig. 25-36. Iodoform gauze and Dentalone solution used to treat alveolitis.

Procedure	Rationale
Irrigation	Removes accumulated debris in the alveolus.
Gauze pack	Helps to prevent food from being packed into the alveolus.
Iodoform	Iodoform in the gauze is a topical antiseptic that helps prevent infection.
Dentalone solution	Contains obtundent medications that soothe the nerve endings in the exposed bone.
Frequent recall	Keeps the wound clean and freshens the medications, which diminish in their effect quickly.

Systemic analgesics are often prescribed to relieve pain until the exposed bone is covered sufficiently by a layer of cells as a result of healing (granulation tissue).

DENTAL ASSISTANT'S ROLE
Suture removal (Fig. 25-37)

Suture removal can be a task for dental assistants where state laws permit. After the extraction site is

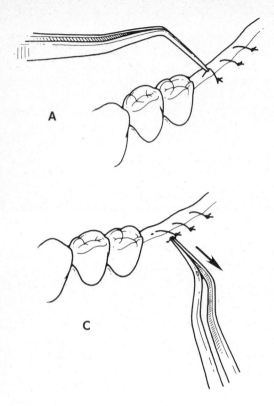

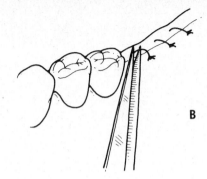

Fig. 25-37. Suture removal.

inspected by the dentist, the assistant can remove the sutures as follows:

Armamentarium
Mouth mirror
Cotton pliers
Suture scissors
2 × 2 inch gauze

Procedure

1. Locate and account for all the sutures placed during the surgical appointment.
2. Lift each suture with the cotton pliers so that the beak of the scissors can fit under the suture material (Fig. 25-37, *A*).
3. The suture should be cut as close to the tissue as possible so that a minimum of material has to be pulled through the tissue (Fig. 25-37, *B*).
4. Grasp the knot of the suture and pull the suture material from the tissue (Fig. 25-37, *C*).
5. Recheck the wound to be sure all sutures have been removed.

SUMMARY

Oral surgery is truly a four-handed procedure. Access and visibility are critical to the success of the process. The ability to perform standard chairside duties and to understand the basic surgical fundamentals just described makes the assistant a critical link in successful oral surgery.

BIBLIOGRAPHY

Calhoun, N.R.: Dry socket and other postoperative complications, Dent. Clin. North Am. **15:**337-348, 1971.
Kruger, G.O.: Textbook of oral and maxillofacial surgery, ed. 6, St. Louis, 1984, The C.V. Mosby Co.
Schoen, M.H.: Frequency of tooth loss in relation to the dentist's ability to prevent the necessity of extraction, Dent. Clin. North Am. **13:**741-755, 1969.
Schram, W.R.: A manual of oral surgery techniques, Philadelphia, 1962, W.B. Saunders Co.

CHAPTER 26

PROSTHODONTICS _____

A prosthesis is an artificial body part. Artificial limbs, eyes, heart valves, and teeth are just a few examples of some common prosthetic devices.

In the strictest sense, any type of dental restoration is a prosthesis. Common usage of the term *prosthodontics* (prosthetics in dentistry) refers to that area of dental practice that deals with the extensive reconstruction of existing teeth and the replacement of missing teeth with various dental restorations and appliances. Generally speaking, operative restorations are not considered a part of prosthodontics. Prosthodontics is a broad term that encompasses crown and bridge procedures (fixed prosthodontics) and both complete and partial denture services (removable prosthodontics). There is a tendency among many dentists to group these dental services into operative dentistry, crown and bridge procedures, and prosthodontics (denture services). For purposes of discussion in this chapter, the term prosthodontics will be used to describe the fabrication of removable prosthetic appliances such as complete and partial dentures.

The utilization of chairside assistants in the area of removable prosthodontic services has not been as well developed as in the other areas of dental practice. This is probably because constant use of four hands during a prosthetic appointment is unnecessary. The assistant's role in prosthodontics is primarily limited to operatory preparation, laboratory duties, and preparation of impression materials. Prosthetic dentistry does not require a lot of the instrument exchanges and constant oral evacuation that are associated with other dental services.

A general understanding of denture construction will be of value to the clinical dental assistant so that appointments, surgical and restorative services, and laboratory phases can all be coordinated properly.

Three common prosthetic services will be described in this chapter to provide the assistant with some of the fundamentals of prosthetic services—fabrication of a removable partial denture, fabrication of an immediate complete denture, and a denture reline.

FABRICATION OF A REMOVABLE PARTIAL DENTURE: CLASS I EXAMPLE

A removable partial denture is a prosthetic device used to replace missing teeth. Since it is used to replace only a part of the dentition while some natural teeth remain, it is called a partial denture. The bridge restoration discussed in Chapter 20 is also called a fixed partial denture because it is cemented in place and cannot be removed by the patient. The removable partial denture can and must be removed by the patient for cleaning. There are several instances in which the dentist has to decide to replace missing teeth with either a fixed or removable partial denture. Such factors as number and location of missing teeth, periodontal status, condition of the remaining natural teeth, occlusal relationships, esthetics, and economics all play a role in this decision. In other instances, the dentist has no choice and must use a removable partial denture.

There are several edentulous situations in which a removable partial denture can be used. Table 26-1 outlines the Applegate-Kennedy system of classifying these situations.

A typical appointment schedule for the fabrication of a removable partial denture is shown in Table 26-2. As with virtually all dental procedures, there are several methods used to construct both partial and complete dentures. The methods to be described are only examples of common techniques currently used.

Preliminary steps

The first step in all dental treatment is to gather all the information necessary for an accurate diagnosis and treatment planning. A complete medical-dental history, oral and radiographic examination, and study

Table 26-1. Applegate-Kennedy classification system for partially edentulous situations

Class	Definition
I 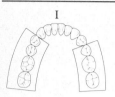	An edentulous situation in which all remaining teeth are anterior to the *bilateral edentulous areas*.
II 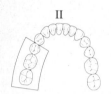	An edentulous situation in which the remaining teeth of either the right or the left side are anterior to the *unilateral edentulous area,* with all teeth (except third molars) of the opposite side remaining.
III 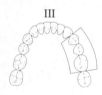	An edentulous situation in which the edentulous area is *bounded by teeth unable to assume total support* of the necessary prosthesis. These abutments require the aid of teeth remotely located, so that the principles of cross-arch splinting (and counterleverage) can be utilized to resist the lateral tilting forces to which these abutments will be subjected.
IV 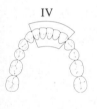	An edentulous situation in which the *remaining teeth bound the edentulous area posteriorly* on both right and left sides of the median line.
V 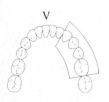	An edentulous situation in which teeth bound the edentulous area anteriorly and posteriorly but where the *anterior boundary tooth is not suitable for abutment service* (as the lateral incisor).
VI 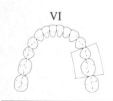	An edentulous sitation in which the *boundary teeth are capable of total support* of the required prothesis.

From Applegate, O.C.: Essentials of removable denture prosthesis, ed. 3, Philadelphia, 1965, W.B. Saunders Co.

Table 26-2. A typical appointment schedule for the fabrication of a Class I removable partial denture (clasp-type)

Appointment	Treatment
1	Complete oral and radiographic examination Dental prophylaxis Alginate impressions for study models
2	Case presentation; discussion of planned treatment and fee estimates
3	Mouth preparations; may require several separate appointments if periodontal or restorative treatment is required
4	Final impressions for master casts on which denture framework is made Occlusal registration
5	Try-in and adjustment of framework
6	Final impression of edentulous ridges on which denture base will rest Reestablish or verify occlusal registration Tooth shade selection
7	Delivery of denture Initial denture adjustments as needed
8	Denture adjustment appointments as required

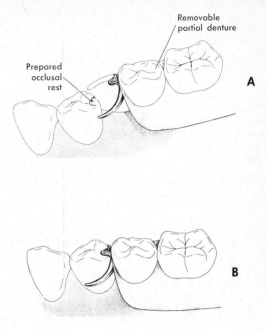

Fig. 26-1. A, Clasp of removable partial denture and prepared abutment tooth. **B,** Clasp in place on abutment tooth.

models are essential elements in achieving this goal.

A thorough dental prophylaxis should be done before the examination and impression taking for study models.

After all diagnostic information has been obtained, the dentist formulates a treatment plan and designs the partial denture on the study models. The patient returns for a case presentation, in which the treatment plan is explained and fee estimates given.

Before a partial denture is constructed, the foundation on which it will rest must be healthy and sound. Therefore the mouth has to be prepared as needed to create a favorable foundation. This preparation may include operative dentistry, extensive restorative procedures, periodontal treatment, and oral surgery, depending on the condition of the individual.

An important part of mouth preparation for a partial denture is the proper contouring of the teeth where the metal framework of the partial denture rests. The occlusal surfaces of teeth that will support the framework have to be contoured to hold the framework firmly in place and allow clearance between the upper and lower teeth to accommodate the thickness of the framework. The buccal and lingual contours of the

abutment teeth must be favorable to allow the denture to be inserted and removed without binding and be held in place by retention clasps (Fig. 26-1). If such contouring cannot be accomplished by minimal grinding of the enamel of these teeth, the teeth have to be recontoured by placing crown restorations on the teeth involved. This is a rather common requirement in partial denture construction. Once the mouth has been prepared, final impressions can be taken.

Steps in the fabrication of a removable partial denture: Class I example (Fig. 26-2)

Final impressions

1. Once mouth preparations are complete, final impressions are taken for construction of master casts (models).
2. These impressions must be very accurate, since the metal framework will be cast in the laboratory on a duplicate of the master cast.
3. It is recommended that the teeth be polished with a rubber cup and pumice and rinsed thoroughly with mouthwash just before the impression, for greater accuracy.
4. Final impressions can be taken with any of the elastic impression materials (alginate, mercaptan, silicone, agar hydrocolloid) prepared in the usual manner.

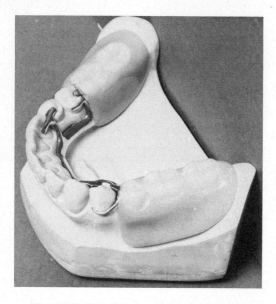

Fig. 26-2. Class I removable partial denture.

5. If agar hydrocolloid is used, stock trays have to be selected to fit the patient. A custom acrylic tray is recommended for use with any of the other materials for improved accuracy. (This can be made from the study models before the final impression appointment.)

6. Gingival retraction is *not* needed for these impressions. However, the syringe-tray technique offers some advantage in eliminating voids in the impression around the abutment teeth and rest areas for the framework. The use of alginate foregoes this advantage.

7. Once the impressions are obtained, they should be poured with improved stone immediately to make the accurate master casts.

8. The impressions should be poured with the two-stage pouring technique. The impression is filled and allowed to rest upright on cotton rolls until the stone reaches its initial set (loses its glossy surface) (Fig. 26-3, *A*). A new mix of stone is prepared, and the impression is inverted onto a pile of the stone on the laboratory bench (Fig. 26-3, *B*). This is allowed to harden for 45 minutes before removing the impression from the stone and trimming the models.

Bite registration

1. A wax bite registration may be necessary to articulate the upper and lower models accurately in the laboratory.

2. One method is to have the patient bite into a sheet of pink baseplate wax that has been warmed in hot water and folded in half. The patient is instructed to bite down just enough to form tiny imprints in the wax.

A

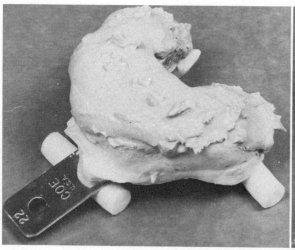

B

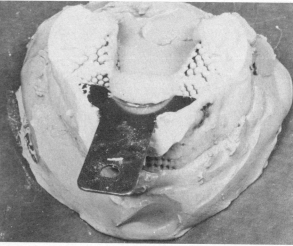

Fig. 26-3. Two-stage method of pouring models. **A,** Impression is filled with improved stone and allowed to remain upright until material reaches its initial set. **B,** Filled impression is then inverted onto pile of stone to form base of model.

3. The wax is removed from the mouth and trimmed so that an excess of ¼ to ½ inch of wax extends buccally and labially beyond the imprints.
4. The area of the imprints is heated with an alcohol torch (Fig. 26-4, *A*) and reinserted in the patient's mouth. The teeth are closed firmly into the imprints so that the teeth penetrate through the wax.
5. The excess wax along the facial aspects of the teeth is pressed against the teeth to achieve a better imprint in the wax.
6. The wax is cooled in the mouth before removal with the air-water syringe and the oral evacuator (Fig. 26-4, *B*). (NOTE: The dentist operates the evacuator while cooling the wax on the right side of the patient's mouth and the syringe while cooling the wax on the left side.)

Shade selection

1. If the denture is to be made entirely on the master cast without a corrected impression of the edentulous ridges, a shade is selected at this time. Conventional shade guides are used for this purpose.
2. The patient is dismissed.

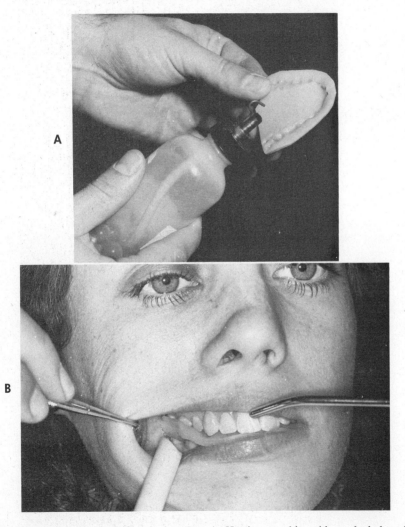

Fig. 26-4. Taking an occlusal (bite) registration. **A,** Heating wax bite with an alcohol torch along area of imprints made by patient's teeth. **B,** Cooling wax bite after it is reinserted in patient's mouth and teeth are closed together tightly.

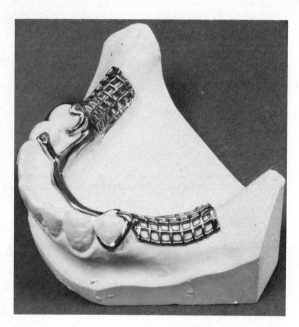

Fig. 26-5. Metal framework.

Laboratory phase

1. The master casts are trimmed and sent to the laboratory along with the study models, the bite registration, the shade, and the laboratory prescription.
2. The study models are used to describe the partial denture design. The dentist can sketch the design on the model as well as describe it in the laboratory prescription. The laboratory prescription will be discussed later in this chapter.
3. The laboratory will cast the metal framework according to the dentist's design and return it to the dentist.
4. In partial denture designs that do not require an additional impression of the edentulous ridges, the entire partial denture is fabricated and returned to the dentist for delivery to the patient.

Framework try-in

1. After the cast framework has been received from the laboratory (Fig. 26-5), it is fitted to the patient's mouth.
2. Adjustments are made as needed to adapt the framework to the teeth and to establish proper occlusion.

Edentulous ridge impression

1. In cases such as a Class I partial denture design in which the denture is supported principally by the edentulous ridges, a separate impression of the ridges is desirable. This permits the dentist to contour and adapt the denture base to the edentulous areas more accurately.

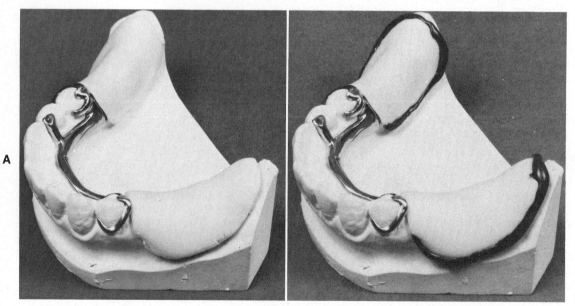

Fig. 26-6. A, Acrylic "saddles" added to framework to be used to take impression of edentulous ridges. **B,** Border-molded saddles.

2. Small acrylic "saddles" are added to the framework, using custom acrylic tray material (Fig. 26-6, *A*). These saddles are used as miniature impression trays for the ridges.
3. The dentist can adjust the size of the saddles by adding softened compound around the border of the acrylic and trying it in the patient's mouth. This is called border molding (Fig. 26-6, *B*).
4. Once the size of the saddles is established, an impression is taken of the ridge areas by coating the tisse surface of the acrylic with impression material and inserting the framework-saddle assembly in the patient's mouth. The impression materials commonly used for this purpose are mercaptan (rubber base), silicone, zinc oxide–eugenol paste, or impression wax.

   The occlusion can be rechecked at this appointment.

Laboraory phase

1. The impressions and master casts are returned to the laboratory along with a laboratory prescription.
2. The laboratory technician sets the denture teeth to the predetermined occlusion and fabricates the denture base with denture acrylic.

Denture delivery

1. The completed partial denture is returned from the laboratory and delivered to the patient (Fig. 26-7).
2. Adjustments in fit and occlusion are made as needed at this appointment.
3. The partial denture is designed to slide on and off the remaining teeth in a specific direction. This is called the path of insertion (and removal). Patients must be instructed in the proper insertion and removal method before being dismissed.
4. Patients should be instructed in oral hygiene procedures

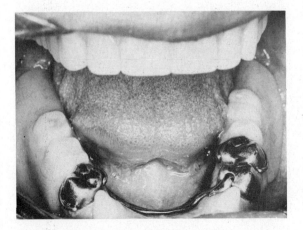

Fig. 26-7. Completed removable partial denture.

and maintenance of the partial denture. Caries, periodontal disease, and mouth odors can develop rather quickly if plaque is allowed to accumulate on the partial denture framework and on the remaining natural teeth.
   a. Partial dentures should be removed and rinsed with tap water after eating.
   b. Twice daily the denture should be scrubbed with a toothbrush and a mild soap in a basin of lukewarm water and rinsed thoroughly.
5. The patient can expect some adjustment period to learn to speak and eat with the new appliance. Excessive salivation is common for a time after insertion of the denture. Patients are encouraged to begin using the denture on soft-textured foods until they become accustomed to the new appliance. Sticky foods, nuts, and foods with tiny seeds should be avoided, since they can be unpleasant for the denture wearer. Candies and caramels tend to stick to the acrylic denture, and seeds work under the denture base and are most uncomfortable for the patient.

Adjustment phase

1. Postinsertion evaluation of the patient is needed to check (a) fit of the denture, (b) occlusion, (c) oral hygiene and denture maintenance, and (d) patient's problems encountered wearing the denture.
2. Adjustments are made on the denture as required to achieve maximum comfort and function for the patient. Patients may require several adjustment appointments to achieve this goal.

FABRICATION OF A COMPLETE DENTURE (IMMEDIATE METHOD)

Patients who have all their teeth removed and replaced with complete dentures are faced with unique and difficult problems. Although some people are successful denture wearers, many are not. No denture can duplicate the comfort, efficiency, and dependability provided by a well-maintained healthy natural dentition. A common misconception regarding complete dentures is that they are a way to solve all dental problems. In truth, dentures often mark the onset of problems for many people. Dentures are prosthetic devices that replace a body part, but they do not completely restore normal function any more than does an artificial leg. Patients who are "successful" denture wearers simply have a greater ability to adapt to a prosthesis. They either accept or overcome the problems associated with wearing a prosthesis.

Successful denture wearing depends on several factors, including the following:
1. The jaw relationship of the patient
2. The size and shape of the edentulous ridges

3. The coordination of the patient's oral musculature
4. The attitude of the individual patient
5. Personal diet and oral habits of the individual
6. The quality of the construction of the denture itself

Prospective denture patients often comment that they have a friend or relative who wears dentures and has no problems at all. The fact is clear that people vary widely in these factors just listed. With these variables in mind, there is little reason to expect that one person should be as successful as another in wearing dentures. Unfortunately, no one knows how well a patient will be able to function with complete dentures until after the individual has worn them awhile. By then it is too late. The natural teeth are gone forever, and dentures are the only alternative. It is not surprising that a majority of dentists try to do everything possible to save natural teeth to avoid this dilemma for their dental patients. Since the emphasis on preventive and restorative dentistry and periodontal therapy has increased during the past 20 years, there has been a corresponding decline in the number of dentures made annually in the United States.

Table 26-3. A sample appointment schedule for fabrication of immediate complete dentures

Appointment	Service
1	Examination and treatment planning (includes radiographs, medical history, study model impressions, and possibly photographs)
2	Extraction of posterior teeth on one side of mouth
3	Extraction of posterior teeth on other side of mouth (Wait approximately 3 to 4 weeks until next appointment.)
4	Preliminary impressions of remaining anterior teeth and edentulous ridges (alginate)
5	Final impressions of remaining teeth and edentulous ridges
6	Recording jaw relationships with occlusal rims and selecting proper shade and mold for denture teeth
7	Extraction of remaining anterior teeth and delivery of complete dentures
8	First postoperative visit (preferably on day after extractions)
9	Adjustment appointments as needed

Techniques that are used to fabricate complete dentures vary widely between dentists. The following is a discussion of a common method used to construct complete dentures that will be inserted at the surgical appointment when the last remaining teeth are removed. This method is commonly called the immediate denture technique. A typical appointment schedule for this procedure is shown in Table 26-3.

Preliminary steps

Careful diagnosis and treatment planning are just as important in the fabrication of complete dentures as they are in all other dental services. The dentist must carefully plan the needed surgery and design of the denture. The patient's health status, age, habits, jaw relationships, and jaw discrepancies are important considerations. Study models are useful aids in treatment planning for complete dentures. A thorough study of the size and shape of the remaining teeth and jaws can be made from the models to enhance the accuracy of denture design. Photographs of the patient's teeth and facial contour are also of assistance to the dentist in creating favorable esthetics for the patient.

After treatment planning, the first step in construction of an immediate denture is to remove the posterior teeth in both arches and perform the necessary alveoloplasty to shape the edentulous ridges to a favorable contour. The idea of the immediate denture is to leave the anterior teeth to preserve some esthetics and speech quality until the dentures are ready for delivery at the surgery appointment when these remaining teeth are removed. The advantage of this technique is that patients are never completely without teeth while making the transition from natural to artificial teeth.

Steps in construction of the immediate denture

Preliminary impressions

1. Generally, a 3- to 4-week period is required after the removal of the posterior teeth for adequate healing to take place for the taking of alginate impressions of the partially edentulous jaws.
2. These impressions are taken with "stock" alginate trays.
3. Work models are made from the impressions.
4. Custom acrylic trays are then made on these work models.

Final impressions

1. The patient returns for more accurate impressions using the custom acrylic trays (Fig. 26-8).

2. The borders of the tray are adjusted to the proper length with stick compound. The compound is heated with a Bunsen burner and fused to the edges (periphery) of the tray. Then the tray is dipped in vary warm water. The tray is inserted in the patient's mouth, and the lips, cheeks, and tongue are manipulated to form accurate lengths of the tray fingers. This is called border molding or muscle trimming.

3. Once the tray has been prepared with compound (border molded), several holes should be drilled through the tray on the dental lathe and the tissue surface painted with an impression-material adhesive.

4. A "tray-consistency" mercaptan impression material is available for denture impressions. The mercaptan material is mixed in the same manner as described for the heavy-bodied material used in the fabrication of gold restorations.

5. The tray is filled with the impression material, and the patient's mouth is rinsed thoroughly.

6. The tray is inserted in the mouth and removed after the material has set completely.

7. The same procedure is repeated for the opposite arch.

8. The patient is then dismissed.

9. The impressions are poured in dental stone to make the master casts.

Determining jaw relationships

1. In a natural dentition the teeth determine how the lower jaw relates to the upper jaw when the mouth is closed. In the closed position with the teeth clenched together, the distance between the upper and lower jaws is determined by the length of the crowns of the posterior teeth (Fig. 26-9, *A*). This distance between the upper and lower jaws is called vertical dimension. The natural teeth also determine how the mandible relates to the maxilla in both an anterioposterior direction and a lateral (side-to-side) position (Fig. 26-9, *A* and *B*). This jaw relationship is called centric occlusion. In other words, centric occlusion is the normal position of the jaws when the teeth are meshed together.

2. Since the natural posterior teeth have been removed, the patient no longer has the natural guides to determine either vertical dimension or centric occlusion (Fig. 26-9, *C* and *D*). The dentist has to substitute artificial spacers in place of the missing teeth to determine these jaw relationships. These spacers are the wax occlusal rims that are mounted on temporary denture bases called baseplates (Fig. 26-10). This assembly is fabricated in the laboratory on the master casts.

3. The dentist can reestablish the proper vertical dimension by adding or removing wax from the rims as needed. The occlusal rims are repeatedly tried in the patient's mouth until proper vertical dimension is established.

4. Centric occlusion can be determined by a variety of techniques that include tracing devices mounted on the occlusal rims and various manipulations of the mandible during closing exercises.

Tooth selection

1. Once jaw relationships are taken on the occlusal rims, the denture teeth have to be selected. The proper shade is determined with the use of shade guides to compare with the patient's remaining natural teeth and the complexion of the facial skin. Age is a factor in shade selection, since natural teeth darken somewhat with age. A very light–shaded tooth would not look natural in an older patient's mouth. The size and shape (mold) of the denture teeth are important in achieving natural esthetics for the denture wearer. This can be done by comparing tooth mold guides with the remaining natural teeth if they are sufficiently intact. If these teeth are substantially destroyed by caries or fracture, the shape of the patient's face is used as a guide to selecting the proper shape of anterior teeth. There is a general correlation between the shape of a patient's face and the shape of the anterior teeth. For example, a person with a long, narrow face will have longer, more slender anterior teeth.

2. Obviously, patients are concerned about the esthetics of their new denture as well as with function. Creating natural-appearing complete dentures for a patient calls on the artistic skill of the dentist and the laboratory technician. Vertical dimension, shade, size, shape, and the arrangement of the teeth all play a role in esthetics. Patients are very apprehensive regarding the appearance of their dentures. The use of study models, photographs, and accurate measurements are helpful in achieving a natural-appearing denture (Fig. 26-11).

3. After all measurements are taken, appointments are made for the removal of the patient's remaining teeth and the insertion of his new dentures.

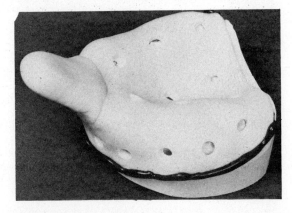

Fig. 26-8. Border-molded custom acrylic impression tray used for final impression.

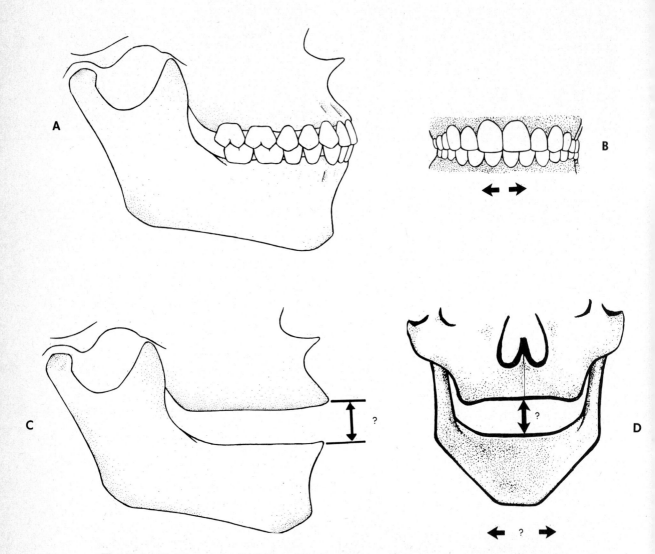

Fig. 26-9. Components of vertical dimension. **A** and **B,** Natural dentition. Vertical dimension (**A**) is determined by lengths of crowns of upper and lower teeth. Centric occlusion is also determined by natural dentition. **C** and **D,** Edentulous ridges. Completely edentulous ridges or those missing only posterior teeth lose natural determination of vertical dimension and centric occlusion.

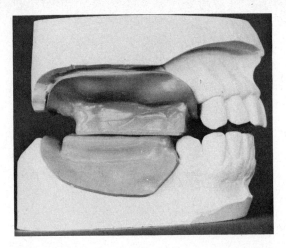

Fig. 26-10. Occlusal wax rims mounted on baseplates. Excessive height exists initially so that dentist can adjust height to proper vertical dimension.

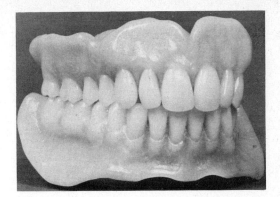

Fig. 26-12. Set of complete dentures.

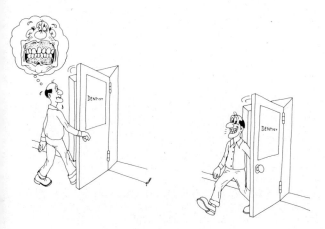

Fig. 26-11

Laboratory phase

1. The master casts, occlusal rims, shade guide, mold, study models, and photographs are sent to the laboratory where the denture is made.
2. The finished denture will not fit the anterior portion of the dental arches precisely, since the denture is made before the teeth in this area are removed. However, this approximate fit does suffice until complete healing occurs.

Delivery of the denture (Fig. 26-12)

1. The remaining anterior teeth are removed, any necessary alveoloplasty is done, and sutures are placed.

2. The dentures are removed from a bath of disinfecting solution and rinsed.
3. The dentures are inserted, and adjustments are made as necessary to improve fit and the occlusion.
4. Denture adhesives are often used to hold the denture more firmly on the edentulous ridge until the patient adapts to the new prosthesis.
5. Patients should be given postsurgical instructions and asked to return the next day. Patients are not to remove the dentures until then.

First postsurgical appointment

1. The patient is asked to return the day after surgery so that the denture can be removed and cleaned.
2. The dentist can carefully clean the surgical site.
3. Additional adjustments on the denture may be made at this time.
4. Detailed instructions on diet, eating methods, and speech exercises are given.
5. The patient returns 4 to 6 days later for suture removal.

Postinsertion adjustments

1. The need for adjustments on a denture varies with each patient.
2. Denture adjustments may include minor alterations of the occlusion or relieving small areas of acrylic on the tissue surface of the denture base. These areas cause excessive pressure on the underlying soft tissue, resulting in "denture sores."
3. Adjustments are accomplished with small grindstones and acrylic burs in the straight handpiece.

DENTURE RELINING

After a complete or partial denture is worn for a period of time, it is common for the edentulous ridge to undergo a generalized reduction in size. This

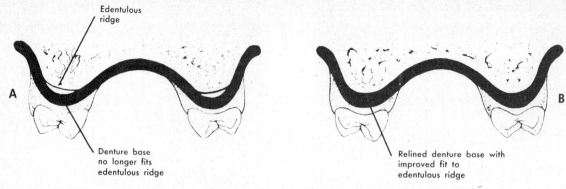

Fig. 26-13. A, Frontal section across maxillae demonstrating poor fit of denture base to edentulous ridge. **B,** Relining denture readapts it to edentulous ridge.

"shrinkage" results from initial healing of the ridges, and later reduction occurs in response to excessive force being placed on the dentures. Regardless of the cause of edentulous ridge reduction, the problem that results is the same—the denture no longer fits the ridge (Fig. 26-13, *A*).

A technique to compensate for ridge reduction has been developed that allows the dentist to add new acrylic to the tissue surface of the denture base. This is called relining the denture. By placing a new layer, or lining, of acrylic inside the denture, the dentist readapts the denture to the now smaller ridges, thus improving the fit without remaking the entire denture (Fig. 26-13, *B*).

Two basic methods are used to reline a complete or partial denture: the chairside reline and the laboratory-processed reline.

Chairside reline

"Chairside reline" is a common way of referring to a technique that allows the dentist to add a new acrylic lining to a denture as a chairside procedure without any laboratory phase. The advantage of this technique is that the entire procedure can be accomplished in one appointment, so that the patient does not have to be without a denture for any period of time. The disadvantage of this procedure is that the lining is generally not as durable as can be achieved with the laboratory-processed lining materials.

Preparing the denture
1. The denture to be relined is removed.
2. The tissue surface of the denture base is roughened with an acrylic grindstone.

3. The tissue surface of the denture base is cleaned for a few minutes in the ultrasonic cleaner.

Preparation of the material
1. Several brands of self-curing acrylics are available to use as relining material. They are available also as either hard or semisoft liners.
2. The material is dispensed and mixed according to the manufacturer's instructions and added to the clean denture. The entire tissue surface of the denture base is coated with the material.

Patient preparation
1. The patient is instructed to rinse the mouth with a mouthwash to remove saliva from the tissue surface.
2. The denture is inserted and positioned properly. The patient is asked to bite gently with the teeth in proper occlusion until the material reaches its initial set. The patient should be cautioned that there may be a burning sensation from the acrylic during the initial setting time.
3. Then the denture is removed and allowed to completely harden.

Finishing the denture
1. After hardening, the excess acrylic can be trimmed away, and the denture polished before returning it to the patient.
2. The denture is reinserted and adjusted as needed. The patient is then dismissed.

Laboratory-processed reline

The laboratory-processed relining procedure involves a laboratory phase whereby the patient has to part with a denture for a period of time. It is common to schedule the two-appointment procedure so that the

LABORATORY COPY 266902

NAME _____ D.D.S. _____

ADDRESS _____ PHONE _____

CITY _____

DATE: _____ LAB CASE NO. _____

PATIENT'S NAME & NUMBER _____ AGE _____
SEX _____

TIME WANTED:

☐ TRY IN   FINISH _____

METAL: **BASE MAT.**   MOULD _____

☐ GOLD   ☐   SHADE _____

☐ CHROME ALLOY   ☐   MAKE _____

TYPE AND DESCRIPTION OF CASE PLEASE GIVE COMPLETE INSTRUCTIONS

DESIGN CASE HERE

UPPER   LOWER

RIGHT   LEFT   LEFT   RIGHT

DENTIST'S SIGNATURE _____ D.D.S. LICENSE NO _____

This form designed and approved by the Michigan State Board of Dentistry In compliance with Michigan Act. No. 198, 1961.
4 H2307   SUPERIOR SYSTEMS FORMS, INC., DETROIT, MICH.   48235

Fig. 26-14. Laboratory prescription form. (Courtesy Superior Systems Forms, Inc., Detroit, Mich.)

patient will not have to be without teeth more than 1 day, especially in complete denture cases.

Preparing the denture

1. The denture is prepared in the same manner as was described for the chairside procedure.

Impression

1. An impression of the edentulous ridge is made with mercaptan, silicone, or wax impression material. Mercaptan is one of the most popular in use today. It is available in a ''tray consistency'' for this purpose. The prepared denture is used as an ''impression tray'' for the mercaptan.

2. The prepared denture is painted with mercaptan (rubber base) adhesive over the entire tissue surface of the denture base.
3. The mercaptan is dispensed and mixed in the usual manner and placed in the denture, covering the tissue surface. Excess material should be avoided to reduce the possibility of gagging the patient.
4. The denture is inserted and positioned properly. The patient is asked to gently close the teeth in occlusion while the material sets.
5. After the impression material sets, the denture is removed, and the patient is dismissed.

Laboratory phase

1. The denture lined with the mercaptan impression is sent to the laboratory where the mercaptan is replaced with either hard or semisoft acrylic that is fused to the denture base.

Delivery of the denture

1. The patient returns to receive the relined denture the day after the impression was made.
2. Adjustments are made as needed, and the patient is dismissed.

The immediate denture patient usually requires a reline 3 to 12 months after initial insertion of the denture. This is because of the rather dramatic reduction in ridge size during the healing process.

LABORATORY PRESCRIPTION

The laboratory prescription is a legal authorization for a dental technician to fabricate a dental appliance, restoration, or device for a patient after all the intraoral procedures have been done by the dentist. This document is similar to that used in prescribing medications for a patient at a pharmacy.

Not only does the prescription authorize the work to be done, but it should also describe in detail what is wanted by the dentist. Fig. 26-14 demonstrates a conventional form that is used. Carbon copies are essential to assure both the dentist and the technician that communications are precise. Note the information that is included on the prescription. The assistant should use this form as a checklist to be sure all information, materials, models, and shade guide directions are included before sending the case to the laboratory.

Most states require the signature and license number of the dentist on the prescription form.

BIBLIOGRAPHY

Applegate, O.C.: Essentials of removable denture prosthesis, ed. 3, Philadelphia, 1965, W.B. Saunders Co.

INDEX